Textbook of
LAPAROSCOPY

Textbook of
LAPAROSCOPY

Second Edition

Jaroslav F. Hulka, MD

Department of Obstetrics and Gynecology
Division of Reproductive Endocrinology and Infertility
University of North Carolina School of Medicine
Chapel Hill, North Carolina

Harry Reich, MD

Wyoming Valley Gyn-Ob Associates
Kingston, Pennsylvania

W.B. SAUNDERS COMPANY
A Division of Harcourt Brace & Company

PHILADELPHIA   LONDON   TORONTO   MONTREAL   SYDNEY   TOKYO

W.B. SAUNDERS COMPANY
A Division of
Harcourt Brace & Company

The Curtis Center
Independence Square West
Philadelphia, Pennsylvania 19106

Library of Congress Cataloging-in-Publication Data

Hulka, Jaroslav F.

Textbook of laparoscopy/Jaroslav F. Hulka, Harry Reich.—2nd ed.

   p.   cm.

Includes bibliographical references and index.

ISBN 0–7216–3643–8

  1. Laparoscopy.   2. Gynecologic examination.   3. Generative
organs, Female—Endoscopic surgery.   I. Reich, Harry.
II. Title.

[DNLM: 1. Peritoneoscopy.   WP 141 H912t]
RG107.5.L34H843   1994

618.1′45—dc20

DNLM/DLC   92–48883

TEXTBOOK OF LAPAROSCOPY (2/E)   ISBN 0–7216–3643–8

Printed in the United States of America

Last digit is the print number: 9   8   7   6   5   4   3   2   1

Dedication

To our wives,

Barbara Hulka

and

Liz Reich

and to the memory of

Sue Parker

Contributors

Joel M. Childers, MD

Clinical Assistant Professor, Division of Gynecologic Oncology, Department of Obstetrics and Gynecology, University of Arizona, Tucson, Arizona

Chapter 28: Laparoscopic Para-Aortic Lymphadenectomy

Avram M. Cooperman, MD

Professor of Surgery, New York Medical College, Valhalla, New York; Director of Surgery, St. Clare's Hospital and Health Center, New York, New York

Chapter 29: Cholecystectomy

William Droegemueller, MD

Chairman, Department of Obstetrics and Gynecology, University of North Carolina School of Medicine, Chapel Hill, North Carolina

Foreword

Charles J. Filipi, MD

Assistant Professor of Surgery, Creighton University; Faculty Staff, AMI Saint Joseph Hospital, Omaha, Nebraska

Chapter 30: Laparoscopic Herniorrhaphy

Robert J. Fitzgibbons, Jr., MD, FACS

Professor of Surgery, Creighton University, Department of Surgery; Chief, Division of General Surgery, AMI Saint Joseph Hospital, Omaha, Nebraska

Chapter 30: Laparoscopic Herniorrhaphy

Jouko K. Halme, MD, PhD

Former Clinical Associate Professor of Obstetrics and Gynecology, University of North Carolina School of Medicine, North Carolina; currently in private practice, Cary, North Carolina.

Chapter 21: Laparoscopic Management of Persistent Ovarian Masses

Charles A. Herbst, Jr., MD

Professor of Surgery, Department of Surgery, University of North Carolina School of Medicine, Chapel Hill, North Carolina

Chapter 31: Laparoscopic Appendectomy

Jaroslav F. Hulka, MD

Professor of Obstetrics and Gynecology, University of North Carolina School of Medicine; Fellow, Carolina Population Center, University of North Carolina at Chapel Hill, North Carolina

Nicholas R. Kadar, MD, Grad. IS, MRCOG

Associate Professor of Obstetrics and Gynecology, University of Medicine and Dentistry of New Jersey, Robert Wood Johnson Medical School, New Brunswick, New Jersey; Director of Gynecologic Oncology, Jersey Shore Medical Center, Neptune, New Jersey

Chapter 27: Laparoscopic Pelvic Lymphadenectomy

Mark J. Koruda, MD

Assistant Professor, Department of Surgery, University of North Carolina School of Medicine; Chief of Gastrointestinal Surgery, University of North Carolina Hospitals, Chapel Hill, North Carolina

Chapter 31: Laparoscopic Appendectomy

David H. Moore, MD

Associate Professor of Gynecology/Oncology, Indiana University Medical School, Indianapolis, Indiana

Chapter 21: Laparoscopic Management of Persistent Ovarian Masses

Harry Reich, MD

Surgeon, Wyoming Valley Gyn-Ob Associates, Kingston, Pennsylvania

Chapter 27: Laparoscopic Pelvic Lymphadenectomy; Appendix A: Instruments and Equipment for Laparoscopy

Giovanni M. Salerno, MD

Research Fellow, Department of Surgery, Creighton University, Omaha, Nebraska

Chapter 30: Laparoscopic Herniorrhaphy

Foreword

The introduction of laparoscopy into operative gynecology has dramatically changed the clinical practice of our discipline. Initially, the ability to perform tubal ligation for the outpatient via laparoscopy has made surgical sterilization of women the most common contraceptive method in the United States. Subsequently, women with acute and chronic pelvic pain, ectopic pregnancy, and endometriosis were managed via the laparoscope. However, during the past 5 to 7 years, the field of laparoscopic surgery has witnessed a revolutionary new emphasis. Innovations have occurred exponentially in instruments and technical equipment. The recent scientific literature reflects this rejuvenated enthusiasm in operative laparoscopy. With the exception of the great vessels, it is difficult to name an intra-abdominal or pelvic organ that has not been operated on via the laparoscope.

Dr. Jerry Hulka has been a leader in the development of innovative surgical techniques and instruments for the past 25 years. The Hulka clip and uterine elevator are the two instruments most widely known. Dr. Hulka is a superb teacher and has shared his wide clinical experience in lectures and demonstrations throughout the world. In this second edition, he is joined by Dr. Harry Reich, a private practitioner, who has been a pioneer and innovator in the revolutionary field of advanced gynecologic laparoscopy.

This monograph comprehensively covers the subject of modern laparoscopy. The excellent illustrations of John Parker complement the practical teachings of Drs. Hulka and Reich. The bibliographies at the end of each chapter are extensive and up to date.

I know that the second edition of the *Textbook of Laparoscopy* is timely. It will be a valuable resource for medical students, residents, practicing gynecologists, and general surgeons.

WILLIAM DROEGEMUELLER, M.D.
Chairman, Department of Obstetrics and Gynecology
University of North Carolina School of Medicine
Chapel Hill, North Carolina

Preface

It has only been a decade since the American Boards of Obstetrics and Gynecology and Surgery required residencies to provide endoscopic training. When the first edition of *Textbook of Laparoscopy* appeared in 1985, the techniques and instrumentation for diagnostic laparoscopy and laparoscopic sterilization had stabilized, and the field of endoscopy was tranquil. However, the therapeutic use of the laparoscope was just beginning as gynecologists used it to lyse adhesions, remove ectopic pregnancies, and deal with ovarian cysts and endometriosis. This expansion exploded in the late 1980s when laparoscopic cholecystectomy was demonstrated to be feasible in surgery. With this came another explosion in training courses in operative laparoscopy. Use of the first edition of this textbook in training courses exhausted the first printing, which had rapidly become obsolete with these fast-moving developments. The basic sciences needed for laparoscopy had expanded with the use of lasers, video monitoring, and electrosurgery, as had the surgical skills needed to dissect and excise tissues never before approached by laparoscopy.

The second edition reflects these dynamic changes in our field. Two authors, both experienced in teaching laparoscopy, have again put into (many more) words and pictures what they believe that physicians now need to know.

Understanding the basic science of the physics of lasers and electrosurgery is as necessary in this new field as understanding the basic techniques of operative laparoscopy. Specific procedures are described in technical detail in gynecology and surgery, and the controversial ones have been presented in a "pro and con" manner so that the reader may be the judge. We are cheerfully aware that many of the descriptions of instrumentation and procedures will be obsolete soon, but we hope that the basic science and surgical techniques described will endure in both gynecology and surgery.

Acknowledgments

The authors wish to acknowledge gratefully the contributions of many institutions and individuals who made this edition possible:

— Our wives and children for their support—Barbara Hulka, M.D., Carol Hulka, M.D., Gregory Hulka, M.D., and Bryan Hulka; Liz Reich and Jonathan, Justin, and Timothy Reich

— The University of North Carolina at Chapel Hill for its generosity in the use of time and space in the Department of Obstetrics and Gynecology

— The Carolina Population Center, University of North Carolina at Chapel Hill, for making its skilled research and editing staff available, as well as providing an office in which this edition was compiled

— Lynn Moody Igoe, whose professional editing of the manuscript at the Carolina Population Center was as cheerful in this edition as in the first

— Laurie Leadbetter, reference librarian at the Carolina Population Center, who performed utterly reliable research in verifying the references used in this edition, as well as numerous "jack of all trades" help, with grace and good humor

— Fred J. Spielman, M.D., Associate Professor of Anesthesiology at the University of North Carolina School of Medicine, for reviewing and correcting the chapter on anesthesiology

— Steven M. Kurtzer, D.V.M., of Medical Concepts Incorporated, Goleta, California, who kindly and patiently reviewed the accuracy of our television descriptions

— Roger C. Odell, of Electroscope, Boulder, Colorado, whose continuing efforts to educate the authors as to the physics of electrosurgery are, we hope, incorporated in the basic science section

— The representatives of Coherent Laser and Surgilase, laser generator manufacturers, who supplied us with details as to waveforms, output characteristics, and frequencies not commonly available

— The Richard Wolf and U.S. Surgical companies for their cooperation in illustrating the numerous instruments that they manufacture

— Tina Ashley and Linda Hurysz, Dr. Hulka's administrative secretaries, who kept the whirl of travel, surgery, writing, and teaching in manageable order

— Fran McGlynn, C.R.N.P., whose help was indispensable for Dr. Reich in manuscript preparation

— Lisa Sekel, C.S.P., who proved to be as invaluable in photograph editing and instrument identification as she has always been in surgery with Dr. Reich

— Ellen Coyle, whose administrative skills have maneuvered Dr. Reich through his travels, teaching, and surgery to this manuscript

— Bridget Evans and Gail Nieczykowski, of the Wyoming Valley Gyn-Ob Associates office staff

— Eileen Finnegan, Mary Jane Hargadon, Karen Joseph, Ayleen Landon, Lois Russell, and Karen Williams, valued members of Dr. Reich's operating room team

— Bernie Kastelansky, Terry McGinley, and Len Romanowski, skilled anesthesia personnel in Dr. Reich's operating theater

— Staff members at W.B. Saunders who guided this book from its early stages to fruition: editors Joan T. Meyer, Lisette Bralow, Avé McCracken, and formerly Martin J. Wonsiewicz; our copyeditor, Marjory I. Fraser; Megan C. Guenthardt, our production manager; and designer Paul Fry

About the Authors

Dr. Jaroslav F. Hulka is Professor of Obstetrics and Gynecology at the University of North Carolina School of Medicine at Chapel Hill (UNC-CH); Professor of Maternal and Child Health at the School of Public Health at UNC-CH; and a Fellow of the Carolina Population Center at that university. In his research career, he has performed extensive animal studies and clinical trials evaluating alternative methods of sterilization. He was one of the first physicians in the United States to use laparoscopy for elective sterilization. He developed the spring clip with a mechanical engineer, George Clemens, to avoid the known complications of electrocoagulation sterilization. As the chairman of the Complications Committee of the American Association of Gynecological Laparoscopists, he has monitored all endoscopic complications to learn how to prevent them and is a recognized authority in the field. He has also taught laparoscopy throughout the world. This book places emphasis on the knowledge and skills he has found to be necessary in his long experience teaching basic and advanced laparoscopy.

Dr. Harry Reich is in private practice in Kingston, Pennsylvania, and brings to his gynecologic surgery his early training as a general surgeon with interest in oncology. His command of pelvic anatomy and lifelong interest in surgery led him to become one of the American pioneers in advanced laparoscopic surgery. He was the first American to apply many of the European principles of managing pelvic abscess, ectopic pregnancy, and adhesiolysis in his practice. He continues to develop and evaluate new laparoscopic techniques that are considered to be controversial by many. He has an extensive library of video tapes of his own surgery, including complications and their management, and has documented the rationale for these procedures in many publications. For these reasons, he is in great demand as a teacher of courses on advanced laparoscopy. For this book, he has written many of the concerns that he had developed in this extensive teaching experience, emphasizing critical details of theory, anatomy, and technique.

Both authors have vast experience in the performance and teaching of laparoscopy. *Textbook of Laparoscopy* represents a blending of the research and world teaching background of Dr. Hulka and the private practice and workshop experience of Dr. Reich to the aim of this book: to teach the knowledge and skills necessary for safe and effective laparoscopic surgery.

About the Artist, John Parker

John Parker began his college education at George Washington University as a zoology major, but his sketches of specimens were so incredibly lifelike that his instructors urged him to consider a career as a medical illustrator. That career is a distinguished one, with posts at the National Institutes of Health, the University of Minnesota Medical School as Chairman of the Department of Medical Art and Photography, and as the architect for the extensive audiovisual facility of the Pennsylvania State University School of Medicine in Hershey. He has since chosen free-lance illustration so he can be closer to his family and his church, to which he is devoted. Parker's accuracy, clarity, and gracious style transform his illustrations into texts themselves in this book and convey anatomic and surgical concepts that cannot be expressed by photographs or words.

Atlas Contents

Contents

Atlas

The following photographs have been selected to illustrate principles of diagnostic and operative laparoscopy. Photographs 1–2, 5–16, and 22 are by Hulka; photos 17–21, 23–26, and 31 are by Reich. Outstanding photographs from a number of contributors are gratefully acknowledged.

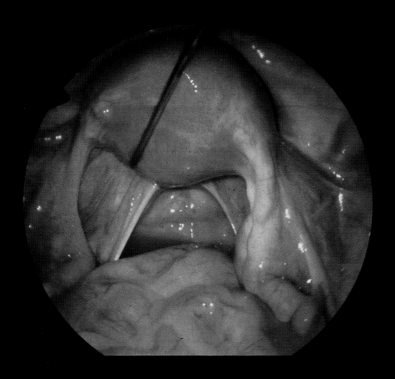

NORMAL FINDINGS

PLATE 1 Panorama

This view should be part of any photographic record of pelvic findings. The uterus should always be anteverted so that the cul-de-sac can be seen and the adnexa are free. Note that without a second-puncture manipulator of adnexa, no left ovary and only a portion of the right ovary would be seen. For recording purposes, the uterus should skim the top of the field and the tube at the bottom of the field, such as in the panoramic view.

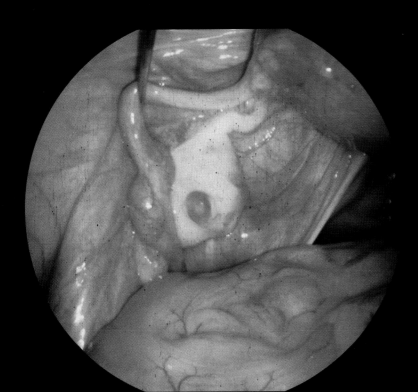

PLATE 2 Adnexa

A close-up of an adnexum should show a portion of the uterus for orientation, and the ovary should fill less than half of the available field. A second-puncture manipulating instrument is necessary to elevate the tube away from the ovaries to expose it. Important negative observations are the absence of adhesions or endometriosis. In this photograph, the follicle on the surface appears approximately on days 7 to 8 of the cycle.

STERILIZATION TECHNIQUES

PLATE 3 Clip Application

A second-puncture instrument has just applied the clip correctly within 1 to 2 cm of the uterine fundus. The tubal serosa in the clip is stretched upward near the hinge between the upper and lower jaws (Kleppinger "envelope" sign), indicating that the isthmic tube is secure within the jaws. During application, the optics should always be kept at this distance from the applicator in order to observe details of the application. (Plate by Kleppinger.)

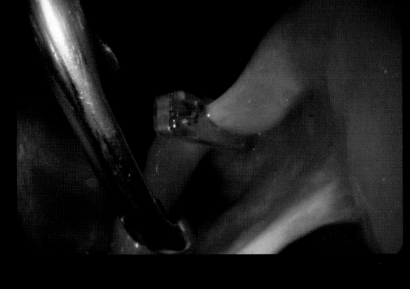

PLATE 4 Bipolar Coagulation

Using Kleppinger bipolar forceps, the surgeon has finished coagulating the isthmic-ampullary junction of this tube in three contiguous places. A 1- to 2-cm segment of isthmus remains to minimize the risk of fistula formation and possible subsequent ectopic pregnancy lodging in the distal remnant of this tube. Note that 2 to 3 cm of tube are destroyed. Again, the optics should be kept at this distance during coagulation in order to observe details of coagulation and desiccation. Despite what is seen, the endpoint of coagulation is the cessation of current flow as seen on an ammeter monitoring current flow. (Plate by Kleppinger.)

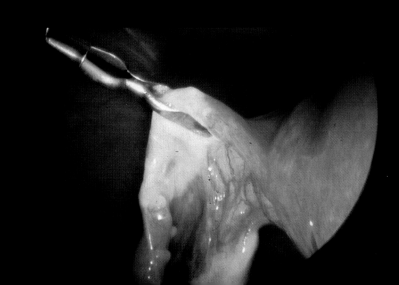

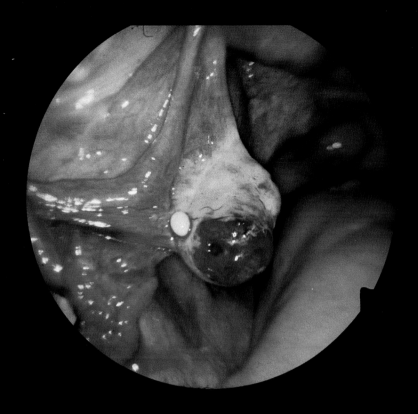

OVULATION

PLATE 5 Normal Corpus Hemorrhagicum with Stigma

Diagnostic laparoscopy for infertility is ideally timed for 2 to 4 days after presumed ovulation. This allows the surgeon to look for a normal corpus hemorrhagicum (a vascularized corpus luteum) that contains a hole or stigma through which the ovum has escaped. This stigma is seen as a 1- to 2-mm dark cavity on the surface of the corpus hemorrhagicum and is believed to remain for 1 or 2 days after ovulation. (Disregard the white fibroma on the surface of this ovary.)

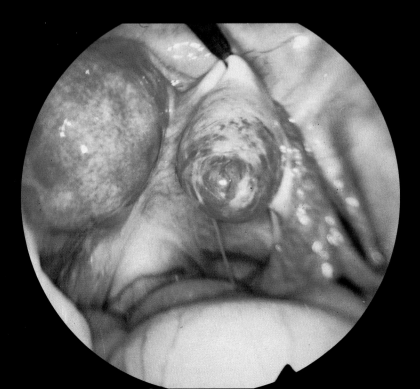

PLATE 6 Luteinized Unruptured Follicle (LUF)

On day 16, after induction of clomiphene citrate and a rise in basal body temperature, a well-vascularized corpus hemorrhagicum is seen; however, there is no stigma, suggesting that the ovum may not have left this structure that has enlarged the ovary. Note that a grasping forceps on the utero-ovarian ligament is necessary in this patient to mobilize the ovary sufficiently to make this observation.

INFERTILITY

PLATE 7 Healed Clip
The clip is completely peritonealized in 4 to 6 weeks after application. Excision of this clip will remove 0.5 to 0.7 cm of tube and allow an isthmic-isthmic anastomosis with good prognosis of pregnancy. In patients seeking reversal of sterilization, a laparoscopy is indicated if the sterilization was performed by electrocoagulation techniques, but not by mechanical methods such as clip or Pomeroy, because adequate tubal tissue has been a consistent finding after mechanical sterilization. Note at the tip of the clip the blue stain that may represent endometriosis.

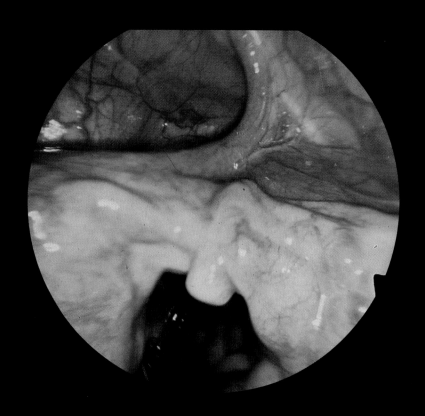

PLATE 8 More Extensive "Minimal" Endometriosis
This plate shows extensive endometrial implants on the peritoneum, uterus, and tubal surface. The peritoneum is hyperemic. It is difficult to assess the extensiveness of endometriosis unless the surgeon has in mind clear and specific criteria for "normal findings" and clear mental definitions for endometriosis, including white areas and red areas, as well as the traditional black spots of old hemorrhagic implants.

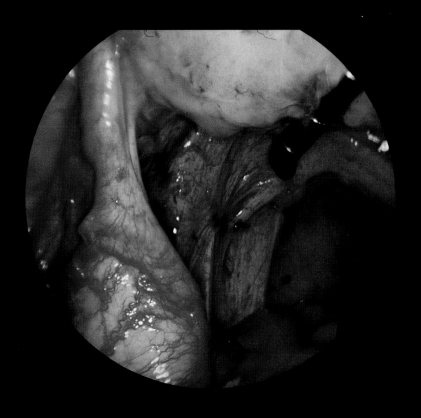

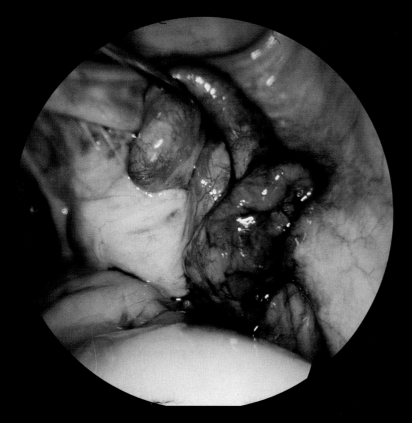

TUBAL OCCLUSION

PLATE 9 Normal Patent Tube

As the tube is elevated to visualize the fim-briae, indigo carmine is instilled into the uterus and should fill the tube promptly with minimal distention of the ampulla. It should then quickly spill over the surface of the fimbriae, which are seen here stained blue. Both tubes should be rapidly visualized to identify spillage from both fimbriae.

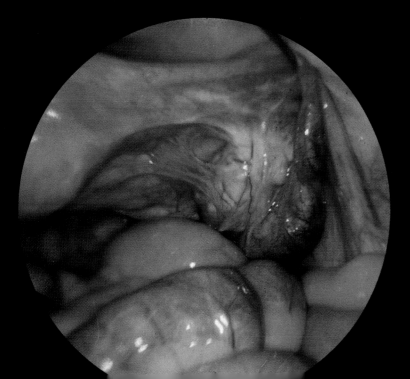

PLATE 10 Hydrosalpinx Stage III

Dye insufflation fills the hydrosalpinx without spillage. Less than half the ovarian surface is visible through dense adhesions that do not stretch. Although these adhesions can be lysed, they will probably form again. The prognosis for this stage III tubal occlusive disease is poor. If these findings are bilateral, we would recommend direct in-vitro fertili-zation (IVF), rather than attempting lysis of adhesions and laparoscopic salpingostomy

ADHESIONS

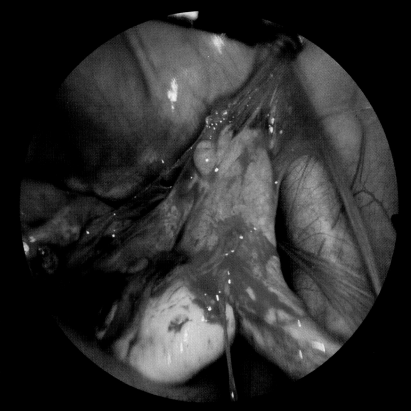

PLATE 11 Stage I

The manipulating forceps can stretch the adhesive systems around this right tube to show how thin and avascular they are. More than 50% of the ovary is visible, making this a stage I classification. After laparoscopic lysis of adhesions, the prognosis for a term pregnancy based on this side is favorable.

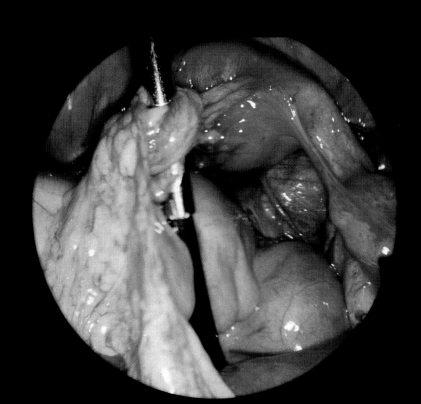

PLATE 12 Stage III

In the same patient as above, the left adnexum was so thoroughly covered with dense adhesions that this photograph was the best one possible of this adnexum. No ovarian surface was visible, making this a stage III classification. No stretching of the adhesions was possible, making these adhesions "thick." Laparoscopic lysis of these adhesions would undoubtedly result in their re-formation. This patient was, nevertheless, placed in a stage I category with a good prognosis, because her right adnexum (Plate 11) showed favorable findings.

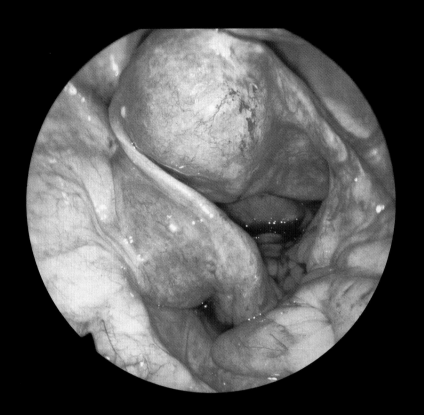

SECOND LOOK: ADHESION REFORMATION

PLATE 13 Findings After Standard Right Salpingo-oophorectomy and Microsurgical Lysis on the Left Side

This patient had extensive endometriosis in her right adnexum, requiring that a standard salpingo-oophorectomy be done. No attempt at reperitonealization of this side was attempted because of the extensive raw surfaces left behind. On her left side, extensive microdissection was carried out to free the ovary from its peritoneal and tubal adhesions. Four weeks after this surgery, her right adnexum is strikingly free from adhesions, but her left ovary has become covered by them again.

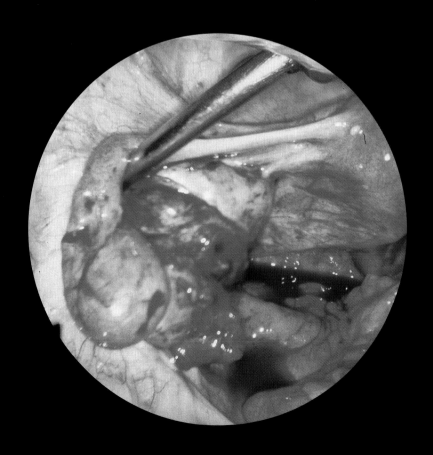

PLATE 14 Results After an Attempt to Relyse Adhesions

The ovarian adhesions in Plate 13 that had formed again were so densely involved with the tube that extensive attempts at dissection were abandoned at the point illustrated in this photograph. Although the fimbriae are open, the tube is distorted and densely adherent to the ovary. Although tubal surgery was technically successful and patency was established, the nature of the ovarian adhesions turned out to be the deciding prognostic factor in determining subsequent success: No pregnancy occurred in this patient.

FINDINGS WITH PAIN

PLATE 15 Posthysterectomy
This patient had chronic pelvic pain after vaginal hysterectomy, and a laparoscopy was performed to look for adhesions or residual disease. This remarkable photograph shows a beautifully healed vaginal vault, adnexal stumps well attached to the vault, normal tubes and ovaries, and no adhesions or disease at all. The pain was thought to be psychogenic in origin.

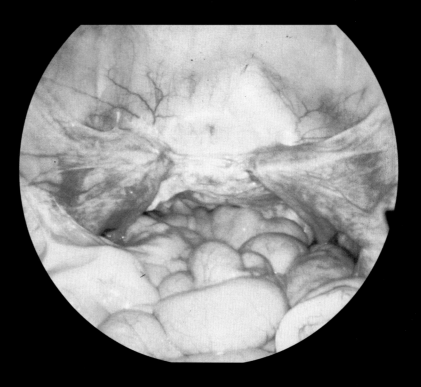

PLATE 16 Acute Pelvic Inflammatory Disease
The tube is edematous, erythematous, painful, and causes a rise in temperature—these features constitute the four classic signs of inflammation. Although there is a dense adhesion between the tube and the pelvic wall, the ovary up to this point has been spared. A day 10-11 follicle is present, indicating normal endocrine function. Further surgery is contraindicated in this case; antibiotics and possibly corticosteroid therapy will minimize inflammatory destruction of this tube.

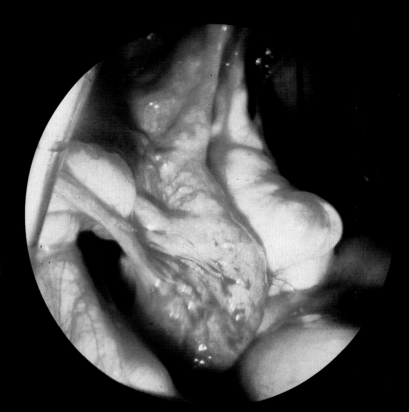

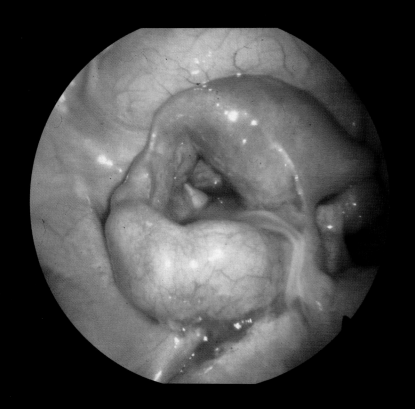

PELVIC ABSCESS

PLATE 17 Drainage of Pelvic Abscess

This patient had a suspected tubo-ovarian abscess that was referred for laparoscopic management. Gentle, blunt dissection of the loosely adherent bowel to the uterus led to the spillage of exudate as seen in this plate. Extensive aspiration of this exudate, dissection of fibrinous exudate, and copious lavage postoperatively led to the findings below.

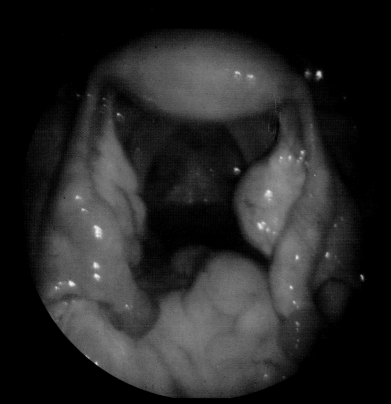

PLATE 18 Postoperative Findings (at 6 Weeks)

At second-look laparoscopy, the tubes and ovaries are remarkably restored to normal, despite their inflamed appearance as seen above. Both European and American experience is documenting the more rapid resolution of tubo-ovarian abscess by laparoscopic drainage, with less prolonged use of costly antibiotics and hospitalization.

ECTOPIC PREGNANCY

PLATE 19 Pitressin Injection of Mesosalpinx

Salpingotomy can be performed with the use of a mesosalpingeal injection of pitressin in a dosage of 5 to 20 units (1 ampule) in 30 ml (1 standard vial) of saline. See Figure 19–3: this photograph is similar and shows the best technique for pitressin injection. The mesosalpingeal surface is presented, twisting the tube to obtain this exposure. A 22-gauge spinal needle (introduced through a disassembled Veress needle as a guide) can be used to inject a 5-ml bleb in the subperitoneal area after aspiration to ensure that the needle tip is not in a venous channel. The same is repeated on the opposite side of the mesosalpinx (see Fig. 19–3). The tube will remain blanched for 1 hour.

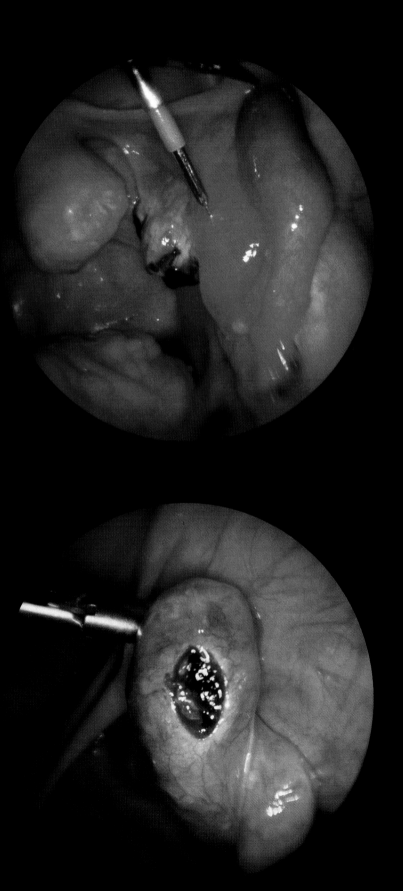

PLATE 20 Salpingotomy

With good vasopressin hemostasis, the thinnest portion of the distended tube, usually opposite the mesosalpinx, is presented for surgery. As in Figure 19–4, an incision is made with minimal bleeding just large enough to allow evacuation of the clot and ectopic gestation. This can be accomplished with scissors, knife, needle unipolar electrosurgery (as seen in this case), or with CO_2 laser. Use of a laser has the technical advantage of allowing one to follow the irregular curve of the tube with ease. The clot and gestation can then be aspirated or flushed out with aquadissection (see Fig. 19–4); the vasopressin should kill any remaining trophoblast by anoxia. Closure of the salpingotomy is not necessary, because suturing may even provoke adhesion formation.

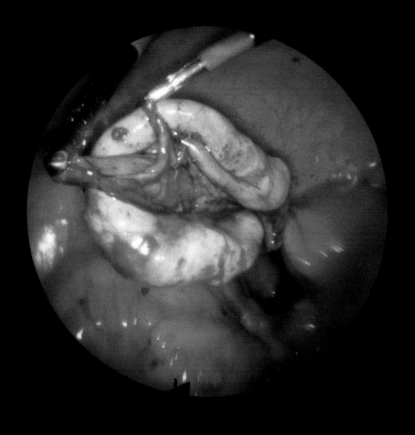

GYNECOLOGIC SURGERY

PLATE 21 Endometrioma Cystectomy

A large endometrioma has been drained; the cyst wall has been identified; and the brownish cyst wall is being pulled out to the left from the inside of the normal ovary. Once the correct plane of cleavage is identified, the endometrioma lining can be stripped bloodlessly as shown. Note also that as the cyst wall is being stripped, the normal ovary begins to curl upon itself, and within minutes of the complete removal of the cyst, the ovary usually curls up and reconstructs itself without suturing being required. See Figure 17–3G and H for a diagram of this remarkable process.

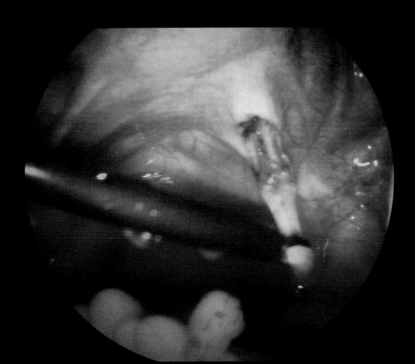

PLATE 22 LUNA

The uterus is elevated and put on a stretch to highlight the uterosacral ligament. In addition, a grasping forceps can grip the uterosacral ligament and elevate it, further defining this structure and bringing it away from underlying vessels and the ureter. A laser can then transect this structure with safety. Alternatively, bipolar coagulation can desiccate the structure, which is then divided to achieve the same result.

HYSTERECTOMY

PLATE 23 Ureteral Dissection

The left ureter has been identified by watching for peristalsis before extensive surgery has occurred. It is then grasped with an atraumatic forceps and deflected medially, with sharp scissor dissection entering and spreading the peritoneum lateral to the ureter. Bleeding is controlled with well-insulated bipolar forceps.

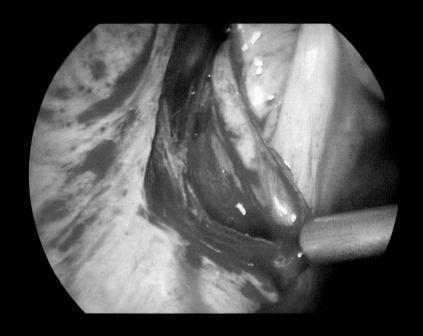

PLATE 24 Round Ligament Entry

The round ligament is desiccated with bipolar forceps and then divided with a spoon electrode at 150-W cutting current. Bleeding can be controlled with bipolar forceps or a fulgurating current at 30-W cutting current. The vesicouterine peritoneal folds are divided with scissors, and the bladder is also mobilized sharply.

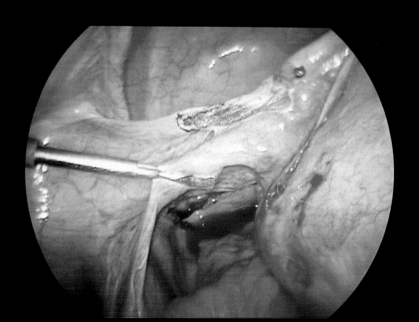

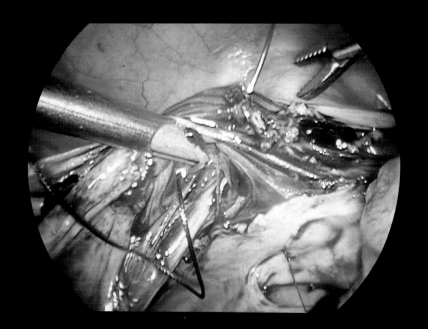

PLATE 25 Uterine Artery Ligation

After dividing the ovarian blood supply, the uterine vessels are skeletonized. A CT-1 needle is inserted just above the unroofed ureter and rotated with a needle holder to bring it around the uterine vessel pedicle well away from the uterus. A single suture at this location identifies the ureter and watches over it for the rest of the procedure, as well as diminishing uterine arterial bleeding.

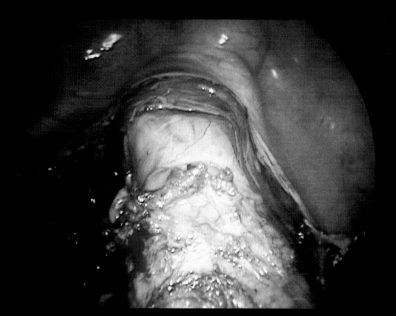

PLATE 26 Vaginal Entry

The bladder has been mobilized well below the cervix to the white vaginal fascia. This has included dissecting the bladder pillars from medial laterally for maximal ureteral mobility. At this point, the vagina can be entered from above or below to complete the hysterectomy.

CHOLECYSTECTOMY

PLATE 27 Abdominal Ports

This is a view of the abdominal wall with the large ports in place for laparoscopic cholecystectomy. See Figure 29–1 for the external landmarks for these entries. (Plate by Cooperman.)

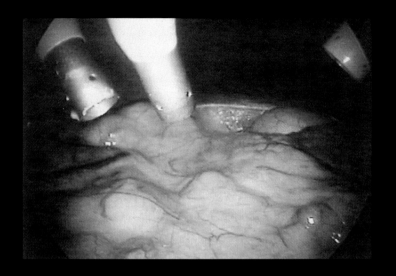

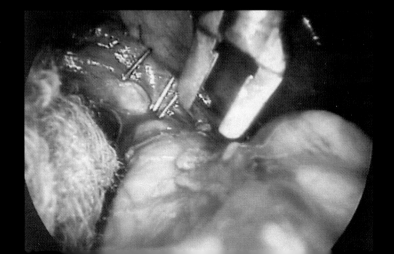

PLATE 28 Cystic Duct

Dissection has identified and isolated the cystic duct for clip occlusion and division (see Fig. 29–3 for a diagrammatic view). (Plate by Cooperman.)

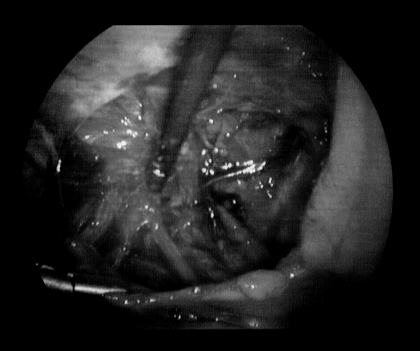

HERNIA

PLATE 29 Peritoneal Dissection

In this recurrent, direct left inguinal hernia, completed sharp and blunt dissection of the peritoneum from the underlying tissue has resulted in the exposure of the structures in and near the hernia: Cooper's ligament, spermatic cord, testicular vessels, and epigastric vessels. The hernial defect has been sutured closed. The peritoneum has been left as flaps above and below this dissection. See Figure 30–6a for a sketch of the structures and Plate 32 for the preoperative anatomic appearance. (Plate by Arregui.)

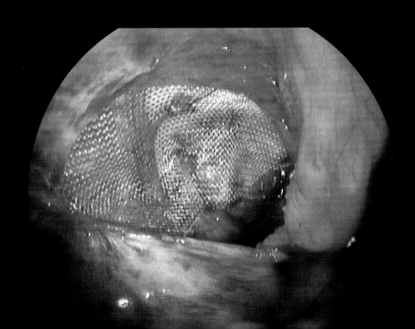

PLATE 30 Polypropylene Onlay

In this repair, a 6 × 5.5 cm polypropylene mesh patch (Prolene, Ethicon, Inc.) is fixed in place over the peritoneal defect and closed hernial defect as shown, using a laparoscopic stapling device (Proximate ES, Ethicon, Inc.). See also Figure 30–6d for a sketch of this procedure. The peritoneum is then replaced and sutured over this defect, making the repair in effect a preperitoneal onlay technique that is performed laparoscopically. (Plate by Arregui.)

COMPLEX ANATOMY

PLATE 31 Pelvic Lymphadenectomy
This photograph shows the end result of a right pelvic lymphadenectomy. The ureter is seen at the left of the dissected area, covered with peritoneum. The isolated structure to the right of and adjacent to the ureter is the superior vesical artery. Deeper in the middle of the field of view is the obturator nerve, parallel to the ureter. Just lateral to the obturator nerve is the obturator internus muscle fascia. The external iliac artery with the external iliac vein beneath it is at the outer limit of this dissection. More laterally, the psoas muscle is exposed with the genitofemoral nerve passing over it.

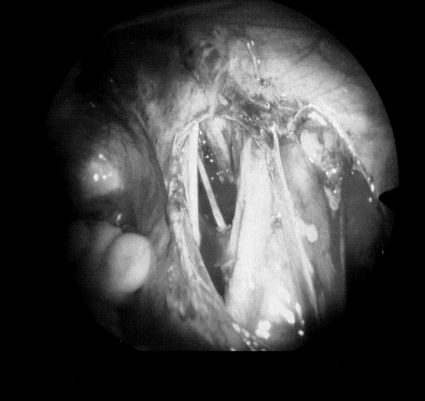

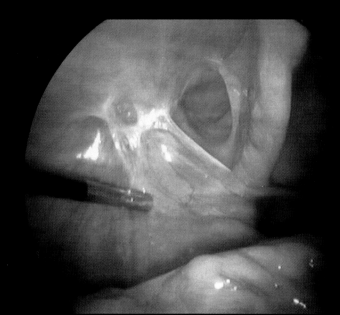

PLATE 32 Recurrent Hernia
This photograph is a recurrent direct left inguinal hernia distorting the tissue and challenging the surgeon for anatomic definition. This is the same patient whose dissection and repair is shown in Plates 29 and 30. See also Figure 30–6a for a sketch of the normal anatomy underneath. (Plate by Arregui.)

BASIC CLINICAL SCIENCES

Laparoscopy uses physics in unique ways in surgery: sophisticated light transmission systems, television, laser, electrocoagulation, instillation of fluids under pressure, and insufflation of the abdominal cavity with gas. Most good practitioners are not aware of the basic physics involved or of the interaction of these physical forces with the biology of the patient. Serious, sometimes fatal, mistakes can be made because of lack of such an understanding. Although doctors spend 2 years before medical school and an additional 2 years in medical school studying the biochemistry of drugs, only 1 year of general physics is required as a premedical course. This section is written to explain the history of how and why all these developments have occurred, and the current physical and physiologic aspects of laparoscopy that the clinician needs to know to avoid complications or to manage them knowledgeably.

History

Those who cannot remember the past are doomed to repeat it.

—George Santayana,
The Life of Reason,
Vol 1

At the turn of the century adventurous physicians began to explore the body visually with specula and optics. At the German biologic and medical society meeting in Hamburg in September 1901, the Dresden professor Georg Kelling reported his examination of the stomach and esophagus. He inserted a cystoscope into the abdomen of a living dog and viewed the viscera, first creating a pneumoperitoneum with air filtered through sterile cotton. He published his report 1 year later and devoted 25 lines to the celioscopic method. Kelling (1902) described the entire procedure, instruments, and future possibilities of this method; peritoneoscopy was born.*

In 1901, D.O. Ott, a Petrograd gynecologist, described ventroscopy by which he inspected the abdominal cavity of a pregnant woman with the help of a head mirror and a speculum introduced into a culdoscopic opening.

In 1910, H.C. Jacobaeus of Stockholm published a discussion of the inspection of the three great body cavities: peritoneal, pleural, and pericardial. This publication was based on his own efforts with humans and described the first method as laparoscopy. A month later Kelling rapidly reported his performance of peritoneoscopy

on two patients, and 2 years later Jacobaeus described 45 laparoscopic examinations on humans, noting liver changes, tumor, and tuberculosis. In 1911, Bertram M. Bernheim first used laparoscopy in the United States, using a half-inch diameter proctoscope and ordinary light for illumination.

The technique of abdominal entry was varied and controversial. Unlike Kelling, Jacobaeus introduced the trocar directly without a prior pneumoperitoneum. In 1938, Janos Veress of Hungary described a new needle for inducing pneumothorax (for the treatment of tuberculosis). This instrument is the one that is now most frequently used for creating pneumoperitoneum.

Because most patients undergoing laparoscopy had liver disease with the possibility of periumbilical varices and enlarged livers in the right upper quadrant, most of the early techniques described left upper quadrant incisions or those well below the umbilicus to avoid the risk of introducing the needle for pneumoperitoneum into the periumbilical varices or liver, causing air embolism. Abdominal pressure was not monitored, although intra-abdominal volume was carefully regulated by slow introduction of gases through a large syringe. Local anesthesia was used consistently, since these examinations were office procedures done for diagnosis.

There were many laparoscopic innovators in Europe and America. H. Kalk in Germany devised a new lens system for oblique viewing (135 degrees), published

---

*The emphasis in this chapter is on the physicians who developed various techniques and the date of these developments. Instead of giving specific citations for these developments, the reader is directed to the references list at the end of this chapter.

extensively, and can be considered the founder of the German school of laparoscopy for the diagnosis of liver and gallbladder disease. The American internist John C. Ruddock made another major contribution; in 1934 he described a good optic system including a built-in biopsy forceps with electrocoagulation capacity.

In 1937 an American surgeon, E. T. Anderson, suggested coagulation for laparoscopic sterilization (Anderson, 1937), and in 1941, two gynecologists, Frank H. Power and Allan C. Barnes, reported performing tubal sterilization by electrocoagulating the cornual portion of each tube. The physicians abandoned this work because of the urgent medical needs of World War II, although Barnes later became a leader of American concern about the world population problem.

The vaginal route was favored in America for gynecologic endoscopy for diagnosis. In 1939 Richard W. TeLinde attempted endoscopy by a culdoscopic approach in the lithotomy position, but he abandoned this technique because of the constant presence of small intestines in this position. In 1944, Albert Decker introduced pneumoperitoneum through the cul-de-sac into patients in the knee-chest position and called the procedure culdoscopy, to be performed under local anesthesia. This method became the standard for gynecologic endoscopic examination in the United States well into the 1970s.

Also in 1944, Raoul Palmer of Paris began a gynecologic examination using peritoneoscopy, but adopting the Trendelenburg position to bring the air up into the pelvic cavity. He described a uterine cannula to manipulate and elevate the uterus, giving better access to the tube and ovary with the patient in lithotomy and a Trendelenburg position. Palmer also designed a forceps for ovarian biopsy and stressed the importance of monitoring intra-abdominal pressure. His techniques were painful and were done under general anesthesia in his private clinic; he used a standard rubber-apron clean but not sterile technique.

In Germany the gynecologist and engineer Kurt Semm incorporated new techniques of fiber optics and careful control of intra-abdominal pressures into instrumen-

tation widely used. Hans Frangenheim, another German gynecologist, also designed instruments and techniques for gynecologic laparoscopy in use today.

In the 1960s the British gynecologist Patrick Steptoe adapted the techniques developed on the continent and began performing laparoscopy in the operating room using sterile techniques. In his book, *Laparoscopy in Gynaecology*, he described for the first time in the English literature the complete instrumentation and techniques for gynecologic laparoscopy and described and illustrated the technique of laparoscopic sterilization with a two-puncture technique and electrocoagulation with division, using the Palmer biopsy drill forceps.

Steptoe's book was published just at the time when world concern about population was growing. His description of laparoscopic sterilization caught on in England and caused the rebirth of interest in laparoscopy as a gynecologic technique in the United States. In 1972 Clifford R. Wheeless, Jr., described outpatient sterilization, using an efficient combination of scheduling and local anesthesia with rapid recovery to allow the outpatient to undergo surgery and go home the same day. Using the Jacobs-Palmer operating laparoscope, this single puncture approach had worldwide appeal because of its rapidity and apparent simplicity.

With wide dissemination of this technique to many inexperienced operators and hospitals, complications rapidly developed. In response to this emergence of worldwide interest and concern about complications in laparoscopic sterilization, Jordan M. Phillips founded the American Association of Gynecological Laparoscopists in 1971. This organization provided rapid and widespread dissemination of all information concerning techniques and complications of laparoscopy in the 1970s. Its annual complications surveys served the same purpose as maternal mortality committees by analyzing causes of complications and deaths to learn how to prevent them. In the mid-1970s, the British performed a prospective survey of more than 50,000 laparoscopies, adding significant insights into complications and techniques (Chamberlain and Brown, 1978). In the late 1970s, the Centers for Disease

Control in Atlanta began including as its charge the surveillance of laparoscopic mortality in the United States and overseas, since by the mid-1970s a quarter of a million laparoscopic sterilization procedures were being performed in the United States annually.

The combination of anesthetic paralysis without intubation, Trendelenburg, and excessive pneumoperitoneum pressure led to deaths from cardiac arrest, later found to be exacerbated by a vagal reflex induced by painful pelvic manipulation. These new anesthetic problems caused Gaylord D. Alexander and John I. Fishburne, Jr., in 1973, working independently, to develop modern techniques of local and general anesthesia suitable for laparoscopy.

Using unipolar circuitry to coagulate tubes led to poorly understood bowel burns and caused major infections and deaths from bowel perforations and peritonitis. The desire to occlude tubes without unipolar coagulation led to the independent development in the 1970s of the bipolar method by Jacques-E. Rioux in Canada, Hans Hirsch in Germany, and Richard K. Kleppinger and Stephen L. Corson in the United States. Kleppinger's technique emerged in the United States as the most popular method for laparoscopic tubal sterilization in use today.

At the same time, nonelectric techniques were explored. Tantalum clips had been applied by the culdoscopic route extensively in Mexico, but subsequent pregnancy rates as reported in the United States were high. Jaroslav F. Hulka and George Clemens examined the previous use of clips and developed a spring-loaded clip for laparoscopic application to avoid the recanalization problems of rigid tantalum or silver clips. Coy L. Lay and In Bae Yoon independently developed a similar band, and Yoon applied it directly to humans. Yoon's band technique was adopted by the United States Agency for International Development (USAID) to substitute for the unipolar technique that it had previously promoted widely throughout the world.

The rare but grave risk of injuring major blood vessels during blind entry with the Veress needle or trocar led to the exploration of minilaparotomy under local anes-

thesia as an alternative to laparoscopic sterilization. Also, Harrith M. Hasson developed a cannula for open laparoscopy. The acceptance of these alternate methods in developed countries with laparoscopic capacity has not been widespread.

In the United States and England, laparoscopy rapidly replaced culdoscopy as the preferred method of diagnostic pelvic endoscopy. In the 1980s in the United States it also became the second most frequent cause for lawsuits against obstetrician-gynecologists (the leading cause being adverse pregnancy outcome). Bowel burns as grounds for lawsuits were replaced by suits based on subsequent pregnancies. The American College of Obstetricians and Gynecologists (ACOG) issued an official public statement, advising physicians and their patients that the risks of pregnancy after sterilization by any technique were somewhat less than 1:100, to dispel the impression among physicians and patients that sterilization was absolute. Recognizing the widespread use of the technique, the American Board of Obstetrics and Gynecology made laparoscopy training a required component of residency training programs in 1981. Response to litigation concerns led to development of excellent documentation of informed consent for this elective procedure.

Many patients were sterilized in the early enthusiasm of the technique, but later these patients came back to gynecologists and microsurgeons requesting a reversal of the procedure. This further led to the emphasis on counseling with regard to the appropriateness of the technique before surgery as well as the choice of more reversible techniques for young women requesting the procedure. In a 1980 editorial, the *British Medical Journal* recommended the clip as an occlusive device in younger women for these considerations.

Laparoscopy has emerged in the United States as a standard method of female sterilization. It is also enormously useful in the diagnosis of infertility and is recommended after 2 years of otherwise unexplained infertility. Widespread use for this indication has led to new insights into the nature and operability of pelvic adhesions, endometriosis, and ovarian dysfunction.

Several simultaneous but independent developments in the 1980s led to the expansion of laparoscopy into the current therapeutic surgical practice:

1. Steptoe dramatically established aspiration of follicles in 1976 for the retrieval of ova for in vitro fertilization. This therapeutic surgery led American gynecologists to become comfortable with operative laparoscopy, even though Semm in Europe had been advocating and performing "pelviscopic surgery" for years. Laparoscopy for egg retrieval was rapidly replaced by vaginal ultrasonography, as other indications for operative laparoscopy were emerging.

2. Earlier detection of ectopic pregnancies with sensitive pregnancy tests and ultrasonography led Maurice Bruhat in France and Alan DeCherney in the United States to describe successful salpingotomy to remove ectopic pregnancies at laparoscopy. Adhesiolysis, once in the domain of microsurgery, could be performed equally as well through the scope. Salpingostomies for hydrosalpinx, ovarian cystectomies, and extensive endometriosis resections were described in Europe and adopted in the United States.

3. The television industry developed cameras that became increasingly suitable for laparoscopy. Miniaturization through the use of a silicon chip, rather than vacuum tube, was combined with greater light sensitivity and control. These developments led to the adoption of television, first as an operative recording device and then as a monitor for surgeon and assistant to look at while operating. The magnification possible by bringing the laparoscope lens close up to the surgical field compensated for the loss of detail in the electronic image. By multiplying the eyes and hands involved in laparoscopy, "videoendoscopy" made possible more complex and extensive surgery through the laparoscope.

4. Laser surgery increased the new enthusiasm for laparoscopic surgery, allowing safe dissection in areas close to the bowel and ureter, as well as technical ease of ablation and division deep in the pelvis.

5. Suture manufacturers expanded the availability of laparoscopic hemostatic clips and suturing devices. In 1972, H. Courtnay Clarke showed that hemostasis was feasible with suturing; in 1977 Kurt Semm showed that it was feasible with Endoloop suturing; and in 1987 Harry Reich showed that it was practical by desiccating large vessels with bipolar electrosurgery. This newfound ability has made possible extirpative surgery on larger structures such as ovaries, uteri, and gallbladders.

These developments led to the performance of the first cholecystectomy in Lyons by Phillipe Mouret in 1987 (Cushieri et al, 1991). A year later, J. Barry McKernan and William Saye repeated this in the United States, and Eddie Joe Reddick established a course for teaching laparoscopic laser cholescystectomy, drawing general surgeons into laparoscopy. While this edition is written, general surgery is undergoing an explosion in laparoscopy similar to the 1970s revolution in gynecology. Appendectomies, hernias, bowel resections, and other surgical procedures are being developed, and manufacturers are producing better equipment suitable to the needs of general surgeons. Urologists are also evaluating laparoscopic bladder surgery, pelvic node dissection, and ureteral surgery. Many of the procedures presented as being controversial in this edition will no doubt emerge as procedures of choice in the next century.

Because this technique is proving to be so useful in gynecology and general surgery and has survived many criticisms and complications, this textbook is written to describe and instruct in the current techniques and indications and also to lay a solid foundation on which to evaluate those that the future will bring.

REFERENCES

Chamberlain G and Brown JC (eds): Gynaecological Laparoscopy: Report on the Confidential Enquiry into Gynaecological Laparoscopy. London, Royal College of Obstetricians and Gynaecologists, 1978.

Cuschieri A, Dubois F, Mouiel J, et al: The European experience with laparoscopic cholecystectomy. Am J Surg, *161*:385–387, 1991.

FURTHER READINGS

Alexander GD, Goldrath M, Brown EM, and Smiler BG: Outpatient laparoscopic sterilization under local anesthesia. Am J Obstet Gynecol *116*:1065–1068, 1973.

Anderson ET: Peritoneoscopy. Am J Surg *35*:136–139, 1937.

Bernheim BM: Organoscopy: Cystoscopy of the abdominal cavity. Ann Surg 53:764–767, 1911.

British Medical Journal (ed): Female sterilisation: No more tubal coagulation. Br Med J 280:1037, 1980.

Bruhat MA, Manhes H, Mage G, and Pouly JL: Treatment of ectopic pregnancy by means of laparoscopy. Fertil Steril 33:411–414, 1980.

Clarke HC: Laparoscopy: New instruments for suturing and ligation. Fertil Steril 23:274–277, 1972.

Corson SL, Patrick H, Hamilton T, and Bolognese RJ: Electrical consideration of laparoscopic sterilization. J Reprod Med 11:159–164, 1973.

DeCherney AH, Romero R, and Naftolin F: Surgical management of unruptured ectopic pregnancy. Fertil Steril 35:21–24, 1981.

Decker A and Cherry T: Culdoscopy: A new method in diagnosis of pelvic disease: Preliminary report. Am J Surg 64:40–44, 1944.

Fishburne JI Jr, Omran KF, Hulka JF, et al: Laparoscopic tubal clip sterilization under local anesthesia. Fertil Steril 25:762–766, 1974.

Gunning JE: The history of laparoscopy. In Phillips JM and Keith L (eds): Gynecological Laparoscopy: Principles and Techniques. Selected papers and discussion from the First International Congress of the American Association of Gynecological Laparoscopists in New Orleans, Louisiana. New York, Stratton Intercontinental, 1974, pp 57–66.

Hasson HM: Open laparoscopy: A report of 150 cases. J Reprod Med 12:234–238, 1974.

Hulka JF and Omran KF: Comparative tubal occlusion: Rigid and spring-loaded clips. Fertil Steril 23:633–639, 1972.

Hulka JF, Mercer JP, Fishburne JI, et al: Spring clip sterilization: One year follow-up of 1,079 cases. Am J Obstet Gynecol 125:1039–1043, 1976.

Jacobaeus HC: Über die Möglichkeit die Zystoskopie bei Untersuchung seroser Höhlungen anzuwenden. Münch Med Wochenschr 57:2090–2092, 1910.

Kalk H: Erfahrungen mit der Laparoskopie (zugleich mit Beschreibung eines neuen Instrumentes). Z Klin Med 111:303–348, 1929.

Kelling G: Über Oesophagoskopie, Gastroskopie und Koelioskopie. Münch Med Wochenschr 49:21–24, 1902.

Kleppinger RK: Female outpatient sterilization using bipolar coagulation. Bull Post-Grad Comm Med, Univ Sydney, Nov., 1977, pp 144–154.

Lay CL: Experimental use of elastic bands for tubal sterilization. Paper presented to the South Atlantic Association of Obstetricians and Gynecologists, Miami, January 30, 1974.

Lay CL: Preliminary report on use of Silastic band in laparoscopy. Presented to the American Fertility Society, San Francisco, April 4, 1973.

Ott DO: Ventroscopic illumination of the abdominal cavity in pregnancy. Zh Akush I Zhens Bolezn 15:7–8, 1901.

Palmer R: La coelioscopie. Bruxelles Med 28:305–312, 1948.

Power FH and Barnes AC: Sterilization by means of peritoneoscopic tubal fulguration: Preliminary report. Am J Obstet Gynecol 41:1038–1043, 1941.

Reich H: Laparoscopic oophorectomy and salpingo-oophorectomy in the treatment of benign tubo-ovarian disease. Int J Fertil 32:233–236, 1987.

Reich H, Freifeld ML, McGlynn F, and Reich E: Laparoscopic treatment of tubal pregnancy. Obstet Gynecol 69:275–279, 1987.

Rioux J-E and Cloutier D: Bipolar cautery for sterilization by laparoscopy. J Reprod Med 13:6–10, 1974.

Ruddock JC: Peritoneoscopy. Western J Surg Obstet Gynecol 42:392–405, 1934.

Semm K: Atlas of Gynecologic Laparoscopy and Hysteroscopy. In Barrow LS (ed): Philadelphia, WB Saunders, 1977.

Steptoe PC: Laparoscopy in Gynaecology. Edinburgh, Livingstone, 1967.

Steptoe PC and Edwards RB: Birth after the reimplantation of a human embryo (Letter). Lancet 2(8085):366, 1978.

TeLinde RW and Rutledge FN: Culdoscopy: A useful gynecologic procedure. Am J Obstet Gynecol 55:102–115, 1948.

Veress J: Neues Instrument zur Aüsfuhrung von Brust- oder Bachpunktionen und Pneumothoraxbehandlung. Dtsch Med Wochenschr 64:1480–1481, 1938.

Wheeless CR Jr: Outpatient laparoscopic sterilization under local anesthesia. Obstet Gynecol 39:767–770, 1972.

Wittman I: Peritoneoscopy, Vols 1 and 2. Budapest, Akademiai Kiado, 1966.

Yoon IB, Wheeless CR Jr, and King TM: A preliminary report on a new laparoscopic sterilization approach: The silicone rubber band technique. Am J Obstet Gynecol 120:132–136, 1974.

Light: Optics and Television

The story of modern endoscopic surgical development follows breakthroughs in optic technology as better, brighter images were seen, first by the eye and then by the video camera. The steady improvement in the quality of video images has enabled surgeons to rely on assistants, also looking at the surgical field, to expose and operate as well as at open laparotomy (and in some cases, better). This chapter presents the major developments in optic and video technologies that have literally shed light on a new era of surgery.

FIGURE 2–1 Anatomy of a single glass fiber

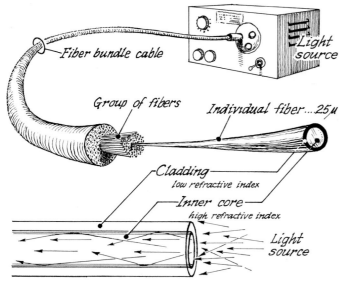

Light wave is reflected by cladding
back into the inner core of fiber.

FIGURE 2–2 Coherent bundles and incoherent bundles

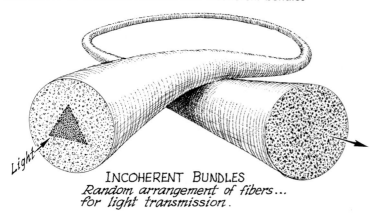

INCOHERENT BUNDLES
Random arrangement of fibers...
for light transmission.

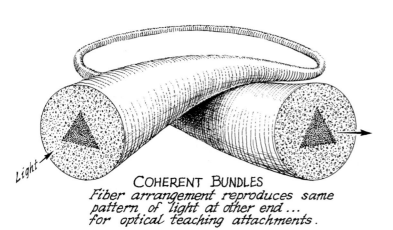

COHERENT BUNDLES
Fiber arrangement reproduces same
pattern of light at other end ...
for optical teaching attachments.

OPTICS

Fiber Optic Cables

Prior to the 1960s, endoscopy used small, hot, tungsten light bulbs inside body cavities. These bulbs did not emit high-frequency (blue) light waves, thus they conveyed a red color to all attempts at photographic documentation. Because the bulbs themselves were hot, they could coagulate bowel and other structures that they touched, and they tended to burn out unreliably in the abdomen. In the 1960s, a major breakthrough in technology occurred in the development of fiber optic cables, which consisted of fibers with an inner core of glass with a relatively high refractive index and a fused sheathing of low-index glass (Fig. 2–1).

FIBER BUNDLES. The coaxial fiber is produced by drawing the core through the sheathing in a furnace so that the sheathing is fused evenly to the core. This procedure would allow visible light (0.4- to 0.7-mm wavelength) to travel in the inner core and be bent back into the core when it reached the interface between the low-index sheathing and the core. Light would enter at one end of the fiber and emerge at the other end after numerous internal reflections with virtually all of its strength. By making the fibers small (usually 10 to 25 μm) and packing multiple fibers together in an "incoherent" bundle with random arrangement of fibers at either end (Fig. 2–2), relatively inexpensive fiber bundles could be constructed that would transmit high-intensity light over the length of the bundle.

COLOR VALUES AND LIGHT LOSS. With the fiber optics system, a light source of relatively high temperature (up to 5500 K [5227°C] containing relatively more blue light) could be focused on a small fiber bundle well outside the body (Fig. 2–3). This heat would be absorbed and dissipated at the source, and relatively little heat would be transmitted into the body cavity. The longer the cable system, the more relative loss will occur at the blue end of the spectrum, so that some systems would still give a more red and yellow appearance.

Light losses within the system (Fig. 2–4) would include about a 6% loss from any reflection at all the air-glass surfaces, such as fiber-end faces at the light source and the interfaces of the coupling of the flexible fiber bundle to the fiber bundle of the optic. The core glass represents only 70% of the surface of the fiber bundle end; the rest of the surface is filler between the round fibers or cladding around the fibers. Thus, 30% of the light is lost at the lamp. Inevitable mismatches at the coupling between the cable and the laparoscope, caused by cable fibers shining onto the filler or cladding of the optic's fiber bundle, account for another 20% loss. The typical light chain thus loses approximately 74% of the generated light as it emerges from the distal end of the optics.

FIGURE 2–3 Endoscopic fiber bundles

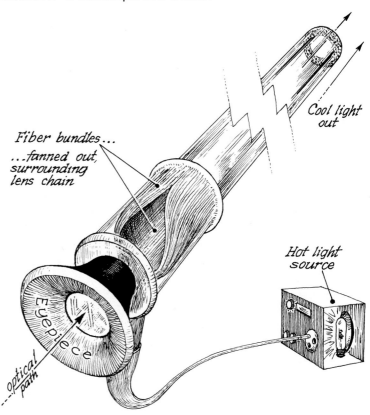

FIGURE 2–4 Normal light loss

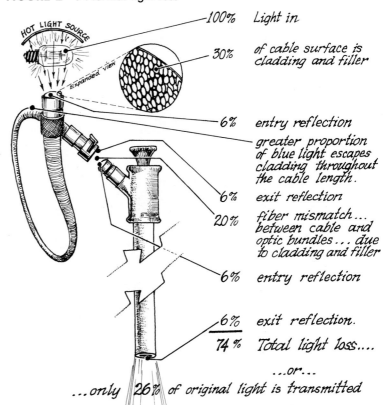

100% Light in

30% of cable surface is cladding and filler

6% entry reflection

greater proportion of blue light escapes cladding throughout the cable length.

6% exit reflection

20% fiber mismatch... between cable and optic bundles... due to cladding and filler

6% entry reflection

6% exit reflection.

74% Total light loss....

...or...

...only 26% of original light is transmitted

FIGURE 2–5 Preventable light loss

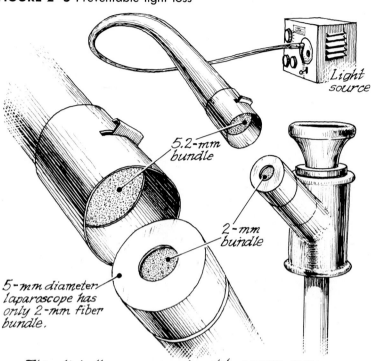

Light source

5.2-mm bundle

2-mm bundle

5-mm diameter laparoscope has only 2-mm fiber bundle.

This clinically common mismatch causes more than 85% of light loss at this point alone.

FIGURE 2–6 Light intensity decreases with distance

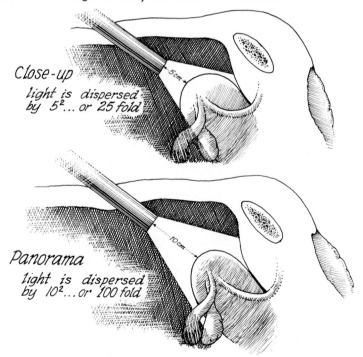

Close-up
light is dispersed by 5²... or 25 fold

5 cm

Panorama
light is dispersed by 10²... or 100 fold

10 cm

Panorama needs four times the amount of light for the same exposure as the close-up.

If the diameters of the fiber cables are different (Fig. 2–5), considerable loss can occur. A 5.2-mm diameter fiber cable attached to a 2-mm diameter endoscope bundle will lose most of its light because of this mismatch, since the 2-mm diameter is less than 15% of the 5.2-mm diameter. Furthermore, since the light source is usually focused intensely on the central fibers of the bundle, in an incoherent bundle these maximum-intensity bundles are scattered at random at the other end, and a 2-mm optic bundle will receive only a small fraction (< 15%) of the light. The human eye is marvelous at adapting to these different levels of brightness; cameras, even modern, sensitive television cameras, are not.

As the light emerges from the endoscope in the pelvic cavity, its intensity decreases with the square of the distance between the endoscope and the organ viewed (Fig. 2–6). Thus panoramic photographs of the entire pelvis or upper abdomen require much more light than do close-ups of ovaries, which are white and highly reflective. The upper abdomen is particularly difficult to photograph because the liver is dark and surfaces are curved away. Extremely high-intensity light flashes are necessary for photography in this area. As light is picked up in the lenses of the endoscope, another series of trade-offs occurs in the optic system. The maximum diameters of the lenses vary from about 1.0 to 5.5 mm, depending on the amount of fiber cable and ancillary channels for forceps, coagulation devices, clip applicators, and so forth, packed into the endoscope (Fig. 2–7). Endoscopes with no operating channel have a maximum combination of fiber bundles in and lens systems out and continue to be the best instruments for photography.

Until the 1960s, lens chains consisted of small lenses interspersed with large distances of air. The total amount of light transmitted by an endoscope is related to the square of the index of refraction of the medium between the lenses (Fig. 2–8). If the medium is air, with an index of refraction of 1.0, the proportional transmission is 1.0. If the medium is glass, however, the index of refraction is between 1.5 and 1.6, and its square is over twice that of air, with therefore more than twice the transmission of light.

Hopkins, a British physicist, realized that light was better transmitted if the air and glass spaces in lens systems were interchanged. This is the basis of the more brilliant Hopkins lens systems of the Karl Storz Company.

Coating the glass surfaces to minimize light reflection as it passes between glass and air surfaces is a modern technique that further reduces light loss. Normally about 4 to 7% of light is reflected from any untreated air-glass surface. For a typical endoscope with 16 lenses, the light loss from these 32 air-glass surfaces could be considerable. A thin film of magnesium fluoride, which is about a fourth of a wavelength thick, is deposited on the glass surface by evaporation in a vacuum. This film decreases the reflection problem throughout the visible spectrum and markedly improves modern lens systems in endoscopes and cameras in use today.

FIGURE 2–7 Lens and fiber bundle sizes

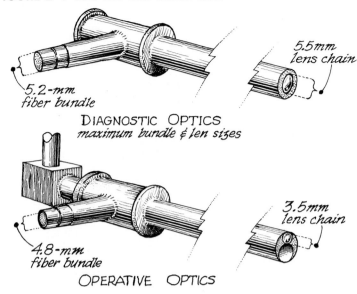

DIAGNOSTIC OPTICS
maximum bundle & len sizes

5.2-mm fiber bundle

5.5mm lens chain

OPERATIVE OPTICS

4.8-mm fiber bundle

3.5mm lens chain

FIGURE 2–8 Lens chain design

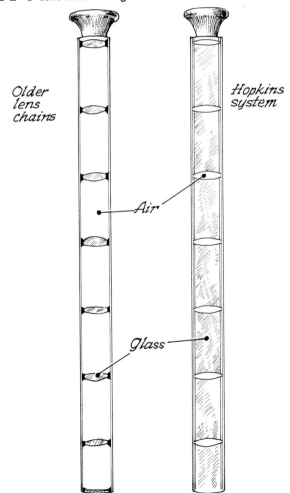

Older lens chains

Hopkins system

Air

Glass

FIGURE 2–9 Viewing angles commonly available

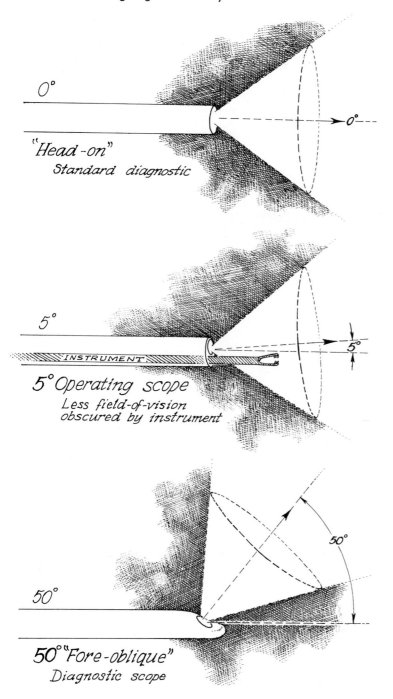

0°

"Head-on"
Standard diagnostic

5°

INSTRUMENT

5° Operating scope
Less field-of-vision
obscured by instrument

50°

50° "Fore-oblique"
Diagnostic scope

Optic Angles

The distal end of endoscopes can have different viewing angles (Fig. 2–9). Most optics have a "head-on" (0-degree deflection), which makes it easy for most physicians to perceive what they are looking at head-on. Some operating laparoscope optics are slightly deviated from the channel by 5 degrees to make the sector blocked by the instrument in the operating channel smaller. Other endoscopes come with large deflections of 50 degrees or more and are more versatile (e.g., a curved versus straight Kelly clamp) and are therefore useful in careful study of adhesions, ovarian surfaces, and other areas in the abdomen. However, they are sufficiently confusing in orientation to most surgeons that they are infrequently used.

Light Sources

Most light sources use a standard tungsten light bulb with a built-in reflector that is identical to those used in most projectors. High-intensity sources use halogen or xenon to produce a more intense light and heat. These high-intensity, continuous light sources may be necessary for cinephotography or television reproduction in endoscopy when the camera or film is not sensitive. Fiber cables carrying such intense light are still capable of generating heat at the end of the bundles. This heat can be high enough to cause paper drapes used for patients to burst into flame, and this has occurred several times. For this reason, cloth drapes should be used with endoscopic procedures to minimize this preventable risk of burning the patient.

Fiber Bundle Problems

If the amount of light entering the surgeon's eye is insufficient, all points along the chain of light transmission should be checked. To see if the fiber bundles are broken, the surgeon can hold one end of the light cable to a light source and look at the other end (Fig. 2–10). Over a third of fiber breakage (caused by rough handling during or between cases) should indicate the need for replacement of the cable.

The lamp end of the cable surface can burn out with use because high temperature inevitably turns even glass surfaces and their plastic packing materials brown from oxidation. A burned-out cable should be replaced. The coupling on the endoscope for the cable may similarly be oxidized because of frequent soakings or gas autoclaving and subsequent oxidation. Even if the scope has survived hundreds of uses, the ends of the fiber light-transmitting cables may not have.

FIGURE 2–10 Fiber bundle wear and tear

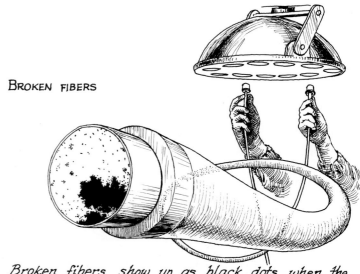

BROKEN FIBERS

Broken fibers show up as black dots when the cable is held against the O.R. light. Replace the cable if over 1/3 of the fibers are broken.

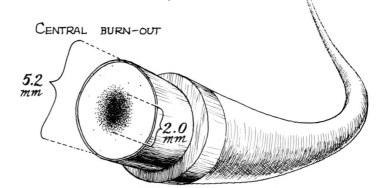

CENTRAL BURN-OUT

5.2 mm

2.0 mm

Central burn-out results from long exposure to heat at the light-source end of the cable. Replace the cable if over 2-mm of the central area is blackened.

FIGURE 2–11 Fiber bundle mismatch

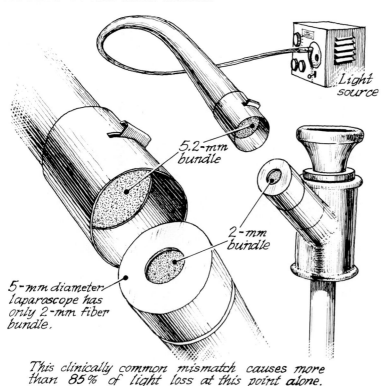

Light source

5.2-mm bundle

2-mm bundle

5-mm diameter laparoscope has only 2-mm fiber bundle.

This clinically common mismatch causes more than 85% of light loss at this point alone.

Mismatch of the cable fiber bundle diameter and optic fiber diameter has been discussed. The problem is easily corrected by purchasing a cable bundle diameter to match the bundles in the optics in use (Fig. 2–11).

Fogging

Endoscopes are high-technology combinations of metals for tubing and glass for light transmission. These materials have different coefficients of expansion when heated (Fig. 2–12). When an endoscope is put into a high-temperature autoclave, the glass and metal expand at different rates and, despite the seals between them, steam may eventually enter the optic chain and result in condensation and fogging within the lens system. Attempts to improve seals between glass and metal or to reduce their different heat expansions have not been completely successful. For this reason endoscopes should not be subject to extremes of temperature if their life span is to be prolonged. "Autoclavable" endoscopes require very careful transitions from the 138°C autoclave temperatures to the 20°C cool stage; dashing in cold water, as is done with autoclaved instruments in most busy operating rooms, will rapidly ruin the lenses by causing more rapid cooling and shrinking of some parts and by allowing water to enter the lens chain. Cold sterilization techniques for expensive endoscopic lens systems are thus safer, because they do not expose the metal and glass to extremes of temperature changes. Gas autoclaving involves temperature ranges to 55°C for 2 hours but requires a 12-hour airing period. Disinfection in alkalinized glutaraldehyde (Cidex) is done at room temperature and is effective in 20 to 30 minutes.

FIGURE 2–12 Glass and metal expansion problems

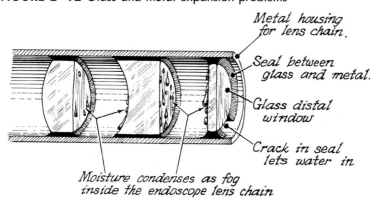

Metal housing for lens chain.

Seal between glass and metal.

Glass distal window

Crack in seal lets water in

Moisture condenses as fog inside the endoscope lens chain

Because the optics are usually at room temperature and the abdominal cavity is at a higher temperature with 100% humidity, cold optics entering the abdominal cavity will fog because of condensation of vapor on the glass surface of the cold endoscope (Fig. 2–13A). This situation can most economically be prevented by having a warm bottle of sterile water or saline (see Fig. 2–13B) at the operating table and by inserting the distal end of the optic into this warm fluid (slightly above body temperature) for approximately 30 seconds just before insertion into the sleeve. Busy endoscopy units use endoscope warmers (see Fig. 2–13C) to heat the entire supply of endoscopes in the operating room under dry and sterile conditions.

Antifogging solutions (see Fig. 2–13D) are available for treatment of proximal and distal lenses; ordinary detergents such as pHisoHex will do the same, causing the droplets of condensed steam to spread themselves rapidly and almost invisibly over the surface of the cold lens. For photographic purposes, heating techniques are much preferable to antifogging solutions, since the extra coating of detergent and condensed water will distort the lens surface sufficiently to blur photographs.

If fogging is still evident after repeated polishing of both lenses, the seal between metal and glass may be cracked and the fogging may be inside the lens system. This situation can be detected by looking (perhaps with magnification) at either end of the endoscope and seeing if there are beads of water inside the first lens on either end.

FIGURE 2–13 A–D, Prevention of fogging

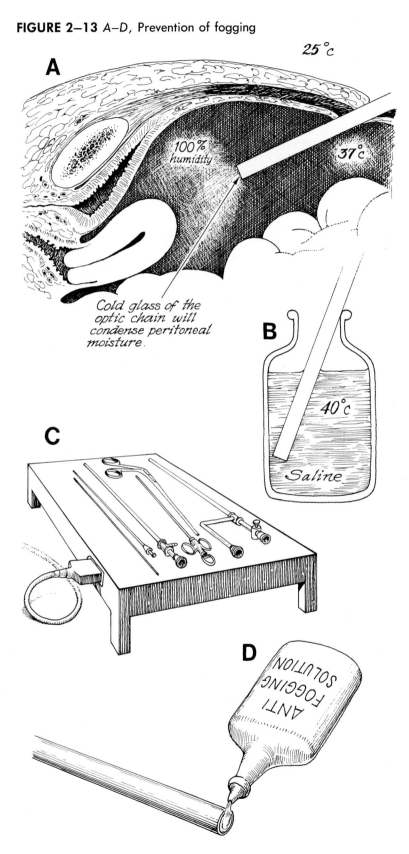

FIGURE 2–14 Treatment of internal fogging

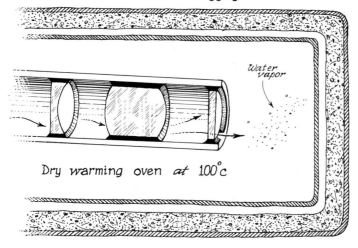

Dry warming oven *at* 100°c

Water vapor can be driven out of the lens chain in a dry warming oven.

FIGURE 2–15 Anatomy of a video signal

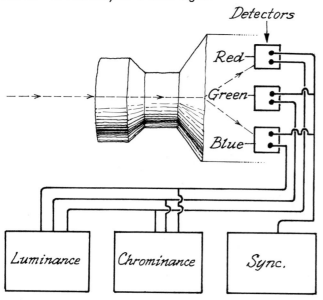

Recording and transmission depends on two characteristics synchronized for each point:
1. Luminance: the brightness (intensity) of the point.
2. Chrominance: the color (mix of red, green and blue) of the point.

If this is the case, the optic may be salvaged for the day by placing it into a warming oven in the operating room, where the dry heat may convert the condensed water to steam and allow it to escape (Fig. 2–14). If this does not work, the optic must be sent back to the factory for disassembly, cleaning, and resealing.

A final word about light sources: Manufacturers have provided excellent backup systems of light sources, so that if one bulb burns out during a procedure, a backup bulb can be substituted instantly. In addition, manufacturers have combined high-intensity light sources (for television or photography) with ordinary light sources for routine diagnostic procedures. Operating room personnel should be thoroughly familiar with the controls of this equipment so that only one of these alternative light sources is being used at any time. The best engineering will be useless if the operating room personnel do not understand the controls.

PHOTOGRAPHY

The original objective of endoscopic photography was to present new techniques and findings at professional meetings, in which high-resolution quality of color slides and prints for publication (see Atlas) were of utmost importance. As endoscopy became widespread throughout gynecology and other fields, the availability of a record of findings for teaching and research purposes has become another objective. The cumbersome technology of still-photography on 35-mm film, which is so important in the development of endoscopy, has been replaced by more convenient video cameras. Modern "chip" video cameras are so small that they interfere little with surgery. They can either record continuously on a video cassette recorder (VCR) tape or capture video images for printing "hard copy" photographs for the medical record. Endoscopy is now like fluoroscopy was just when Roentgen found that he could record x-ray images on plates of film: Transient images seen by one physician can now be recorded reliably for records and study by many physicians. Records on video and print allow findings to be reviewed at conferences leading to rapid insights into endoscopic surgery and pathology.

The 1990s should be the decade for endoscopic teaching and research through video. Also, as we enter into the legal realities of this litigation-prone era in which laparoscopy is still a frequent reason for suing gynecologists, documentation of findings and procedures performed for medicolegal purposes has been found to be a valuable defense appreciated by judges and juries.

TELEVISION

With the advent of miniaturized and highly sensitive television cameras, endoscopy is in a state of revolution. This section covers the minimal amount of physics and technology required to enable the videoendoscopist to choose equipment knowledgeably and use it intelligently. Hospital personnel are not trained in "troubleshooting" this complex equipment, and often a knowledgeable physician needs only to push the right button or wire to turn a system back on to finish the case.

The Chip Camera

Modern endoscopy cameras are marvels of electronic miniaturization. In large top-quality broadcast television cameras, light is split into three beams and passed through a red, green, or blue (RGB) filter to three photosensitive vacuum tubes or silicon chips to record these color values separately (Fig. 2–15). A highly accurate and detailed signal results. At the other end of the quality and expense spectrum are the consumer-grade chip cameras with one photosensitive silicon surface divided into about 500 × 700 separate picture elements *(pixels)*, each capable of reading a light signal (Fig. 2–16). A single-chip camera has each pixel assigned to detect one color by bonding an RGB filter onto each pixel and by clustering them in groups of three. *Three pixels* thus make up *one image bit*. As a result, sharpness in terms of resolution is sacrificed for simplicity and low cost.

FIGURE 2–16 Chips, image bits, and pixels

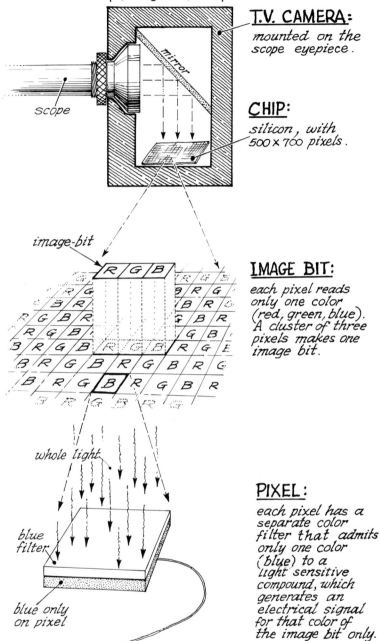

T.V. CAMERA: mounted on the scope eyepiece.

mirror

scope

CHIP: silicon, with 500 × 700 pixels.

image-bit

IMAGE BIT: each pixel reads only one color (red, green, blue). A cluster of three pixels makes one image bit.

whole light

blue filter

blue only on pixel

PIXEL: each pixel has a separate color filter that admits only one color (blue) to a light sensitive compound, which generates an electrical signal for that color of the image bit only.

FIGURE 2–17 Standard signals and their cables

THOSE CONNECTING WIRES

NAME	SIGNAL	RESOLUTION	CABLE	SHAPE	AUDIO
Broadcast grade	RGB	600+	4 wires	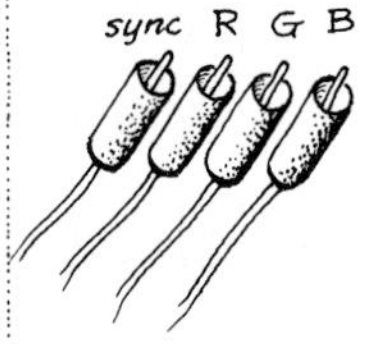 sync R G B	no audio
S-VHS	YC	500	2 wires	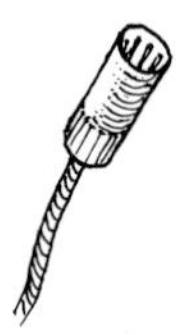	2 more wires for stereo
VHS	Composite	240	1 wire	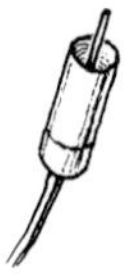	on the same wire

Resolution

To operate off a video screen, the image must be as sharp as possible. Our eyes and brains have evolved with greater side-to-side sensitivity (to view prey and to sense danger on the ground), an acuity called *horizontal resolution*. Video equipment specifies this resolution in terms of how many separate vertical lines can be distinguished when projected on a video screen. Most consumer-grade VCRs and camcorders have 240 lines of resolution, which is adequate for most entertainment purposes. Good television sets have double this resolution, or about 500 lines, which is the standard resolution in American broadcast signals. A modern single-chip video camera, through clever engineering, can display 450 lines of resolution. A three-chip camera displays over 600 lines. The Japanese are developing a wide screen video system with 1200-line resolution.

Color Quality: Luminance and Chrominance

In addition to sharpness, each image bit must have its color values reproduced accurately. Colors are transmitted as composites of the red, green, and blue components. The United States has three standard systems of transmittal (Fig. 2–17):

1. *RGB output.* In some cameras, computer displays, and video monitors, three separate cables carry the information about RGB. These three cables plus a synchronizing cable are needed for high-quality RGB output.

2. *Y-C signals.* Information can also be transmitted at somewhat less cost by electronically combining and encoding color information about one image bit: the Y signal, representing *luminance*, the overall *brightness* of the image bit, and the C signal, representing *chrominance*, the *color* of the image bit as determined by the relative amount of each of the three colors sent by the three pixels. The Y and C information carried on *two* separate wires in the cable is characteristic of *super-VHS* and *hi-band 8-mm* systems.

3. *Composite signal.* In this system, all chrominance and luminance information from the camera (as well as the audio signal) is transmitted on one wire. This system offers the least detailed information, at the lowest cost, and is used in most consumer television and VCR systems.

CLINICAL CHOICES

Monitoring or Recording Endoscopy

For simple monitoring or recording of endoscopy, relatively inexpensive consumer-grade television monitors and VCRs are satisfactory and widely used. A single-chip camera produces a good signal for this system. Consideration should be given to recording cases on two video recorders in the operating room: a VHS copy for the patient and a super-VHS for the surgeon who may consider future editing for presentations (Table 2–1 and Fig. 2–18).

Editing Tapes

For editing tapes (e.g., simple elimination of long, nonsurgical segments) for referring physicians, patients, or conferences, the resolution and color quality deteriorate rapidly with composite signal VHS. Super-VHS equipment is recommended. Some cameras have a recording control switch built into the camera held by the surgeon. Experienced surgeons can do their own editing and narrating into a microphone as they operate.

Videoendoscopy

For videoendoscopy (operating directly off the screen), a three-chip camera with a high-resolution video monitor gives the best quality and resolution. Most of the quality and resolution of this system can be captured on super-VHS or hi-band 8-mm recording systems.

	Type	Camera	Output	Monitor	Recorder-VCR
1.	Standard	1 Chip (240–480)	Composite	Standard (400)	VHS (240)
2.	S-VHS	1 Chip (at 480)	Y-C	High grade (700+)	S-VHS (400+)
3.	Broadcast	3 Chip (600+)	RGB	High grade (700+)	S-VHS (400+)

TABLE 2–1.   MATCHING EQUIPMENT TO CAMERA

Notes: Numbers in ( ) are maximum lines of resolution with this equipment.
For monitoring by operating room staff, use standard consumer grade.
For editing, S-VHS has the best detail retention.
For video surgery, the highest resolution (3 chip) is needed.

FIGURE 2–18 Endoscopy "chip" TV camera

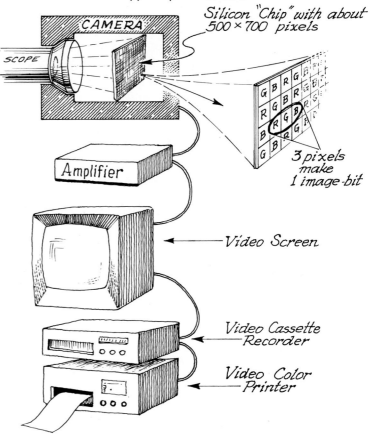

Color Prints

Most American and Japanese cameras scan 525 horizontal lines of pixels 60 times/sec. (These "NTSC" standards are linked to our 60-cycle alternating current; the European "PAL" video standard is linked to their 50-cycle current.) Every *other* line of pixels is scanned once, creating one *field*, and then the alternate line is scanned. These *two fields* create *one frame* with all pixels displayed at 30 frames/sec. Our eyes perceive such a rapid sequence of frames with much greater resolution than actually exists in the individual frames.

When we "freeze a frame" in television, the picture thus looks grainy compared with the live video. A high-resolution camera produces a less grainy color print. Printers can be adjusted to minimize these electronic limitations and are increasingly used to produce reliable prints in the operating room during surgery. These prints are suitable for medical records, referring physicians, and so on.

FOCUSING

Viewing directly through an endoscope allows the surgeon's eye to focus the images coming from various distances between the surgery and the scope. The surgeon's iris also adjusts for variations in light intensity. When working directly off a monitor, however, the video camera must constantly be focused by the surgeon's hand. Thus, the surgeon's right hand becomes his or her eye and not only keeps the surgery in the center of the field and as enlarged as is appropriate but also focused. Variations in light intensity are dealt with by chip cameras automatically dimming a powerful light source mechanically or by varying sensitivity of the chip electronically. The focusing ring on a beam splitter is off to the side of the laparoscope, and focusing is comfortable with the surgeon's arm at his or her side.

A video camera with or without beam splitter attached to the laparoscope enables the surgeon and staff to operate while watching a video monitor. Beam splitters supply 80 to 90% of available light to the video monitor, thus providing an excellent picture. For difficult dissections or anatomic areas, some skilled physicians rely on the clarity that only direct viewing can provide. Beam splitters allowing 10 to 20% light to the surgeon produce considerable eyestrain. Recently, beam splitters have been developed that supply 50% of available light to the operator's eye. These require more sensitive cameras but eliminate the problem of eyestrain.

Power: Electricity and Laser

Electricity is a versatile tool in laparoscopy for sterilization, treatment of endometriotic implants, management of hemorrhage, and division of adhesions. Except for sterilization, the same is true for the laser. It is therefore important for the practicing laparoscopist to be familiar with the biophysical principles involved in both energy sources: electricity and laser.

FIGURE 3–1 Current

CURRENT : *the "flow"*

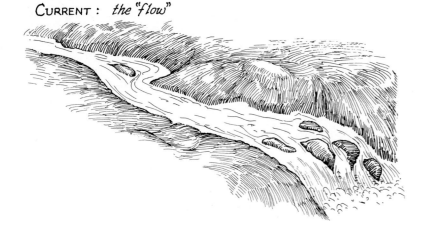

FIGURE 3–2 Ampere

AMPERE : *the "rate of flow"*
the rate of current

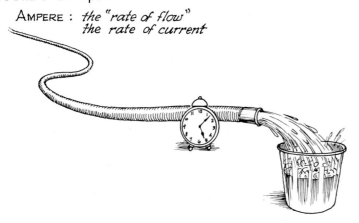

ELECTRICITY

Terminology

Only the most frequently used terms and concepts are defined and explained below. All terms are described with their analogy to a hydraulic system, since physicians are generally more familiar with the physics of fluids than the physics of electricity.

Current. An electrical current is a stream of electrons flowing through a conducting body (Fig. 3–1). Just as water flows through a hose, a certain amount flows under a certain pressure to overcome resistance.

Ampere (André-Marie Ampère, French physicist, 1775 to 1836). An ampere (A) is the amount of current produced by 1 volt (V) applied across a resistance of 1 ohm (Ω) over 1 second (Fig. 3–2). The ampere is a measure of the rate at which current flows, as one would measure gallons per minute coming out of a hose.

Volt (Count Alessandro Volta, Italian physicist, 1740 to 1827). The volt (V) is the unit of electromotive force which, when steadily applied to a resistance of 1 Ω, will produce a current of 1 A (Fig. 3–3). As water flows under so many pounds per square inch (depending on the height of the water column from which it comes), a certain pressure level is reached.

Ohm (Georg Simon Ohm, German physicist, 1787 to 1854). An ohm (Ω) is the electrical resistance equal to the resistance of a circuit in which a potential difference of 1 V produces a current of 1 A (Fig. 3–4). This is equivalent to the resistance of a water wheel. In electrosurgery, resistance is supplied by the tissue.

Watt (James Watt, Scottish engineer, 1736 to 1819). A watt (W) is the rate of work represented by a current of 1 A under pressure loss of 1 V (watts = volts × amperes) (see Fig. 3–4). The concept would be similar to the combination of gallons of water per minute and the water pressure used up as water is applied onto a water wheel to generate work, measured as force times distance. Since the practical purpose of electricity is to generate energy, most electrical appliances, including coagulation generators, are described in terms of watts with voltage and amperage characteristics varying considerably. Work done over time is measured by joules (watts × time) (James P. Joule, English physicist, 1818 to 1889), or British thermal units (BTUs).

FIGURE 3–3 Volt

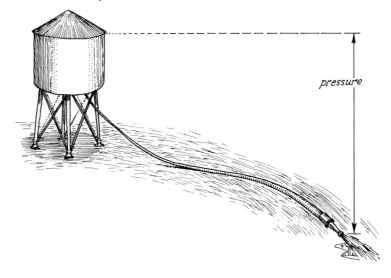

VOLT: *the electromotive force the "pressure" of the current*

pressure

FIGURE 3–4 Ohm and watt

OHM: *the resistance to the flow*
WATT: *the work produced*

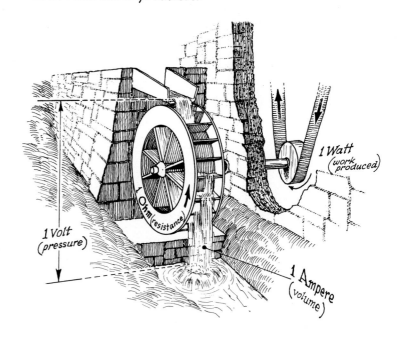

1 Volt (pressure)

1 Ohm (resistance)

1 Ampere (volume)

1 Watt (work produced)

FIGURE 3–5 High voltage

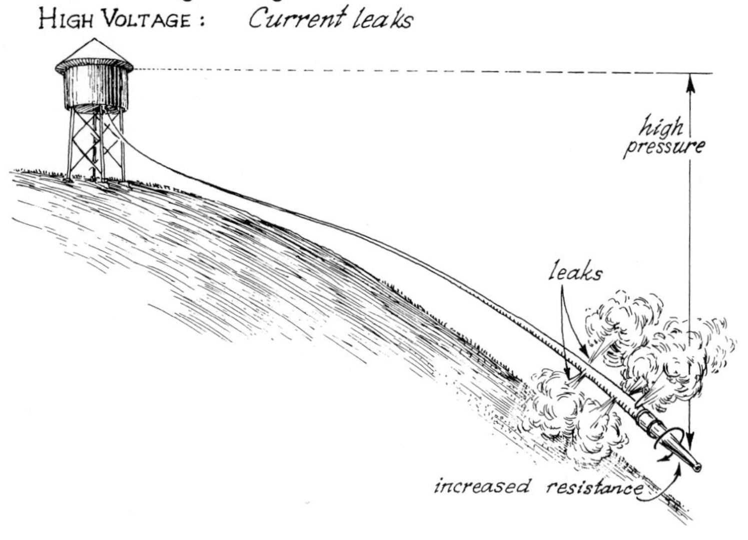

HIGH VOLTAGE : *Current leaks*

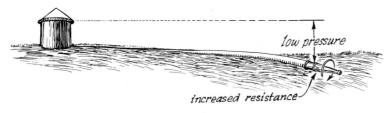

FIGURE 3–6 Low voltage

LOW VOLTAGE : *Current stops*

Clinical Significance

The resistance of tissues in the human body varies between 100 and 1000 Ω. The human fallopian tube has a resistance of 400 to 500 Ω. As tissue is coagulated, water in the cells evaporates, and resistance increases until it prevents further passage of current, similar to turning off the nozzle of a hose. In a system characterized by high-voltage output, when this drying out phenomenon occurs, sparks or leaks through different portions of the instruments can occur (Fig. 3–5; the hose might burst as the nozzle is shut). In systems in which the voltage is low, the amperes vary with the resistance. As the resistance of the tube goes up, the electric flow slows and stops (Fig. 3–6); the nozzle turns off the flow of water at low pressures.

Since the human fallopian tube has a relatively low resistance, it can easily be heated to coagulation with a 25- to 50-W generator. Generators shared with urologists, who need up to 300 W to cut through the prostate under water, subject the gynecologic patient to avoidable risk, particularly if the operating room personnel are unfamiliar with dial settings.

Generators and Circuits

Kinetic energy of water stored behind a dam (Fig. 3–7) (1) drives a turbine that moves a wire through a magnetic field (2) in a hydroelectric generator. Electrons start flowing with energy (3), transmitted with little loss until the resistance of the fallopian tube (4) dissipates the electron's energy as coagulating heat. Electrons then continue to flow through the body to the ground plate (5) into the ground (6), displacing electrons until they are replaced at the other end of the generator wire (7). (In the water analogy, the great water cycle of the Earth involves evaporation into the clouds, rain falling into reservoirs, and man's use of a small fraction of this cycle as the water comes out of the hose.) Electrons are not absorbed by tissue—their energy is. All electrons doing work must return to the ground. These electrons seek the path of least resistance in their journey, just as water does as it flows downhill.

FIGURE 3–7 The Great Electron Circuit

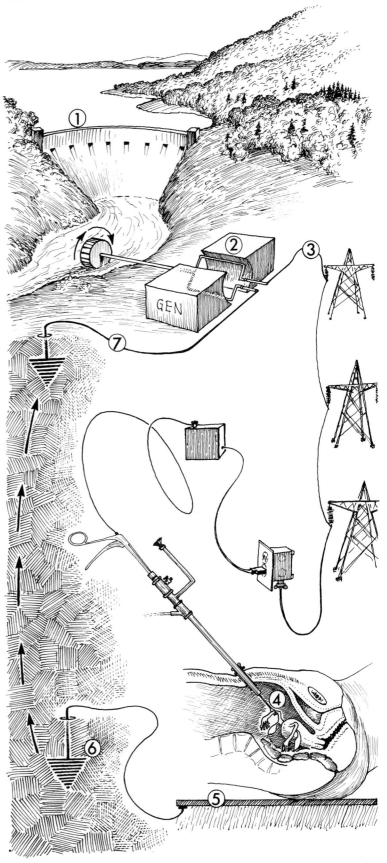

FIGURE 3–8 Anatomy of alternating current

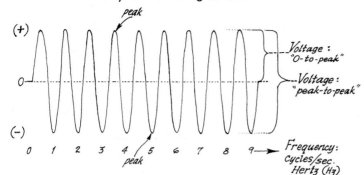

Alternating current flows to and fro, increasing to a maximum voltage in one direction, dropping to zero and increasing to the same voltage in the opposite direction. The United States has settled on electricity supplied as an alternating current of 60 cycles/sec (50 cycles/sec in Europe). The frequency of the waves measured in seconds is described as hertz (Hz) (named after Heinrich Rudolf Hertz, German physicist, 1857 to 1894). One Hz is a frequency of 1 cycle/sec. Voltage is measured from zero to maximum (peak voltage) or from the maximum in one direction to the maximum in the other (peak-to-peak voltage) (Fig. 3–8). The ordinary household (and hospital) power supply is 60 Hz. Because nerves and muscles respond to frequencies below 10,000 Hz, modern electrocoagulation generators convert the 60-Hz house current into high-frequency patterns using solid-state circuits. These generate frequencies between 300,000 and 4,000,000 Hz, with no particular biologic advantage as these frequencies are increased beyond 10,000 Hz. However, at these frequencies tissue impedance (a combination of resistance, inductance, and capacitance) results in biologic effects much more complex than a simple water analogy can explain and beyond the scope of this chapter.

Clinical Currents

In 1928, Harvey Cushing, an American neurosurgeon, described the advantage of using electrical current for control of hemorrhage in brain surgery. The high-frequency current was generated by a unit designed by William T. Bovie; the name Bovie has since become a colloquial term in the operating room for electrosurgical units. These early units were spark-gap units in which transformers boosted the voltage of a current until it could jump across an air gap; regulation of the size of the gap would regulate the characteristics of the current. This "spark-gap" power source was useful to *fulgurate* (intense superficial carbonization and shrinkage of tissue) to create a physical barrier of coagulum to stop bleeding. Spark-gap generators are no longer used in operating rooms but are still sold as small generators to be used in doctors' offices for various minor coagulation purposes.

"CUTTING" AND "COAGULATING" CURRENTS. In modern solid-state generators cutting and coagulating currents are produced by varying either the voltage or the wave patterns. The use of these clinical terms to describe currents has led to much misunderstanding. As Hausner (1989), a biomedical engineer in this field, puts it,

The reason for misconception over which type of current to use lies in the incorrect and greatly antiquated terminology for cutting current and coagulation current. It would be much better to use the correct terminology: modulated current and nonmodulated current. Many accidents originate out of this misconception.

NONMODULATED CURRENT. High-frequency electrical current generates intense heat in tissue when applied through a small contact area such as a needle tip electrode. The resultant high-energy densities turn the tissue water into steam and literally vaporize the cells. This is the nonmodulated wave supplied when these generators are set on "cutting" current (Fig. 3–9).

MODULATED CURRENT. Bursts of electric waves are separated by intervals in which no energy is passing through the tissue. During the "off" period, the heat generated by the bursts of electricity dissipates by conduction into the tissue and heats it up (coagulates); however, the heat does not vaporize it. Current flow less than 10% of the time ("coagulating") is useful for coagulation or hemostasis by desiccation. Higher voltages result in deeper tissue penetration of the heat during the bursts, with more volume of tissue coagulated.

BLENDED CURRENT. Current flow 50 to 80% of the time is useful in cutting through vascular tissue such as muscle. In open surgery in which relatively large amounts of tissue need to be divided quickly, a nonmodulated cutting current with peak voltages of 1200 V is used. A blended current can have peak voltages of 2000 V. Coagulation currents are modulated waves with peak voltages of 5000 V. More precise coagulation, involving good, relatively large surface contact with a ball, the side of a blade, small forceps, and so forth, is actually best accomplished with a nonmodulated wave (set on "cutting" current) of less than 500 V. The current for bipolar coagulation is such a low-voltage, nonmodulated one.

FIGURE 3–9 Clinical currents

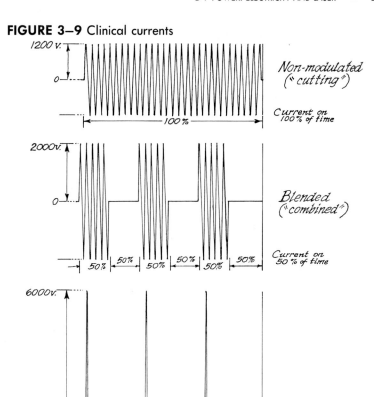

FIGURE 3–10 Unipolar induction of capacitance

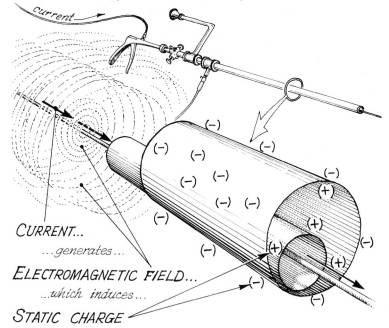

current

CURRENT...

...generates...

ELECTROMAGNETIC FIELD...

...which induces...

STATIC CHARGE

Capacitance

As electrons pass through a unipolar forceps, they generate an electromagnetic field that in turn will create an electrical charge in nearby conductors (Fig. 3–10). In an operating laparoscope, the forceps are completely insulated from the surrounding metal laparoscope and sleeve. In a bipolar forceps, the electrical currents within the forceps running in both directions cancel out each other's electromagnetic fields, and no charge is created in the surrounding metal of the laparoscope. If the laparoscope is not touching any other part of the circuit (e.g., if it is held outside of the body in the air with rubber-gloved hands), this electrical energy in unipolar systems will be stored in the metal tubes as a capacitor, which is defined as any device that can store an electrical charge.

Under normal conditions, when a unipolar electrical current is passed through an operating channel of a laparoscope, the electrical charge of the surrounding laparoscope is rapidly dissipated by contact with a metal sleeve. The sleeve has a relatively large surface in contact with the patient's abdominal wall, and no damage occurs. If, however, the sleeve surrounding the laparoscope is nonconducting, this electrical energy may be released through a relatively small area, such as the laparoscope's accidentally touching bowel (Fig. 3–11A).

In a second-puncture approach, however, inadvertent contact between the live metal electrode and a metal sleeve has led to skin burns at the second-puncture site. This situation can occur as a unipolar instrument is drawn up toward the sleeve for retraction. For this reason, plastic or fiberglass is used for second-puncture sleeves, allowing elevation of tissue away from adjacent structures and touching the forceps to the sleeve without fear of causing a skin burn by such contact (see Fig. 3–11B).

Moreover, a coagulating (modulated) current going through a metal second-puncture sleeve may have about half its power lost through capacitance, requiring dangerously high voltages to achieve unipolar cutting for dissection. An all-plastic or fiberglass sleeve is therefore required for second-puncture electrodissection. With some combinations of disposable instruments and high-frequency generators, thin insulation may allow a potentially hazardous capacitance current to be generated in tissue touching the insulated shaft.

To minimize these risks, Electroscope Inc. has developed a reusable sheath connected to their power source by way of a monitor. When an insulation failure or excess current is detected, the generator is disabled.

FIGURE 3–11 *A and B,* Dangers of metal versus plastic sleeves

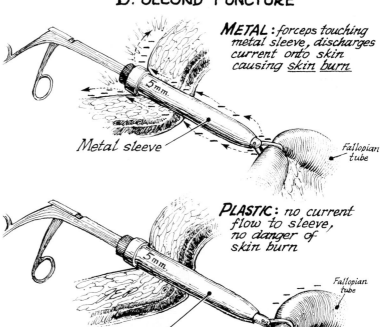

A. OPERATING LAPAROSCOPES

METAL: *the charge is constantly dissipated over a large area of abdominal incision*

Metal sleeve

Bowel

PLASTIC: *the charge may discharge onto bowel on contact with the laparoscope, causing* <u>*bowel burn*</u>

Plastic sleeve

Bowel

B. SECOND PUNCTURE

METAL: *forceps touching metal sleeve, discharges current onto skin causing* <u>*skin burn*</u>

Metal sleeve

Fallopian tube

PLASTIC: *no current flow to sleeve, no danger of skin burn*

Plastic sleeve

Fallopian tube

FIGURE 3–12 Coagulation; desiccation; fulguration; cautery

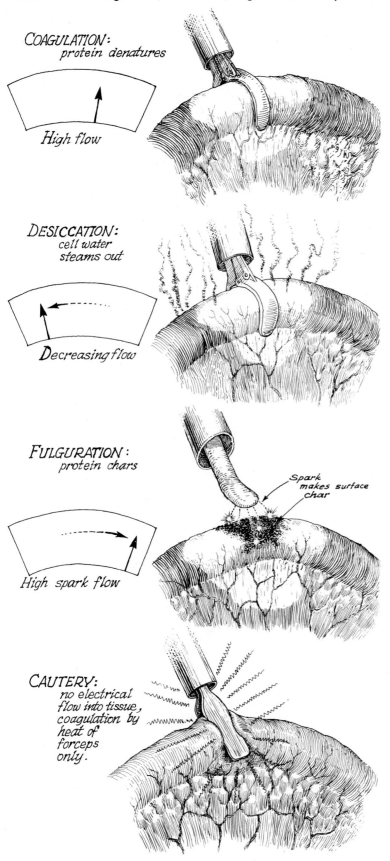

COAGULATION:
protein denatures

High flow

DESICCATION:
cell water steams out

Decreasing flow

FULGURATION:
protein chars

Spark makes surface char

High spark flow

CAUTERY:
no electrical flow into tissue, coagulation by heat of forceps only.

Effects of Current

Electrical currents have several specific effects on tissue:

1. *Coagulation* (Fig. 3–12): denaturation of protein coagulation in tissue from heat (45 to 100 degrees) produced by a current.

2. *Desiccation* (see Fig. 3–12): heating of tissue past coagulation until cellular water has evaporated and the tissue is dry (100 degrees). In the "2075" electric generator designed by Kleppinger for the bipolar system of the Richard Wolf Medical Instruments Corp., an ammeter (measuring amperes, or current flow) initially jumps when the forceps hold the tube and the current is turned on; the tissue turns white (electrocoagulation) with the maintenance of a steady flow of electrical current. The electrical current slowly drops back as desiccation of the tissue causes the resistance of the tube to increase.

When the tube is completely desiccated (dry), there is no electrolytic solution left in the cells to conduct electricity, current flow stops, and the ammeter returns to zero. This is the endpoint for current application. Because the surgeon is usually looking through the scope and cannot see the ammeter, a nurse needs to report the needle position. The Elmed bipolar power source provides an audible tone that lowers its pitch as the current decreases. A unit to indicate current flow of most generators is available (Electroscope EPM-1).

3. *Fulguration* (see Fig. 3–12): allowing sparks to fly from a large electrode to tissue, causing a surface char and coagulum of underlying tissue with little tissue separation. This process is in contrast to cutting, in which a spark is allowed to leap from a fine electrode, rapidly destroying small cells and resulting in separation of tissue and little underlying coagulation.

4. *Actual cautery* (see Fig. 3–12): applying heat to tissue from a heated filament resulting in a direct burn. The term *cautery* is also used incorrectly to describe coagulation, as in bipolar cautery.

GROUNDING SYSTEMS. Since all electrons must eventually seek ground to return to the wire in which they were generated, several different grounding systems are available.

1. In the *traditional grounded system* (Fig. 3–13), the current is delivered through an active electrode to the site required in the patient. The electrons then dissipate through the patient's tissues to a ground plate, usually connected to the thigh, which is in turn connected to a metallic connector in the operating room through which the electrons go into the ground (just as water in a hose flows onto the ground).

2. In the *isolated system* (Fig. 3–14), the current going into the patient returns by way of a return plate, which is not connected to the ground but which returns electrons to the isolated circuit of the generator. The patient forms part of a circuit isolated from the grounded current coming from the wall, as well as the metal in the room connected to the ground. The water-cooling system of an automobile, in which water is recirculated but isolated from the great water cycle of the Earth, is a good analogy for the isolated circuit.

The great safety advantage of this isolated system is that no current will flow if the return electrode is not correctly connected to the circuit, whereas traditionally grounded systems with faulty ground connections will allow electrons to seek the path of least resistance through electrocardiogram (ECG) electrodes or other small areas where the patient's body is in contact with metal during surgery.

FIGURE 3–13 Unipolar grounded system

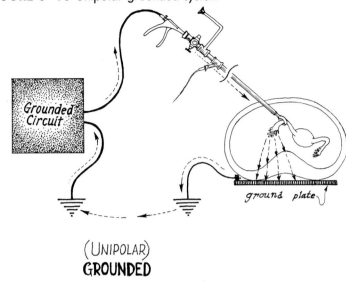

FIGURE 3–14 Unipolar isolated system

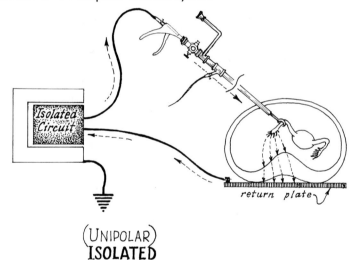

FIGURE 3–15 Unipolar forceps system

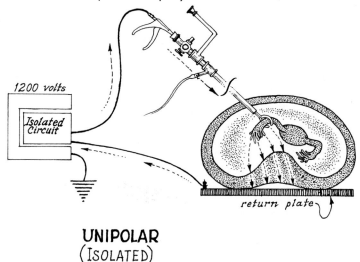

1200 volts

Isolated Circuit

return plate

UNIPOLAR
(ISOLATED)

FIGURE 3–16 Bipolar forceps system

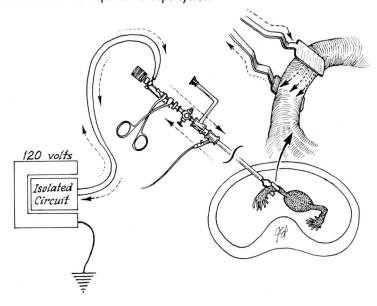

120 volts

Isolated Circuit

BIPOLAR
(ISOLATED)

FORCEPS SYSTEMS. The forceps delivering the electrical energy through the body can be designed in two ways. The *unipolar system* (Fig. 3–15) considers the forceps as one electrode through which the electrical current flows to the ground plate or return plate. This system requires a 1200-V generator. In this arrangement, a large portion of the patient becomes part of the circuit as electrons must flow from the point at which they are delivered by the forceps to the ground or return plate. Risks of accidental burns are higher with this system because electrons seek the path of least resistance, which may be the adjacent bowel, as electrocoagulation desiccates the tube touching the bowel. Because of unexplained bowel injuries by good surgeons using the unipolar technique, alternative mechanical and electrical techniques have been sought.

The *bipolar system* (Fig. 3–16) is essentially a miniaturized isolated circuit, in which one prong of the forceps is the source of the current and the second prong is the return plate. With high-frequency alternating current, both prongs are equal in design and function. The current does not travel through the body to an externally placed return plate, but only through the tissue held between the electrodes. This system requires only a 120-V generator. The patient does not become a part of the circuit, only the tissue between the electrodes does. When the two prongs coagulate the tissue excessively, the prongs come into contact at some point and no current flows through the highly resistant tissue, preferring the low resistance of the metal prongs. For these biophysical reasons, bipolar systems have greatly reduced the hazards of intra-abdominal accidental burns.

Both nonmodulated (cutting) and modulated (coagulation) waveforms can be passed through these electrodes, but a nonmodulated (cutting) low-voltage current is usually recommended. A more uniform desiccation process is obtained using a nonmodulated current, as the steady in-flow of electrons without a change in peak voltage appears to reach the core of the tissue being desiccated before the surface impedance becomes too great. With modulated high-voltage "coagulation" current in the bipolar mode, often the outer layers of tissue in direct contact with the tip become quickly desiccated with superficial resistance developing. This resistance may prevent deeper penetration by the electrons delivered; incomplete desiccation results. Thus, when using bipolar forceps, a nonmodulated waveform should be selected.

Electrode Shape and Electron Density

The amount of heat that an electrical current generates is directly related to the electron density passing through the tissue, which is determined by the metal contact area of the electrode. In the least-damaging configuration (Fig. 3–17), two large metal plates are placed with a sore shoulder or other body part between them, and a diathermy current is passed through the body to generate warmth with no burning. If just the wire to one of those plates touches the skin (Fig. 3–18), the same number of electrons will be flowing into that small area. Electron concentration or density in the skin touching the wire will be great enough to heat the skin to the point of burning.

FIGURE 3–17 Electron density: diffused

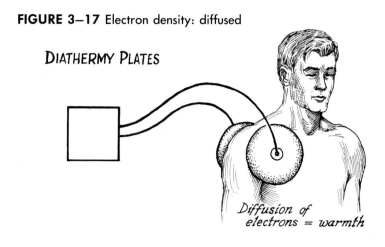

FIGURE 3–18 Electron density: concentrated

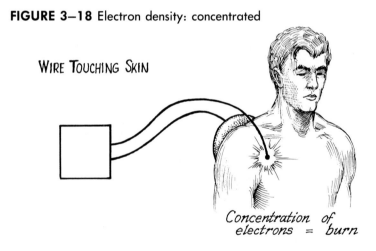

FIGURE 3–19 Unipolar forceps: one small electrode area

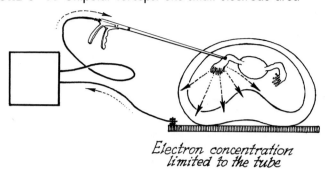

Electron concentration limited to the tube

FORCEPS. The second example illustrates the principle in the unipolar coagulating forceps (Fig. 3–19), where the small electrode area is in a forceps configuration to distribute electrons densely through the tube to coagulate it. The electrons then dissipate into adjacent structures such as the uterus or vessels and thus are no longer concentrated enough to heat these tissues. The bipolar forceps (Fig. 3–20) similarly has a relatively small surface grasping the tube between two prongs, limiting the entire circuit to the tube and allowing electrical current to generate heat between the two prongs to the point of coagulation and desiccation.

FIGURE 3–20 Bipolar forceps: equal electrode area

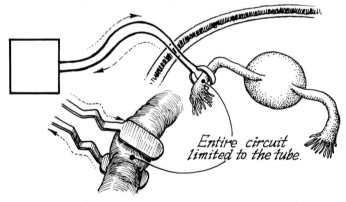

Entire circuit limited to the tube.

In using coagulation to control hemorrhage (Fig. 3–21) (e.g., applying a unipolar, nonmodulated, lower voltage current to a hemostat on a bleeder in an abdominal incision), the rapidity of the coagulation is directly dependent on the amount of tissue grasped in the forceps. A lower density of low-energy electrons is distributed by the forceps over a wider area, and the lower energy load coagulates, rather than evaporates, the tissue. If the area of contact is large (e.g., a large bite or in a pool of blood, which is an excellent conductor), no coagulation or hemostasis occurs because the electrons are dissipated over too wide a surface to generate sufficient heat.

KNIFE OR NEEDLE. If the electrode is reduced to a point (Fig. 3–22) (e.g., an electrocoagulation knife or fine needle in microsurgery), the concentration of electrons and energy at the cells making contact through a spark with the electrode causes these cells to vaporize; the spent electrons then rapidly dissipate into adjacent tissues without further damage. The finer the point (of current exit), the higher will be the power density, thus allowing the surgeon to use less power to dissect with less thermal destruction of adjacent tissue. This principle is the key to microsurgical electrodissection.

FIGURE 3–21 Electron density: coagulating

FORCEPS ELECTRODE

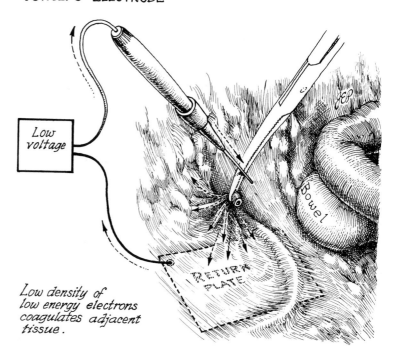

Low density of low energy electrons coagulates adjacent tissue.

FIGURE 3–22 Electron density: cutting

FINE-POINT ELECTRODE

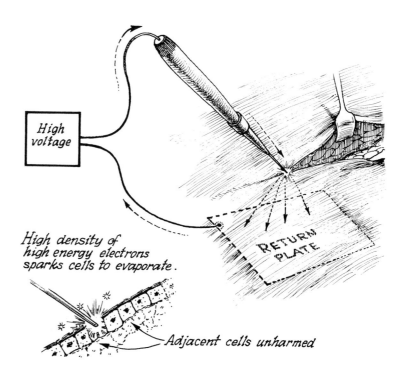

High density of high energy electrons sparks cells to evaporate.

Adjacent cells unharmed

FIGURE 3–23 Timing: cutting

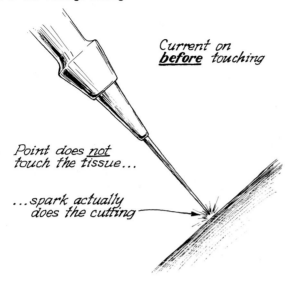

Current on ***before*** *touching*

Point does not touch the tissue...

...spark actually does the cutting

FIGURE 3–24 Timing: coagulating

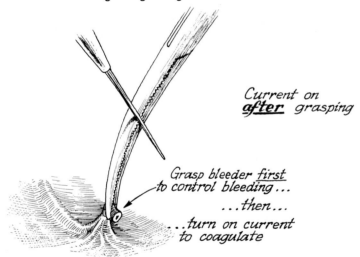

Current on ***after*** *grasping*

Grasp bleeder first to control bleeding...

...then...

...turn on current to coagulate

Timing

Considerations of electrode shape and electron density enter into the timing of applying the electrical current, depending on the surgeon's objective.

In cutting (Fig. 3–23), the electrical current should be turned on before bringing the needle to the tissue to be cut, so that a minimum area of contact exists between the electrode and tissue. (Actually, a fine spark should do the exploding of the cells without the electrodes ever touching the body.) The point of the needle, rather than its side, should be used for cutting, and of course a cutting current should be used. The depth of the incision, degree of lateral damage to tissue, and hemostasis is dependent on a combination of the sharpness of the electrode, the current, and the speed with which the electrode is drawn over the tissue being cut.

For coagulation (Fig. 3–24), on the other hand, the coagulating forceps should be applied first. Mechanical hemostasis is achieved by occluding the vessel between the forceps prongs (or clamps), with a (cutting) low-voltage, nonmodulated current turned on after grasping to ensure coagulation of the vessels gripped within the forceps. Applying the current before firmly grasping the tissue will result in charring of the surface without hemostasis. Beyond these basic physical principles is the "art" of using electrosurgical tools. With a wide selection of currents on the palette and electrodes for brushes, the surgeon perfects the art of electrosurgery just as the painter perfects landscapes.

LASER

The laser beam is another form of energy used in surgery and its use is very similar to that of electricity. The same principles of applying power in different concentrations and forms to cut or coagulate tissue apply. However, the nature of the power delivered to the tissue is uniquely different from electricity and requires separate description.

Laser is an acronym for *light amplification by stimulated emission of radiation.* Certain molecules (e.g., carbon dioxide [CO_2], argon) can be excited inside a "laser tube" by a powerful electromagnetic field so that their electrons jump to a higher energy state. As these electrons decay back to a lower energy state, a *photon* (a unit of energy with a characteristic wavelength) is released. As a photon hits an adjacent molecule, another photon is released with its wavelength exactly in phase with the colliding photon. The cumulative collisions produce a cascading effect, called *stimulated emission.* At either end of a laser tube is a mirror, which reflects these photons back and forth until they emerge out of one mirror. When this beam of photons emerges, it has several unique properties. It is:

- *Monochromatic* (one specific wavelength characteristic of the material)
- *Coherent* (all photons are released in phase with each other so that all waves peak together when they emerge)
- *Collimated* (all waves are parallel and do not diverge over a great distance)

FIGURE 3–25 Laser: different wavelengths

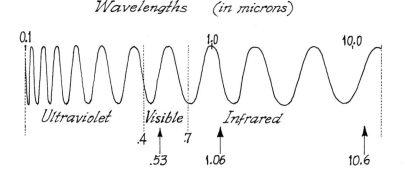

Characteristics	Argon KTP	Nd: YAG	CO$_2$
1. Tissue penetration (cm. water)	30	10	0.5
2. Electrosurgical equivalents	"Coag"	"Blend"	"Cut"
3. Fiber transmission	yes	yes	no

Clinical Lasers

Carbon dioxide in the laser tube results in a wave pattern 10.6 μm in length (Fig. 3–25). This pattern is beyond the visible range, in the far infrared range, and because of its long wavelength this pattern cannot be bent or refracted through fiberglass bundles. It is incapable of penetrating tissue but discharges all its energy on whatever surface (including water) it falls. Thus, it is useful for destruction of superficial cells or adhesions.

Helium-neon (hene) is an inexpensive red beam that is useful to line up the mirrors and instruments required for use of the invisible CO$_2$ laser. This low-energy beam is comparatively harmless to tissues and is also used as a pointer in lectures.

Argon laser is 0.458 to 0.515 μm in length, is visible (green), can be guided easily through fiberglass, and penetrates water up to 30 cm before discharging its energy preferentially into dark-pigmented (green-blue) tissue. This beam is useful in ophthalmology: It can be directed through the cornea, lens, and clear humors of the eye to coagulate the pigmented retina.

Potassium titanyl phosphate (KTP) emits a wavelength of 0.532 μm, similar to the argon wavelength, and is therefore very similar in physical and clinical properties.

Neodymium - yttrium - aluminum - garnet (Nd:YAG) emits a wave that is twice as long as KTP: 1.064 μm. This wave is beyond the visible range in the near infrared, but it can still be guided by fiber bundles. The beam can pass through 10 cm of water, making it useful for deep coagulation of endometriosis and other tissues. However, this poor surface absorption makes it a poor cutting beam without special focusing sapphire tips.

Clinical Laser Waveforms

Laser generators can produce several wave patterns that are similar to those of electro-generators (Fig. 3–26). In contrast to electrons, however, the photons generated by the CO_2 laser do not penetrate tissue but are dissipated into the peritoneal cavity. The biologic effects of different laser waveforms are therefore not the same as the corresponding electrical waveforms.

Continuous wave mode releases energy of a set power (maximum 120 W) constantly from the tube as long as the foot pedal is held. A *single pulse* releases one burst for a specific length of time. A *repeat pulse* releases bursts periodically, with burst time, interval time, and power in watts being a matter of specification by the surgeon. These forms are comparable to nonmodulated ("cutting") current.

Super pulse delivers high power (up to 150 W) at high frequency (250 to 750 pulses per second or pps) but sustained for a brief (10%) part of the duty cycle, so that the total average energy (measured in joules per second) delivered is about one tenth of the maximum (approximately 15 J). This form is comparable with modulated ("coagulation") current.

Power pulse delivers bursts of high power (about 100 W maximum at about 1000 pps) sustained over longer periods (approximately 75% of the duty cycle), so that the duration of contact with tissue is longer and the total average energy (joules per second) delivered is about half the maximum (about 70 J). These forms are comparable to "blended" current.

Ultrapulse (Coherent Co.) delivers high-power (up to 500 W) pulses over a short (<1%) part of a 25-pps duty cycle, allowing longer cooling intervals and vaporization with less char.

FIGURE 3–26 Electricity and laser: modes of power

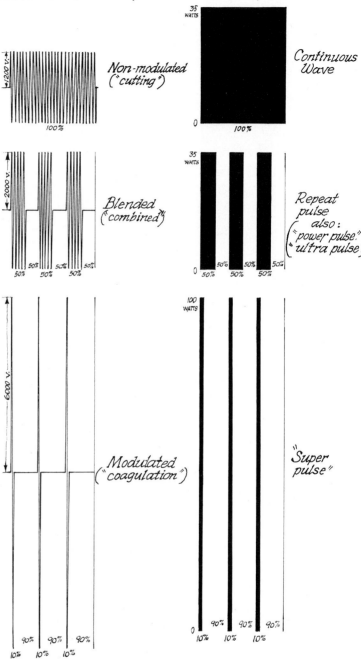

FIGURE 3–27 A–E, Electricity and laser: tissue effects

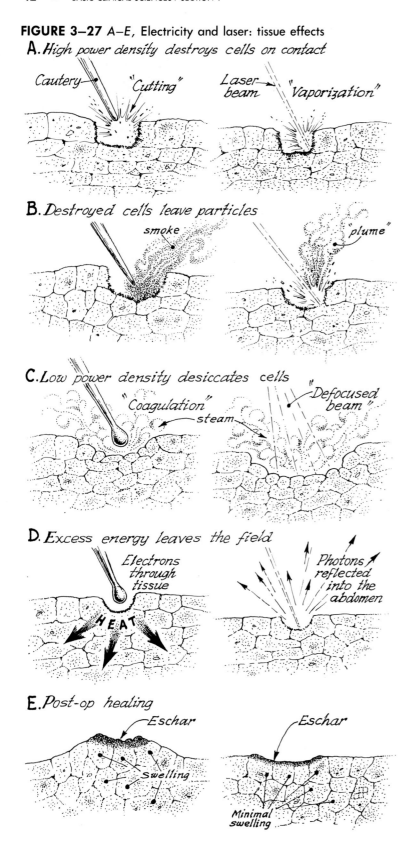

A. *High power density destroys cells on contact*

Cautery — "Cutting"   Laser beam — "Vaporization"

B. *Destroyed cells leave particles*

smoke   "plume"

C. *Low power density desiccates cells*

"Coagulation" — steam   "Defocused beam"

D. *Excess energy leaves the field*

Electrons through tissue   HEAT   Photons reflected into the abdomen

E. *Post-op healing*

Eschar — swelling   Eschar — Minimal swelling

Laser Power Density

Laser power, like electrical power, has different effects on tissue depending on the density with which the power is applied to the tissue. These similar characteristics of electricity and laser are summarized in Figure 3–27. With electricity, the effects are controlled by the size of the contact instrument (e.g., needle, forceps) through which the electrons flow to the tissue. With the laser, this density is controlled by changing the focus of the beam, thus changing the spot size, or area of tissue the photons are striking. A concentrated beam of high-power density cuts tissue or reduces its bulk by *vaporizing* it, with the smoke of the tissue residue going up in a *plume*. A defocused beam, on the other hand, causes coagulation and desiccation of tissue as a low-power density effect.

Cutting

In both electricity and laser, energy delivered is changed into intense heat, which causes cutting or coagulation. The absorbed heat is dissipated into the cavity and into the tissue. When cutting with laser and electricity (see Fig 3–27A), a zone of tissue is coagulated by the heat on the edges of the incision. This can be useful (minimizing bleeding) or harmful (increasing scar formation in healing). The wave pattern, the power density, and the speed with which the surgeon moves through the tissue all affect how deep and wide this zone will be. Beyond this coagulation zone, heat absorption will not coagulate and kill cells but will damage them and will result in postoperative swelling. These outcomes of operative bleeding, postoperative scar, and swelling depend more on the skill of the physician than on the choice of laser versus electricity as the source of power.

SMOKE AND PLUME. High density energy bursts cells, and the cellular debris must go somewhere. This smoke, or plume, is an indicator of the vaporization or destruction of cells (see Fig. 3–27B). The more the smoke, the more tissue is being eliminated. The evacuation of this smoke from the abdominal cavity in laparoscopy makes high-flow gas regulators necessary.

DESICCATION. Lower power density (electricity or laser) does not burst cells but rather heats them past coagulation until the water content is driven out (see Fig. 3–27C). The cells shrink, and in this desiccated state the cells cease to conduct electricity. With bipolar hemostasis, cessation of current flow (desiccation) is the endpoint for current application. This degree of coagulation of tissue usually stops capillary oozing.

Dissipation of Unused Energy

There is an important difference between laser and electricity in how unused energy is dissipated. As electrons discharge their energy in tissue, they flow through tissue to the dispersive electrode (in unipolar electrosurgery) and continue to dissipate energy in the form of low heat. This heat results in postoperative swelling of the viable but damaged tissue just beyond the surgery. Photons, in contrast, are reflected off the tissue that the laser has damaged or destroyed and go back into the cavity in which the endoscopic procedure is being done. There is no heat absorbed by adjacent tissue, thus less postoperative swelling occurs. These photons are of low power and are reflected in a random manner, leading to a clinically nondamaging effect on the cavity (see Fig. 3–27D). This difference is important in neurosurgery, in which postoperative swelling in the confines of the spinal canal or cranium can be life-threatening but is of minor clinical importance in other areas such as tubal surgery (see Fig. 3–27E).

LASER IN LAPAROSCOPY

Use of the CO_2 laser through a laser laparoscope converts the umbilical incision into a portal for performing surgery. The invisible CO_2 laser beam is delivered to the laparoscope through mirrors fixed in an articulating arm. This beam then travels down the 5- to 8-mm operating channel of an operating laparoscope, with a focal point of approximately 2 cm from the end of the laparoscope.

This beam is centered as it travels down the operating channel by adjusting the visible hene (helium-neon) guide beam into a 1-mm spot in the center of the 5- to 8-mm channel. A useful technique is to align the beam and its surrounding symmetrical halo emanating from the laparoscope into the center of the operating channel by using transparent tape or the cuff of the surgeon's glove over the scope tip to identify where the beam exits.

FIGURE 3–28 CO_2 "gas lens"

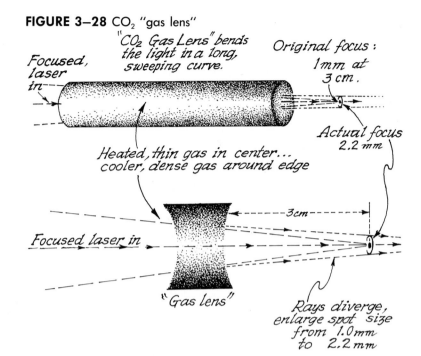

Beam Distortions

The alignment of the articulating arm mirrors requires frequent adjustment to ensure a centralized beam with reproducible tissue effects. Bending of the laparoscope as it traverses through the trocar sleeve causes the centered beam to glance off the channel wall and distort the beam spot. A drop of irrigant on the scope tip, or of rinsing solution inside the channel, acts as a lens and also distorts the beam. Finally, smoke in the peritoneal cavity will block as well as defocus the beam.

Carbon dioxide insufflated through the operating channel is necessary to keep smoke and debris out. However, CO_2 itself distorts the beam (Fig. 3–28). It absorbs between 3 and 19% of CO_2 laser energy in a 5-mm laparoscope channel. This energy heats up the CO_2 in the center of the channel more than at the edges, creating a divergent "gas lens" effect with cool, dense gas at the edges which defocuses the beam. For example, at 50 W of power the spot size increases from 1 to 2.2 mm. This blooming of the spot size occurs at all powers and with all scope sizes and is more noticeable as the power is increased. As a practical result, at 50 W of generator power, 5-mm laparoscopic laser channels have a maximum power density of 732 W/cm². Less than 50-W settings should prove optimal for fine lysis of adhesions. Higher power settings result in larger spot sizes and lower power densities (e.g., at 60 W a spot size of 2.4 mm has a power density of 574 W/cm²) and are suitable for division of vascular tissue such as myomectomy or culdotomy.

Power Reductions

Power produced by the generator is released as an 11-mm beam. As this beam enters the narrower channel of the laparoscope, the laser rays that do not enter the channel are lost as heat in the laser coupler (Fig. 3–29). With high-power settings, the resultant hot coupler can burn the surgeon's hand and require an ice-pack between the coupler and hand to prevent injury. Delivery to tissue is reduced by 30 to 50% with an 8-mm laparoscopic operating channel and by 70% with a 5-mm operating channel. A setting of 40 W in a 5-mm scope thus results in 14-W output at the tissue. In Table 3–1 we present the actual power delivered at a variety of settings by 7.5-mm and 5-mm channel laser laparoscopes.

With these limitations in mind, Reich uses a setting of 35 W in superpulse mode on a Sharplan 1100 laser through a 5-mm operating channel for most procedures (approximately 700 W/cm² at the tissue) and between 80- and 100-W continuous mode for a diffuse hemostatic effect.

FIGURE 3–29 Power loss in laser laparoscopes

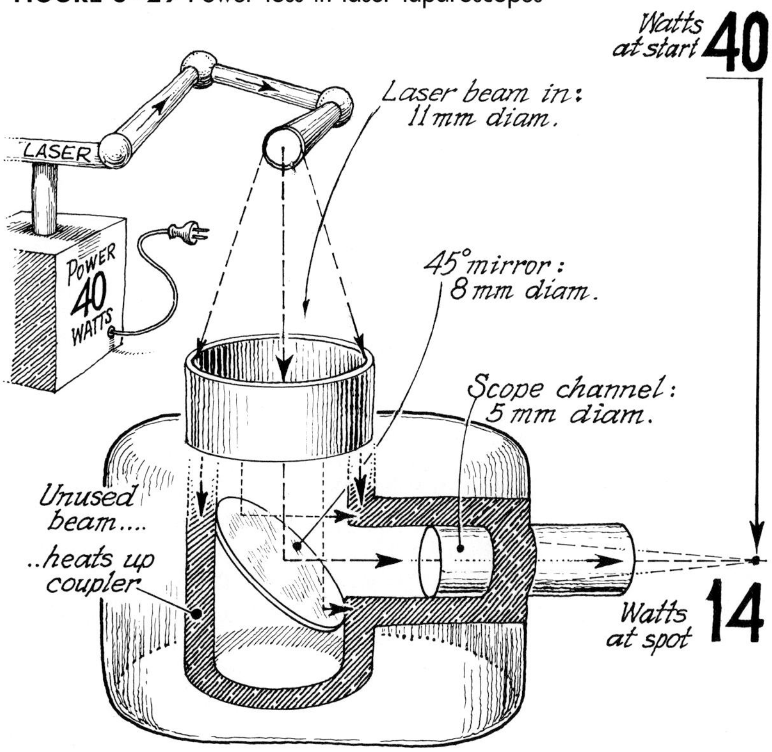

TABLE 3–1.	POWER AT DISTAL END OF SCOPE (CO₂ LASER)*	
Power Entering Laparoscope	Power Leaving Laparoscope (At Tissue)	
Laser Setting	7.5-mm Channel†	5-mm‡
20 W	11 W	5 W
40 W	24 W	14 W
60 W	40 W	20 W
80 W	52 W	27 W
100 W	70 W	32 W

*Sharplan 1100 laser.
†Sharplan or Storz laser laparoscope with 7.5-mm channel.
‡Wolf laser laparoscope with 5-mm channel.

The main effect of the CO_2 laser on tissue is vaporization. This laser can be used for direct vaporization of lesions, but it is more often used for division or separation of adhesions and for excision of tissue in a manner similar to using scissors. As with electrosurgery, blood vessels less than 1 mm in diameter are often coagulated in the process, but application of the beam to an actively bleeding vessel usually results in "boiling, black blood."

The major advantages of the CO_2 laser are:

- Its 0.1-mm depth of penetration, allowing a greater margin of safety when working around the bowel, ureter, and major vessels, with dispersion of heat by the laser plume rather than into the tissue. "What you see is what you get."
- Its ability to reach otherwise inaccessible locations in the deep pelvis perpendicular to the panoramic field of vision while other instruments are used for traction.

Most laparoscopic procedures can be performed without a laser. However, it must be emphasized that laser surgery is associated with a zone of thermal necrosis surrounding treated tissue, and in susceptible patients, adhesions will form. Laser surgery does not result in a reduced rate of adhesion formation when compared with other energy sources. Fiber lasers (KTP, argon, and YAG), in our view, show no advantage over the cutting and coagulation possible with electrosurgery, CO_2 laser, and scissors combinations.

REFERENCES

Hausner K: Electrosurgery—macro vs micro. *In* Laser v. Electrosurgery: Practical Considerations for Gynecology. Addison, IL, Elmed Inc., 1989, pp 7–9.

FURTHER READINGS

ELECTRICITY

Odell RC: Principles of electrosurgery. *In* Sivak MV Jr (ed): Gastroenterologic Endoscopy. New York, Praeger, 1987, pp 128–142.

Rioux J-E and Yuzpe AA: Electrosurgery untangled. Contemp Obstet/Gynecol 4(3):118–124, 1974.

Rioux J-E and Yuzpe AA: Know thy generator. Contemp Obstet/Gynecol 6(4):52–77, 1975.

Semm K: Atlas of Gynecologic Laparoscopy and Hysteroscopy. Philadelphia, WB Saunders, 1977.

LASER

American College of Obstetricians and Gynecologists: Laser technology. ACOG Tech Bull no. 146, September 1990.

Reich H, MacGregor TS III, and Vancaillie TG: CO_2 laser used through the operating channel of laser laparoscopes: In vitro study of power and power density losses. Obstet Gynecol 77:40–47, 1991.

Gas and Pneumoperitoneum

Pneumoperitoneum—the instillation of gas into the peritoneal cavity—is necessary to enhance the surgeon's ability to see inside the cavity. Local anesthesia and laparoscopic laser surgery are two extremes of the requirements for pneumoperitoneum. In this chapter we present the principles underlying correct choices of gases and equipment.

CHOICE OF GAS

Carbon dioxide (CO_2) and nitrous oxide (N_2O) are used for laparoscopy: CO_2 is the gas that is most rapidly absorbed by the blood should an open venous channel lead to CO_2 embolism, and many prefer it for this reason. N_2O is 68% as rapidly absorbed in the blood as CO_2 and has the great advantage of being inert on peritoneal surfaces, causing no pain under local anesthesia for sterilization or diagnostic procedures. CO_2 turns into carbonic acid on the moist peritoneal surfaces and can cause considerable discomfort.

During prolonged laparoscopic surgery, N_2O may leak out into the operating room and affect personnel. Also, although it is not itself an explosive and has been used safely for many years for electrocoagulation sterilization, it supports combustion better than room air. Laser ablation releases carbon particles (smoke or plume) into the abdominal cavity. A combination of this particulate matter, an oxidizing gas, and the high temperatures created when laser energy hits smoke particles can result in an explosion. N_2O should therefore *not* be used for laser ablation.

FIGURE 4–1 Gas-regulating system: schematic diagram

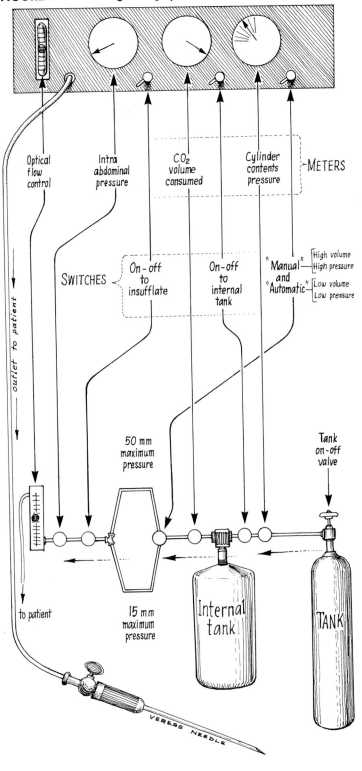

Optical flow control
Intra abdominal pressure
CO₂ volume consumed
Cylinder contents pressure
METERS

outlet to patient

SWITCHES

On-off to insufflate
On-off to internal tank
"Manual" and "Automatic"
High volume / High pressure
Low volume / Low pressure

50 mm maximum pressure
Tank on-off valve

to patient
15 mm maximum pressure
Internal tank
TANK

VERESS NEEDLE

DELIVERY SYSTEM

The most widely used gas-regulator system was designed by Kurt Semm (Fig. 4–1). A CO_2 or N_2O tank (with its own on-off valve) is connected to the regulator that shows the tank pressure. After pressure reduction, gas is allowed into a 10-liter reserve tank by a "fill" switch. A high-pressure (50 mm Hg) or low-pressure (15 mm Hg) maximum out-flow system is chosen by a "manual-auto-matic" switch. The "on-off" flow switch allows gas to enter the abdomen. The vol-ume of gas remaining in the reserve tank, the outflow pressure, and gas flow are mon-itored.

Since it has been observed in air con-trast radiographic studies of the spinal canal that the body can safely absorb CO_2 intra-venously when administered for somewhat less than 1 l/min, pneumoperitoneum should be begun at insufflation rates well below 1 l/min for maximum safety.

COMMON PROBLEMS

Patient Variation

Patients can vary widely in their pressure and volume requirements. The thin, nulliparous, athletic patient with strong abdominal musculature has a small abdominal cavity (Fig. 4–2) that will rapidly be distended to an elevated pressure with a relatively low volume (1 to 2 liters) of gas, especially under local anesthesia. In contrast, a moderately obese, parous patient with relaxed abdominal walls has a larger abdominal cavity (Fig. 4–3) that will require more volume (5 to 6 liters) to distend to an elevated pressure. In markedly obese women with a thick abdominal wall, the thickness of the wall (in centimeters) adds to the baseline intra-abdominal pressure roughly in millimeters of mercury (Fig. 4–4), so that the endpoint of intra-abdominal pressure in these women should be near the upper limits of normal, or about 20 mm Hg. The true intra-abdominal pressure should never exceed 20 to 25 mm Hg, because higher pressures may interfere dramatically with the diaphragmatic excursion in respiration or with central venous return due to vena caval compression. Since the insufflating gas flow usually adds 3 to 7 mm Hg of measured pressure because of the resistance of the insufflation system, the true intra-abdominal pressure can be rapidly determined by turning this flow off for a moment.

Operative laparoscopy requires delivery systems capable of high rates of insufflation (9 to 15 l/min) to compensate for leakage during instrument changes and suction evacuation of smoke from a laser or from electrodissection.

Equipment Difficulties

All commercial insufflating equipment has automatic valves for maintaining safe pressures throughout laparoscopy if the machine is switched to them after induction of pneumoperitoneum. All laparoscopic trocar sleeves have rubber gaskets and valves to keep intra-abdominal gas from leaking out. If the intra-abdominal gas—and therefore visibility—is disappearing, the surgeon can usually find an open valve, a loose connec-

FIGURE 4–2 Volume: thin patient

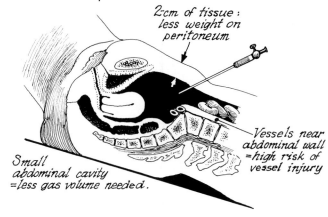

FIGURE 4–3 Volume: fat patient

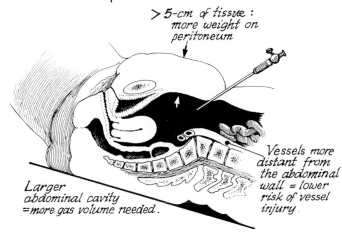

FIGURE 4–4 Intra-abdominal pressure: fat patient

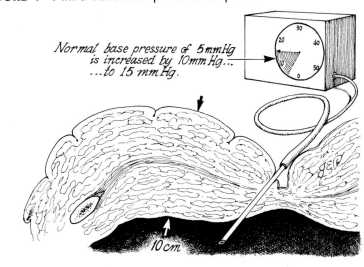

FIGURE 4–5 Avoidance of postoperative pain

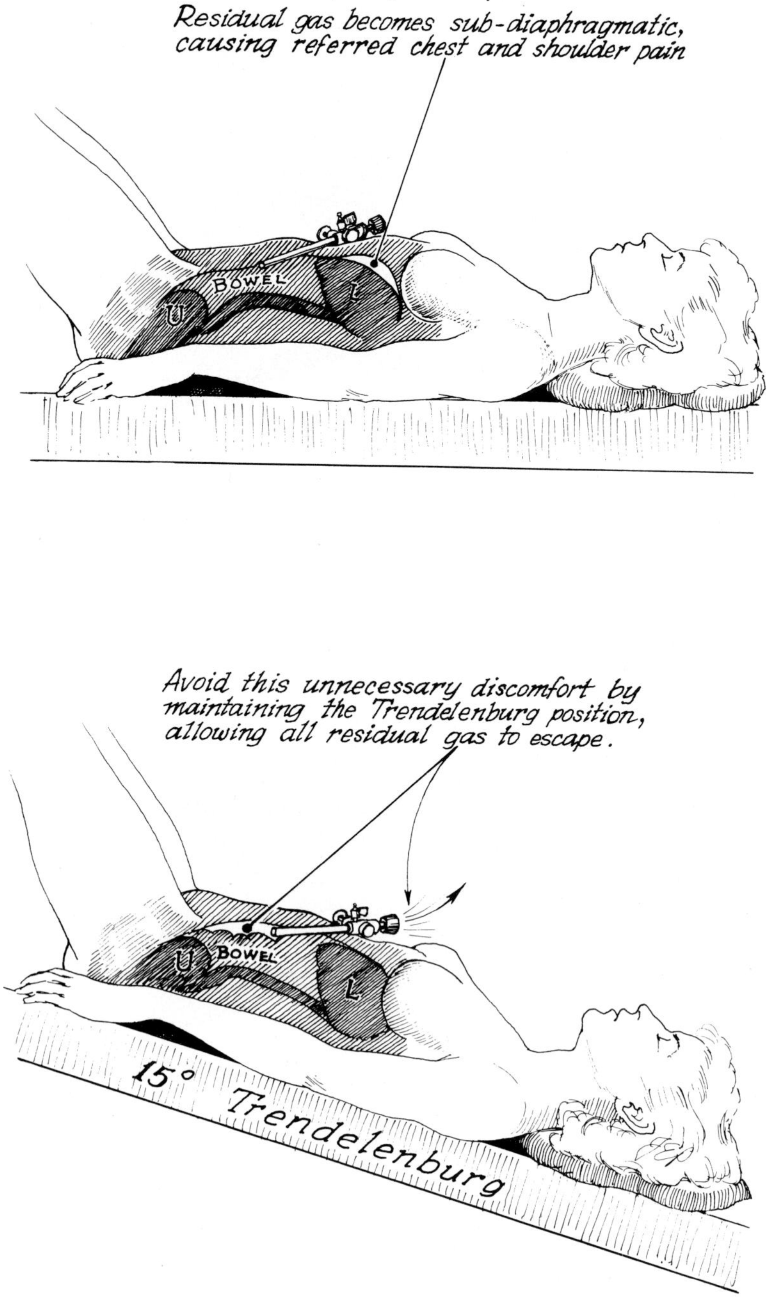

Residual gas becomes sub-diaphragmatic, causing referred chest and shoulder pain

Avoid this unnecessary discomfort by maintaining the Trendelenburg position, allowing all residual gas to escape.

15° Trendelenburg

tion, a cracked gasket, or an empty gas tank. Neither diagnostic nor operative procedures should continue in the presence of such easily correctable flawed equipment.

Postoperative Chest and Shoulder Pain

Residual pneumoperitoneum (Fig. 4–5) causes one of the most uncomfortable parts of the procedure—postoperative chest and shoulder pain caused when gas remains in the abdomen and irritates the diaphragm when the patient sits upright. To avoid this situation at the end of the procedure, keep the patient in the Trendelenburg position with the trumpet valve of the sleeve open to allow gas to be evacuated. Only after the sleeve is removed should the Trendelenburg position be discontinued.

Another strategy to displace abdominal gas is to instill 2 to 3 liters of Ringer's lactate and place a 5-mm blunt probe in the umbilical incision to purge the abdomen of gas. By pushing bowel and omentum away from the incision, gas is released and postoperative pain is markedly diminished.

Because some gas invariably remains, it may be difficult to evaluate possible bowel perforation after laparoscopy since subdiaphragmatic gas is a normal laparoscopic finding for 24 to 48 hours in cases of incompletely evacuated pneumoperitoneum.

Facilities and Equipment

Laparoscopy is best performed in a room sufficiently generous in size to accommodate all tables necessary for the procedure and the endoscopy team. Ideally, laparoscopy should be part of the endoscopy service of an operating room where trained staff technicians can handle the delicate equipment between cases.

OPERATING ROOM PERSONNEL

In most hospitals the rotations of nurses and technicians through the laparoscopy service are such that no particular person is assigned to the maintenance of this equipment. The equipment is cared for in the same manner as other lap packs and instruments. As a result, optics that normally would have a life span of 2000 procedures may have a life span of no more than 500

procedures before someone inadvertently sends them to the steam autoclave and ruins the optics or if the optics fall and break. Also, vital portions of the trocars and accessory instruments can be blunted or lost and need replacement, to the point that disposable trocars and sleeves become cost-effective. Gastroenterologists prefer to perform laparoscopy in their own suites, where they have the same skilled nurses and assistants to handle the equipment properly. Some hospitals have combined the endoscopic needs of orthopedics, urology, surgery, and gynecology in rooms specially designed for videoendoscopy and staffed with technicians skilled in handling these delicate instruments. The savings in costs of repair and replacement with such services more than justifies the hiring of special technicians for such an endoscopy suite.

FIGURE 5–1 Somebody help him!

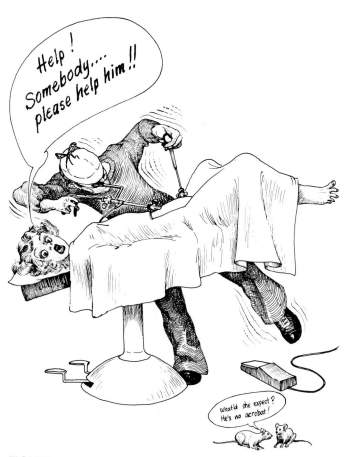

PERILS OF PAUL LEAN M.D.

FIGURE 5–2 Operating room team and equipment

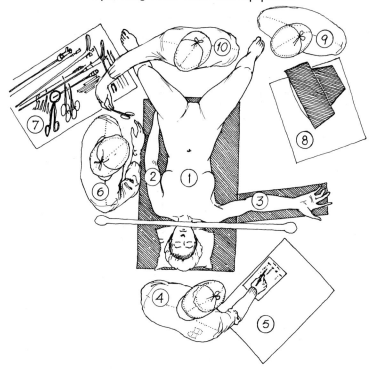

OPERATING ROOM TEAM

There is no more dependent surgeon on Earth than one who has one eye fixed on the view down the laparoscope, one eye shut, one hand holding the scope, the other hand holding a manipulating instrument, one foot on a coagulation pedal, and one foot bearing his or her entire weight. In this position, the surgeon is completely dependent on the skill of the operating room assistants (Fig. 5–1).

The advent of television monitoring has enhanced the use of the laparoscope and made it an extremely useful tool for many operating room teams, since they can look at the television monitor and see what the laparoscopists have been enjoying all these years. Figure 5–2 shows a convenient arrangement of equipment and the operating room team. The patient (1) has her left arm (2) at her side to make room for the surgeon. Her right arm (3) has an intravenous line for the anesthesiologist (4) with monitoring equipment (5). The surgeon (6) is on the patient's left, with sterile equipment (7) behind or beside. Nonsterile "utilities" (e.g., light, gas, electricity, television) (8) are visible across the patient. The nonsterile circulating assistant (9) manages the utilities; the sterile assistant (10) stands at the foot of the operating table to manipulate the uterus and to hand the surgeon instruments from the table (7). The team is vital for the proper selection of equipment before use; the safe and coordinated operation of gas, light, electricity, laser, or coagulation during surgery; and the proper maintenance of equipment after use. For procedures for which access to the uterus is not required and the patient is in the supine position, the assistant (in sterile gown and gloves) can stand on the patient's right side, opposite the surgeon, with an ancillary monitor behind the surgeon. Right-handed surgeons can change places with the assistant quite comfortably with this ancillary monitor, although a period of hand-eye coordination relearning is necessary.

SPECIAL ANCILLARY EQUIPMENT

A narrow operating table with Trendelenburg capacity is required. When the lithotomy position is required for uterine manipulations, the patient's legs should be comfortably supported by padded obstetric leg holders (Fig. 5–3) or Allen stirrups (Fig. 5–4) rather than by the standard leg straps used for dilatation and curettage. This minimizes risk of venous thromboses from prolonged surgery. Strapping the calves onto these stirrups minimizes the risk of the patient's sliding into the anesthetist when the patient is in a steep Trendelenburg position and eliminates the need for shoulder stops, which can cause transient but annoying brachial plexus paralysis.

FIGURE 5–3 Obstetric leg holders

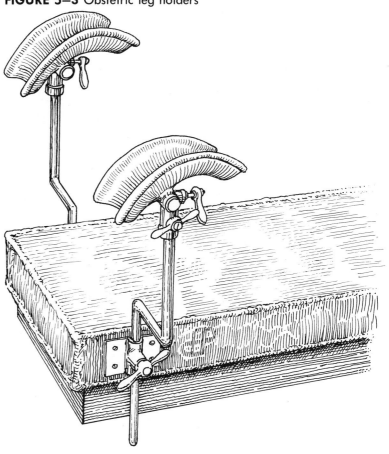

FIGURE 5–4 Allen stirrups

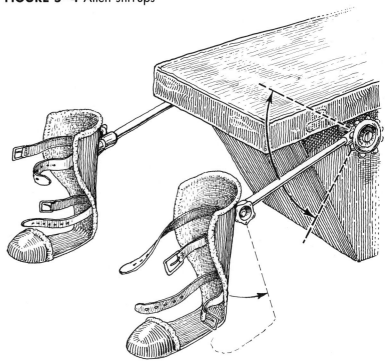

FIGURE 5–5 Single-hinged speculum

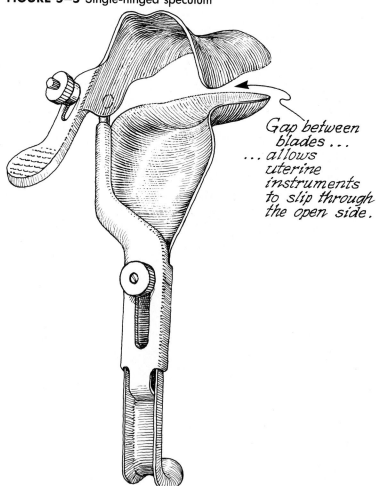

Gap between blades . . . . . . allows uterine instruments to slip through the open side.

To insert uterine manipulators, a *vaginal single-hinged speculum* (Fig. 5–5) with the hinge on the left allows the instruments to be attached to the uterus under direct vision. The speculum can then be removed with ease, thus allowing more room in the pelvis for uterine manipulation, and is more comfortable for the patient under local anesthesia.

A *uterine elevator*, inserted at the beginning of the procedure, is necessary in diagnostic and sterilization procedures to maximize adnexal exposure. The uterus should always be anteverted for laparoscopy. The combined tenaculum and sound (Fig. 5–6) (Hulka controlling tenaculum, made by Rocket, Weck, and Wolf) has a 5-cm–long sound tip deflected almost to a 90-degree angle. This is combined with a tenaculum to hold the sound in the uterus. A button on the handle indicates the direction of the sound.

FIGURE 5–6 Uterine elevator

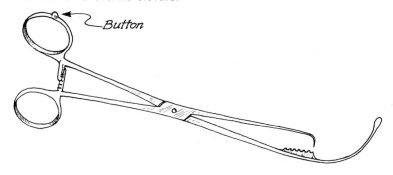

Button

For the occasional combined first-trimester abortion and sterilization, a special *Hulka uterine controlling forceps* (Rocket, Wolf) (Fig. 5–7) is needed to manipulate the recently evacuated pregnant uterus, since standard intrauterine manipulators do not offer maximal uterine control and may lacerate the soft myometrium. If instillation of indigo carmine dye is desired during diagnostic laparoscopy or to check on correct mechanical occlusion of a tube, a standard *hysterosalpingogram spring-loaded cannula,* such as the Cohen-Eder cannula (Eder) (Fig. 5–8) held with a tenaculum, is a simple and secure uterine insufflator but is less versatile for uterine mobility.

FIGURE 5–7 Uterine controlling forceps

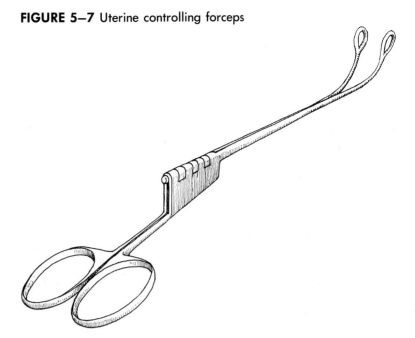

FIGURE 5–8 Uterine insufflator

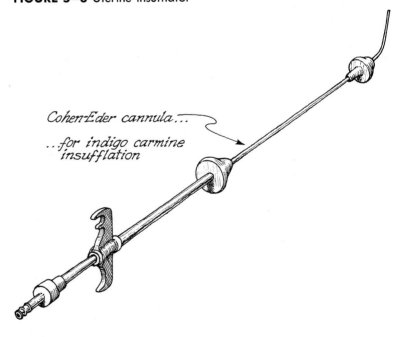

Cohen-Eder cannula...
...for indigo carmine insufflation

FIGURE 5–9 Procedure for retroverted uteri

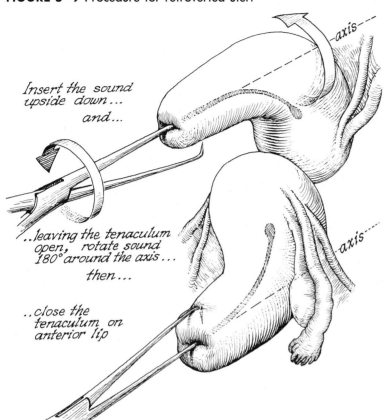

Insert the sound
upside down...
        and...

..leaving the tenaculum
open, rotate sound
180° around the axis...
        then...

..close the
tenaculum on
anterior lip

axis

axis

For retroverted uteri (Fig. 5–9) a uterine elevator can be inserted into the uterus upside down, rotated 180 degrees with the tenaculum open, and secured by the tenaculum in the anteverted position on the anterior lip of the cervix. Recent uterine elevators have been manufactured with a button on the anterior grip of the forceps so that the surgeon can tell by feeling the instrument whether it is properly inserted and also by anteverting the uterus.

The surgeon can use the uterine manipulator to shake down overlying omentum, push up bowel onto the pelvic brim, and elevate ovarian cysts by passing the uterus behind the ovaries and pressing against the pelvic sidewall. In clip application, the isthmus is put on maximal stretch and optimal position by the uterine manipulator.

LAPAROSCOPIC INSTRUMENTS

There should be at least two optics in a hospital providing laparoscopic service. The occasional breakdown of an optic requires sending it off to the manufacturer for repair, during which time the second, backup optic allows the service to continue uninterrupted.

The choice of optics is a highly subjective one, depending on the training of the staff (Fig. 5–10). At least one good *10-mm diagnostic laparoscope* with no operating channel should be available. A *10-mm operating laparoscope with a 5-mm channel* is a good compromise between slightly diminished brightness and flexibility of operating maneuvers.

Physicians doing laparoscopy infrequently will find that a good 10-mm diagnostic laparoscope, combined with a second-puncture sleeve for diagnosis and sterilization, offers the best security in terms of maximum visibility and maximal control of manipulative procedures.

Smaller trocars, sleeves, and instruments are quite satisfactory for diagnostic purposes. In strong men, nulliparous women, children, or patients with a high degree of risk of bowel perforation, a 5-mm sleeve and laparoscope is useful. The 5-mm trocar and sleeve requires a quarter of the force of a 10-mm trocar and sleeve (a quarter of the cross-sectional area and therefore a quarter of the resistance), and 5-mm optics are excellent for direct viewing. Equipment is available to dilate a 5-mm sleeve tract to accommodate a 10-mm sleeve by passing a dilator over a long 5-mm guide.

A 3-mm channel 10-mm operating laparoscope has better optics than a 5-mm channel 10-mm operating laparoscope but accommodates limited equipment, such as an aspirating needle or grasping forceps. A 5-mm channel operating laparoscope is the most versatile and accommodates a variety of instruments (see Fig. 5–10) as well as a bipolar coagulating forceps. A 7-mm channel is required for a clip applicator, and an 8-mm channel is required for a band applicator. Operating laparoscopes for these uses are available.

FIGURE 5–10 Laparoscopes

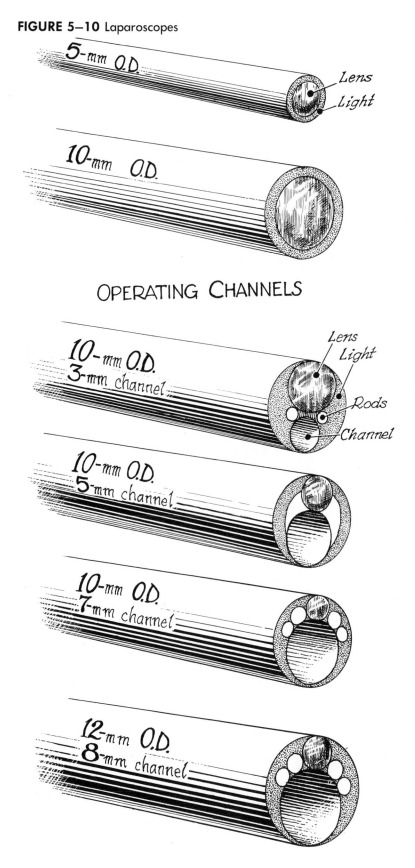

OPERATING CHANNELS

FIGURE 5–11 Manipulating instruments

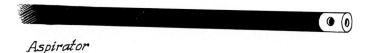

Centimeter probe ... for measuring

Aspirator

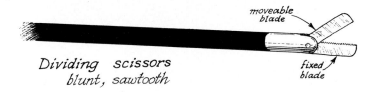

Dividing scissors
blunt, sawtooth

moveable
blade

fixed
blade

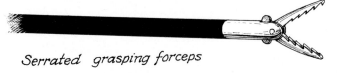

Serrated grasping forceps

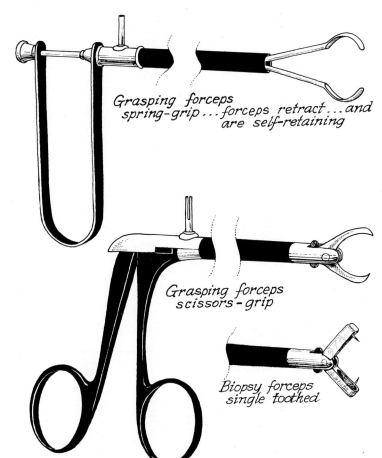

Grasping forceps
spring-grip ... forceps retract ... and
are self-retaining

Grasping forceps
scissors-grip

Biopsy forceps
single toothed

Surgical Instruments

There should be at least one *5-mm second-puncture trocar and sleeve* through which probes can be used for manipulation in diagnostic laparoscopy. Some of the more useful manipulating, grasping, and dividing instruments are illustrated in Figure 5–11. A *centimeter probe* is useful for manipulating and measuring pelvic structures.

An *aspirator* is also a useful tool for clearing abdominal fluid and manipulation and can be adapted to provide suction and irrigation by clever use of a standard three-way disposable stopcock (Fig. 5–12).

Blunt, sawtooth scissors (see Fig. 5–11) are recommended for lysis of adhesions with minimal risk of injuring underlying structures, as occasionally happens with hooked, curved scissors. Since scissors become dull, *disposable scissors* (U.S. Surgical) are useful to ensure sharpness.

Forceps come in a variety of designs. *Serrated alligator* forceps grasp tissue better than any other type but may produce traumatic results. *Self-retaining smooth grasping* forceps are useful for atraumatic manipulation of tubes and bowel during diagnostic procedures. Finally, a *toothed biopsy* forceps, although a poor biopsy remover, is an excellent grasper of strong tissues such as the ovarian cyst wall or peritoneum, and should be used during excision of such structures.

A *Veress needle* (Fig. 5–13) is an important part of most laparoscopy equipment. (This name is often misspelled as Verres; the correct spelling is from the original reference for the needle [Veress, 1938]). The spring should be freely moving between the inner and outer sleeve, and the tip of the inner sleeve should be intact. Often between cases, the tip can be damaged to create a weakness between the outer tip and the lateral hole through which gas escapes. This can lead to difficult insertions of the needle as the tip collapses, or in the inadvertent loss of this tip in the abdomen after successful entry. Also, repeated use dulls the needle tip. Finally, cleaning and reassembling requirements have led many hospitals to use disposable Veress needles to eliminate all these concerns.

The long Veress needle is very useful for aspirating simple ovarian cysts. For simple diagnostic procedures, it can also be used as a second-puncture manipulating instrument. A small nick in the skin with a knife does not require suturing. Ovarian manipulation adequate for diagnosis is possible, and the 5-mm sleeve, trocar, and instruments are not needed.

FIGURE 5–12 "Stewart" system for irrigation-aspiration

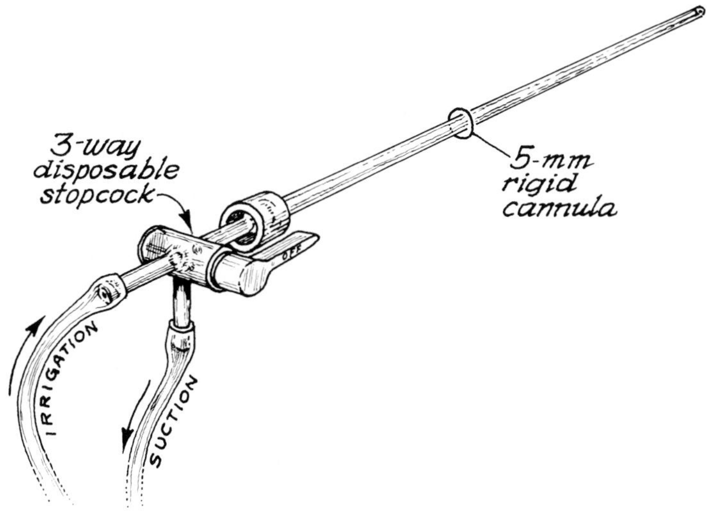

FIGURE 5–13 Veress needle

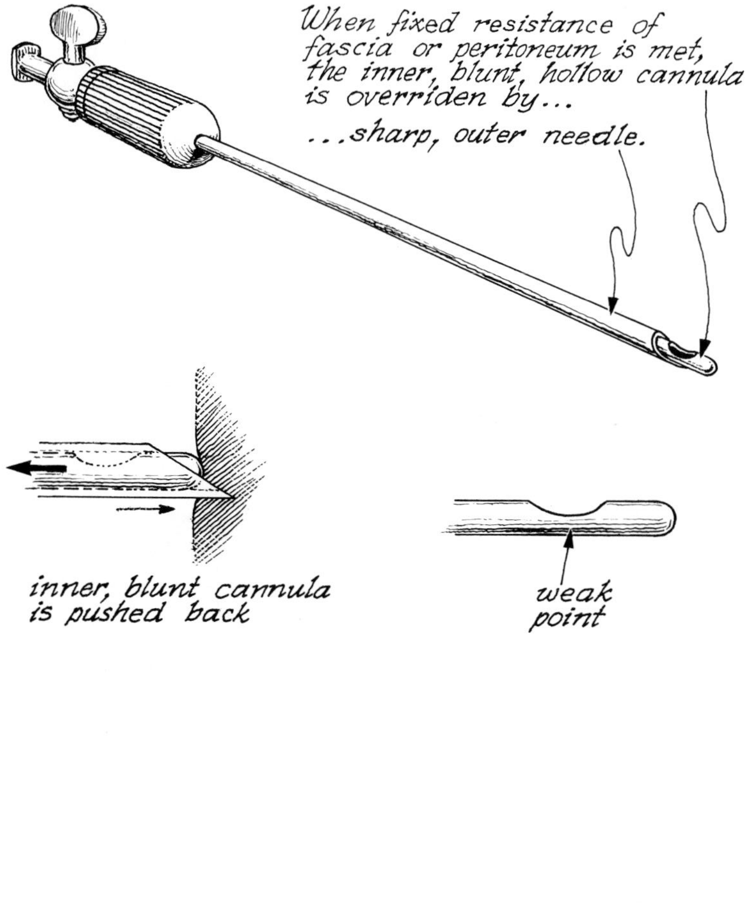

FIGURE 5—14 Bipolar system

Matched generator and forceps:

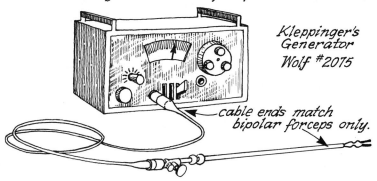

Kleppinger's Generator Wolf #2075

cable ends match bipolar forceps only.

Single-puncture instrument:

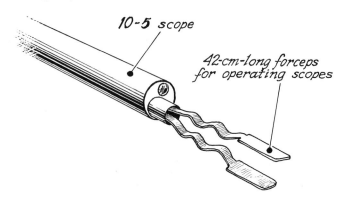

10-5 scope

42-cm-long forceps for operating scopes

Double-puncture instrument:

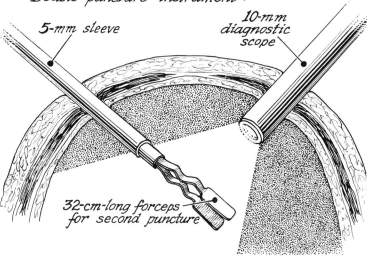

5-mm sleeve

10-mm diagnostic scope

32-cm-long forceps for second puncture

Light, Gas, and Coagulation Sources

A hospital providing laparoscopic capacity should have at least one good light source, gas source, and electrosurgical generator designed for laparoscopic use. Since there is a potential for bleeding with every laparoscopy, functioning electrocoagulation equipment for laparoscopy should be available even though its use is not planned. The Kleppinger biopolar forceps is widely used for hemostasis.

Interchangeability of parts from different manufacturers is an important consideration in purchasing equipment. Manufacturers have agreed upon one standard diameter for the eyepiece to which cameras are attached. Storz fiber cables have end connections that are adaptable to most light sources and optics, although their sleeves and optics are of different diameters. The other manufacturers (e.g., ACMI, Eder, Olympus, Wolf) have standardized diameters of sleeves, optics, and instruments for interchangeability, although their fiber cable end-connectors have not.

Manufacturers have appropriately avoided interchangeability of power cables, to ensure proper matching of forceps and power sources for coagulation (Fig. 5–14). A bipolar forceps must be matched to the appropriate bipolar generator. Mismatches can occur when operating room personnel try to adapt a cable to a power source and may result in too much or too little power flowing through the instruments. If a hospital is switching from unipolar to bipolar, the purchase of an appropriately matched power source is strongly recommended. Finally, if a physician wishes to revert to a unipolar method (e.g., to coagulate endometriosis), the bipolar generator should be replaced with a unipolar generator. Complications from such mismatches have included the incomplete coagulation of the tube leading to subsequent pregnancy, as well as skin burns when excessive wattages are passed through laparoscopes and their sleeves.

Equipment Maintenance

A dull *trocar* may appear to be safe because it diminishes the risk of vessel or bowel injury. On the contrary, a dull trocar markedly increases the force necessary to exert on the abdominal wall during entry. This force depresses the abdominal wall so that the underlying vessels and bowel can be compressed between the wall and the spine, despite the establishment of pneumoperitoneum, and markedly increases the risk of impaling a bowel or blood vessel during entry. Disposable trocars (Rocket), as well as disposable combined trocar and sleeves (U.S. Surgical), eliminate this problem.

Operating room personnel should be instructed to treat the trocars with as much respect as they do knives. Trocars should be inspected periodically for sharpness and should be kept sharp or replaced when dull. Whether a trocar is sharp or not can be determined by holding the edge under a light (Fig. 5–15) and by seeing if light is reflected off the edge. A sharp knife or trocar will not reflect. A thin line of reflected light indicates dullness and the need to sharpen the edge until the light reflection disappears. Many experienced centers are now storing their instruments in a padded but open shelf of a tool chest. The trocar should be stored with a protective covering over its sharp edge. This open-shelf storage allows nurses and physicians to select the instrument that they want for a particular case and to be certain that the equipment they select is in working order before disinfection.

Visual inspection of *insulated* instruments may reveal bare spots (Fig. 5–16) where the sharp edge of a channel has stripped away insulation. The integrity of the entire electric circuit should be tested every day before elective surgery is begun to ensure that the surgery can be completed as planned.

FIGURE 5–15 Checking the trocar for sharpness

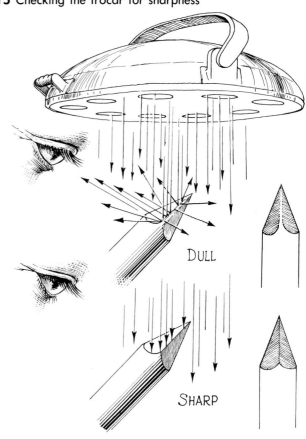

DULL

SHARP

FIGURE 5–16 Stripped insulation

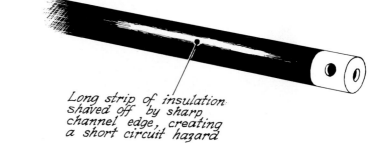

Long strip of insulation shaved off by sharp channel edge, creating a short circuit hazard

FIGURE 5–17 "Bending" of the optic chain

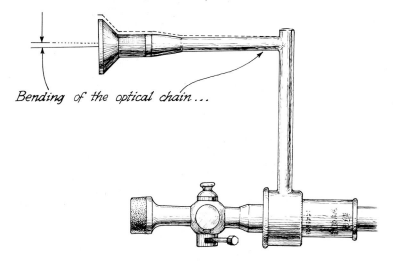

Bending of the optical chain...

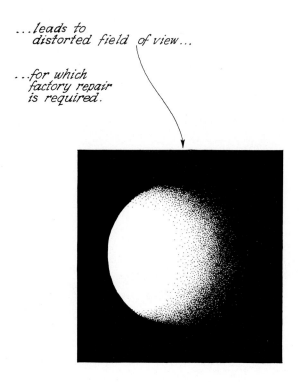

...leads to distorted field of view...

...for which factory repair is required.

The *optics* are the most delicate of the instruments and are most frequently damaged by dropping the scope and bending the optic chain, causing distortion (Fig. 5–17), or by inappropriate heating and chilling, causing internal fogging. There should be at least one backup laparoscope to allow an operating room to continue providing services while a damaged optic is returned to the manufacturer for repairs. There should similarly be a generous supply of all sizes of gaskets and connecting wires for bipolar coagulation.

CLEANING EQUIPMENT. The most effective way to clean optics is to rinse the instruments rapidly in cold water after use and wash thoroughly with soap and a brush. This mechanically removes any bacteria from the surgeon's and patient's skin as well as rinsing away any serum or blood in the scope or sleeve. Simple mechanical instruments should occasionally be disassembled and cleaned. Disassembly after every use may lead to improper reassembly and malfunction; it is not necessary for disinfection (see later).

Most hospitals in the United States are now disinfecting the optics and accessory instruments in alkalinized glutaraldehyde (Cidex) between cases for 20 to 30 minutes. After disinfection, the instruments should be rinsed thoroughly in water, and before storing, the internal channels of the laparoscope should be thoroughly air dried.

All concerned organizations have officially agreed that disinfection with alkalinized glutaraldehyde is not associated with nosocomial transmission of disease. It is nevertheless prudent to recommend that instruments be gas sterilized overnight when feasible and that they be gas sterilized after patients with known active hepatitis, acquired immunodeficiency syndrome (AIDS), or tuberculosis have undergone laparoscopy.

ASSEMBLING EQUIPMENT. Current Association of Operating Room Nurses (AORN) guidelines recommend the disassembly of all equipment for sterilization (Association of Operating Room Nurses Ad Hoc Committee on Infection Control ..., 1980). When this rule is applied to laparoscopic equipment, serious problems arise in the operating room. Technicians and operating room nurses are not familiar with the correct assembly of complex sleeves, gaskets, and forceps with resultant hazardous malfunction of equipment at surgery. To evaluate the bacteriologic need for this disassembly, a series of bacteriologic studies at the Hospital Epidemiology Laboratories of the University of North Carolina at Chapel Hill (Marshburn et al, 1991) demonstrated that exactly the same degree of sterilization was achieved when instruments were disassembled, washed, and assembled (before sterilization) in a central instrument preparation room, compared with sterilizing them unassembled.

We therefore strongly recommend that hospitals provide sterile, correctly assembled laparoscopic equipment to the operating room staff to reduce the very real legal risk of equipment malfunction because of improper assembly.

DISPOSABLE EQUIPMENT. Problems of maintenance, storage, cleaning, disinfecting, and sterilizing laparoscopic equipment have led many hospitals, especially those not used to a high volume of laparoscopic procedures, to rely on disposable products. This is especially useful for instruments that need to be sharp (e.g., Veress needles, trocars, scissors) and are complex to reassemble properly (e.g., sleeves with springs and gaskets). U.S. Surgical Instrument Company is actively developing disposable instruments and kits (e.g., for cholecystectomy, ectopic pregnancy) to meet this practical problem in hospitals that are unfamiliar with laparoscopy.

REFERENCES

Veress J: Neues Instrument zur Ausführung von Brust- oder Bauchpunktionen und Pneumothoraxbehandlung. Dtsch Med Wochenschr 64:1480–1481, 1938.

EQUIPMENT STERILIZATION

Association of Operating Room Nurses Ad Hoc Committee on Infection Control in the Handling of Endoscopic Equipment: Guidelines for preparation of laparoscopic instrumentation. AORN J 32:65–76, 1980.

EQUIPMENT MAINTENANCE

Marshburn PB, Rutala WA, Wannamaker NS, and Hulka JF: Gas and steam sterilization of assembled versus disassembled laparoscopic equipment: Microbiological studies. J Reprod Med 36:483–487, 1991.

SUGGESTED READING

Soderstrom RM: Safeguards in laparoscopy: Education, equipment care, and electron control. Contemp Obstet/Gynecol 11(3):95–107, 1978.

Wound Healing

One reason why laparoscopy has proved to be so safe in a wide variety of clinical situations is that the body's response to the injuries the procedure induces is usually successful and complete. A brief description of these responses will be useful in understanding the normal uneventful healing course and some of the complications which may arise.

FIGURE 6–1 Bacteria and macrophages

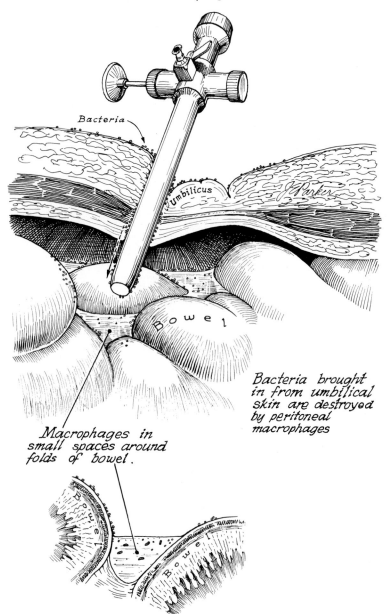

Bacteria

Umbilicus

J. Parker

Bowel

Bacteria brought in from umbilical skin are destroyed by peritoneal macrophages

Macrophages in small spaces around folds of bowel.

BACTERIA AND MACROPHAGES

The umbilical skin cannot be cleansed of all bacteria, even with modern iodophor solutions. Corson and associates (1979a and 1979b) demonstrated that bacteria introduced into the abdomen at laparoscopy come mostly from the abdominal skin (Fig. 6–1). As a sharp trocar makes its way through fascia, fat, and the peritoneum, it separates well-vascularized tissue by a combination of pulling cells apart as well as by cutting through some of them. Tissue destruction (leaving behind dead tissue) is thus minimal, and the bacteria introduced do not have many dead cells to act as a culture medium. When the sleeve is removed, viable tissue with its blood supply falls back together, and normal defense mechanisms rapidly destroy the few bacteria that have been introduced. When blood vessels are torn in entry, a small hematoma can act as a culture medium, and abdominal wound infections can then occur. Similarly, when sutures are placed to close the skin, they act as the focus for the inevitably introduced bacteria and can cause a superficial wound infection. These umbilical sutures, when left long, can act as a wick to encourage bacterial entry. Thus, in most cases, umbilical sutures should be inverted with the knot below the skin.

In the abdominal cavity the bacteria introduced are left on the peritoneal surface, where blood supply combined with the peritoneal cavity's extensive macrophage defense system makes the bacteria rapidly disappear. For these reasons, laparoscopy has been performed with remarkably little infection in situations throughout the world where sterile technique has been impossible.

HEALING OF THE ABDOMINAL WOUND

As soon as the 1-cm sleeve is removed, the tissues of the peritoneum, fascia, and skin come together, usually in their original relationships. If the skin incision site has been carefully chosen in a fold, a skin suture may not even be needed. An unsutured wound will heal by secondary intention, if it is clean, has a good blood supply, is free from pressure, and is surrounded by mobile tissue. Normal wound healing will generate sufficient strength for the patient to proceed with normal strenuous activities in 72 hours, although nonstrenuous daily activities can resume the day after surgery. If there are episodes of increased intra-abdominal pressure (e.g., coughing, sneezing, or vigorous exercise within 72 hours), it is possible for omentum or bowel to make its way through the peritoneal wound and create an adhesion that may not reduce itself despite the motion of the abdominal contents against the wall during breathing.

In very thin patients, the short distance between the peritoneum and fascia may lead to a true hernia formation of omentum or bowel if the fascia is not closed (Fig. 6–2). These events usually follow episodes producing very strong intra-abdominal pressure and can be treated with direct reduction by pushing the hernia back through the fascial defect if the patient presents herself within 24 hours. To avoid these rare complications, the thin patient is best advised not to undertake any strenuous activity for 2 or 3 days after laparoscopy.

FIGURE 6–2 Herniation

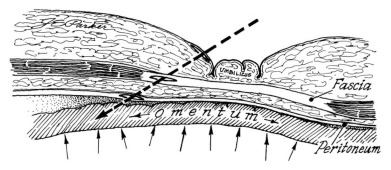

In normal body walls, peritoneal opening is not opposite the fascial opening nor the skin opening. Herniation is not likely.

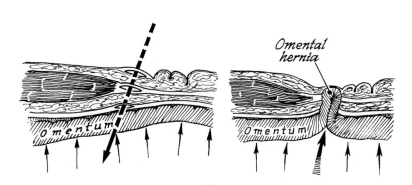

In very thin body walls, these openings may be more nearly aligned. Postoperative intra-abdominal pressure may force omentum out through aligned openings and create a herniation.

FIGURE 6–3 Wound healing.
A–C, Peritoneal healing.

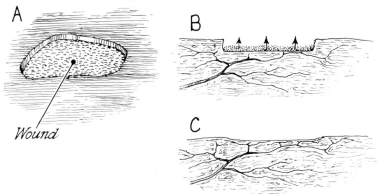

Cells and vessels repair from the "bottom up". Regardless of size, no contraction.

D–F, Skin healing

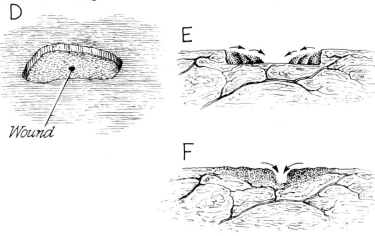

Cells and vessels repair from the edges to the center. Large defects take longer and involve contraction.

HEALING AFTER LYSIS OF ADHESIONS

Recent studies have revealed that adhesions tend to re-form less frequently when lysed by a laparoscopic approach than by open laparotomy (Luciano et al, 1989; Lundorff et al, 1991; Operative Laparoscopy Study Group, 1991). It thus becomes necessary for the laparoscopist to understand the current principles behind adhesiolysis to prevent a recurrence. Several new theories concerning the re-formation of adhesions have evolved from human and animal studies.

Peritoneal Healing

Wound healing of the peritoneal surface has been intensely studied in animals and humans to develop materials to minimize adhesion re-formation. The subject has been reviewed in detail (diZerega, 1990; Drollette and Badawy, 1992).

After an abdominal surface is denuded of peritoneum, macrophages (either from underlying vessels, mesenchymal tissue, or the peritoneal fluid) cover the surface and initiate a process of peritoneal regeneration from the "bottom up," rather than from the "edges in" as in skin healing (diZerega, 1990) (Fig. 6–3). If there are no damaged cells (see below) in this denuded area, no adjacent structures will become adherent. Figure 6–4 is a summary of the healing process as it occurs during the days after surgery: vascularization begins in about 7 days; collagen deposition begins on about day 11. An important surgical implication is that reperitonealization by suturing is not necessary. Robbins, Brunschwig, and Foote (1949) first reported experimentally and clinically on reperitonealization in 1949. It has recently been amply documented in clinical experiments when adhesion formation was found to be identical whether the abdominal wall incision underwent peritoneal closure or not (Ellis, 1971; Tulandi et al, 1988). Stretching a devitalized sheet of peritoneum over a surface may do more harm than good (Buckman et al, 1976). The use of materials (e.g., Interceed) to minimize adhesion re-formation on damaged peritoneal surfaces is being currently evaluated. Corticosteroids, antihistamines, and peritoneal fluid expanders (e.g., Hyskon) have not been consistently documented as effective.

Ovarian Surface Healing

Controversy exists concerning the important problem of ovarian surface healing. The ovary is the pelvic structure most likely to re-form adhesions after lysis (Trimbos-Kemper et al, 1985) and the degree of ovarian surface covered by adhesions is a major prognostic factor after adhesiolysis for infertility (Hulka, 1982). Since the ovary is not covered by true peritoneum, the materials used to prevent adhesion re-formation on the peritoneal surfaces may not work on the ovary. Indeed, animal and human observations suggest that the ovary heals best (with minimal adhesions) without attempts at reapproximation by suturing (Brumsted et al, 1990; Wiskind et al, 1990). The achievement of hemostasis appears to be a sufficient endpoint of ovarian surgery to minimize adhesions.

Plasminogen

Fibrinolysins are normally present in tissue; the concept of their being reduced in damaged tissue resulting in adhesions from persistent fibrinous attachments (Buckman et al, 1976; Gervin et al, 1973; Thompson et al, 1989) has led investigators to study the role of plasminogen activators (PA) in the prevention of adhesions. These studies showed that grafts or tight sutures can make peritoneum ischemic, reducing PA, and that abraded or inflamed peritoneum also resulted in reduced PA activity. The common insult in these experiments was the creation of damaged or hypoxic cells.

FIGURE 6–4 Normal peritoneum healing timetable.

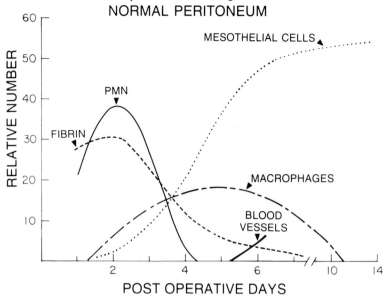

(Adapted from diZerega GS: The peritoneum and its response to surgical injury. In diZerega GS, Malinak LR, Diamond MP, and Linsky CB [eds]: Treatment of Post Surgical Adhesions: Proceedings of the First International Symposium for the Treatment of Post Surgical Adhesions. Phoenix, AZ, September 15–17, 1989. © 1990. Reprinted by permission of John Wiley & Sons, Inc.)

FIGURE 6–5 Adhesion formation by damaged cells

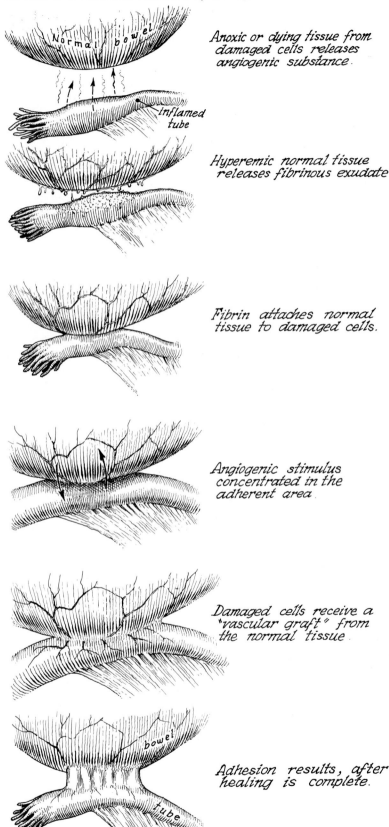

Anoxic or dying tissue from damaged cells releases angiogenic substance.

Hyperemic normal tissue releases fibrinous exudate

Fibrin attaches normal tissue to damaged cells.

Angiogenic stimulus concentrated in the adherent area.

Damaged cells receive a "vascular graft" from the normal tissue.

Adhesion results, after healing is complete.

Hypoxic Cells

Damaged cells release angiogenic factors (probably a fibroblast growth factor—βFGF) that stimulate vascular growth and hyperemia in adjacent normal tissues (Fig. 6–5). These hyperemic areas in turn can release a fibrinous exudate that attaches the normal tissue to damaged tissue. Stimulus of these factors is concentrated on a specific area of the normal tissue, generating vascularization. A permanent adhesion is formed, probably to supply blood by a "vascular graft" and minimize cellular death (Ellis, 1980). Similarly, a suture around a large pedicle leaves devitalized anoxic cells in the pedicle and partially anoxic compressed cells near to the suture (Fig. 6–6). These cells also release angiogenic factors and may lead to adhesions marked by a nonabsorbable suture after all nonviable cells are absorbed.

Absorbable suture material provokes a similar hypervascularization response to promote digestion and absorption of the suture. In this theory, it follows that totally dead cells (e.g., those that have been electrocoagulated to the point of desiccation) and nonabsorbable materials do not provoke a vascular response and therefore do not provoke adhesions.

These concepts seem to be supported by careful clinical observation. The implications for surgical techniques to minimize adhesion formation or re-formation are important:

1. Minimize use of absorbable sutures for hemostasis: adhesions are invariably found on surfaces where absorbable sutures were used. Inert metals and plastics are reperitonealized with minimum adhesions.

2. Sharp dissection, which causes minimal cell destruction, is preferred on surfaces where adhesion re-formation should be avoided. A well-focused CO_2 laser or cutting with electrocoagulation minimizes bleeding but damages more cells.

3. Less meticulous hemostasis during dissection allows normal clotting to control most tissue bleeding. Blood itself does not cause adhesions (Nisell and Larsson, 1978), although the combination of drying of tissue and blood may (Ryan et al, 1971). Routine hemostasis by fulguration or defocused laser coagulation, which damages surface cells, should be avoided. Any large vessel bleeding requires immediate bipolar compression and electrodesiccation. Surfaces bleeding after 5 minutes need minimum electrocoagulation with compression or defocused laser coagulation, keeping in mind that the surface cells damaged in the process will stimulate adhesion re-formation.

4. Peritoneal fluid will dilute angiogenic factors and minimize the risk of stimulating vascular growth in nearby tissues. This is the theory behind leaving 1000 to 2000 ml of lactated Ringer's solution in the peritoneal cavity after surgery. Lactated Ringer's solution has been shown to be superior to Interceed or Gore-Tex in the prevention of adhesions in an animal model (Pagidas and Tulandi, 1992).

FIGURE 6–6 Adhesion formation by a large pedicle

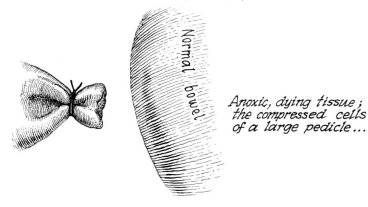

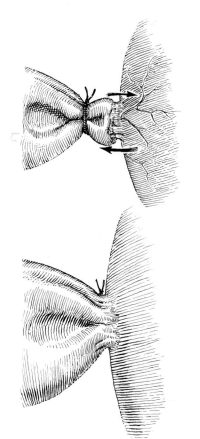

Anoxic, dying tissue; the compressed cells of a large pedicle...

...stimulate "vascular graft" adhesion.

End result is adhesion at the suture site.

FIGURE 6–7 Healing after bipolar coagulation

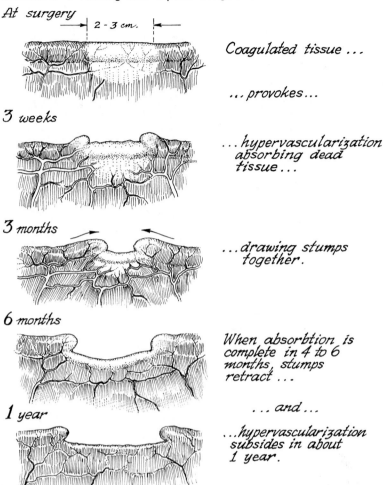

At surgery

Coagulated tissue . . .

. . . provokes . . .

3 weeks

. . . hypervascularization absorbing dead tissue . . .

3 months

. . . drawing stumps together.

6 months

When absorbtion is complete in 4 to 6 months, stumps retract . . .

1 year

. . . and . . .

. . hypervascularization subsides in about 1 year.

FIGURE 6–8 Inadequate coagulation

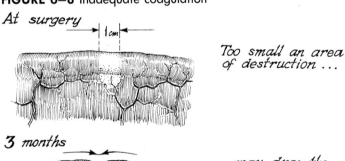

At surgery

Too small an area of destruction . . .

3 months

. . . may draw the stumps together, allowing recanalization in 3 months.

HEALING AFTER COAGULATION

Tubal electrocoagulation to the point of desiccation also coagulates all bacteria in the affected tissue and, therefore, results in a sterile, devitalized area of tissue. Secondary infections of this dead tissue from uterine bacteria or from perforated bowel are possible but rare. The body reacts to this devitalized tissue by increasing the vascularization around the wound, gradually absorbing it (Fishburne and Hulka, 1976) (Fig. 6–7). Hysterographic venograms, as well as direct visualization of tubes within 3 weeks of coagulation, have also demonstrated this hypervascularization. The proximal and distal stumps of the tube gradually approach each other as the intervening tissue is absorbed during the 3 to 6 months after coagulation. When absorption of the dead tissue is complete, usually at 6 months, the stumps fall apart, and the hypervascularization subsides in about 1 year. This process is asymptomatic in that no pelvic pain or menstrual irregularities have been detected during this stage.

Coagulation of 2 to 3 cm of tube without division has been demonstrated to be as effective as coagulation and division. Division in the past has led to a significant incidence of complications of bleeding from underlying blood vessels that were not occluded during coagulation. Today's better understanding of bipolar compression and desiccation for large vessel hemostasis enables us to avoid or immediately treat these complications. Spontaneous recanalization may result in about 3 months if only a small portion of the tube is coagulated (e.g., only one bipolar coagulation per tube) (Fig. 6–8). A bridge of peritoneum can cover the dead tissue and hold the two stumps in approximation. For this reason more extensive tissue destruction is necessary with coagulation alone than with coagulation and division, in which the proximal and distal stumps are not drawn together.

CLIP OCCLUSION

The spring clip was designed to allow a gap of 1 mm between the upper and lower jaw at the time of application (Fig. 6–9). This gap allows the tissue to be squeezed and held firmly by the surrounding spring but does not force the tissues to be squeezed to zero gap, which in some situations can lead to hemorrhage from transection (Hulka, 1975). Teeth in the jaws prevent the tissue from rolling out during or after application, so the clip always remains where it was applied. Another gap prevents vessels in the mesosalpinx from tearing and bleeding. Over the next 24 to 48 hours, the spring compresses the upper and lower jaw and exerts sufficient pressure to squeeze out the fluids in the cell to ensure complete necrosis, since the springs deliver a pressure equal to twice that of normal arterial pressure to the tissue within the jaws. During this time, nerves in the tube are also compressed and may cause postoperative cramps. This occurrence is in contrast to electrocoagulation, in which the nerves are destroyed at the time of coagulation thus causing no further pain.

Epithelialization and healing are complete in 6 weeks, at which time the cells of the endosalpinx form a pouch-like seal on either side of the occluding clip, biologically as well as mechanically separating the uterus from the ovary. The amount of tube destroyed is 0.5 mm. Over 4 to 6 weeks, the clip itself is gradually covered by peritoneum going over it from the edges of the adjacent viable tubes. Since the clips are made of biologically inert materials—Lexan (Lexan Products Division, General Electric) plastic and a gold-plated surgical-grade stainless steel spring, this reaction is limited to reperitonealization of a foreign body.

Clips that have been handled with starch or talcum powder or have picked up lint from operating drapes have stimulated granulomatous reactions.

FIGURE 6–9 Healing after spring clip application

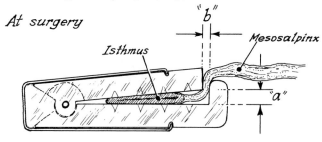

At surgery

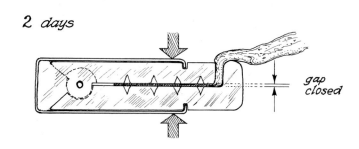

2 days

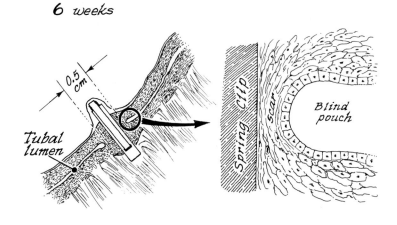

6 weeks

FIGURE 6–10 Right and wrong location of clip

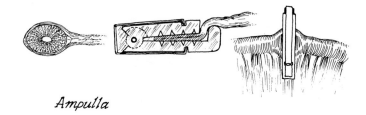

Isthmus

Ampulla

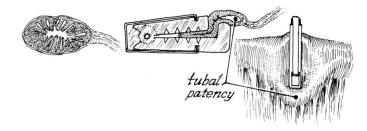

tubal patency

We are aware of two cases in which patients with probable gold allergy underwent clip sterilization and subsequently had sufficient pelvic pain to warrant removal of the clips with pathologic findings of small lymphocyte reaction around them. Adhesions between the clip and other structures occasionally occur because omentum, ovary, or bowel may become attached to these surfaces in the process of reperitonealization. These adhesions are usually asymptomatic and are detected incidentally at the time of subsequent surgery for either anastomosis or hysterectomy.

The clip was designed to crush the isthmus of the tube with its thick musculature and narrow lumen (Fig. 6–10). Incorrect application on the ampullary part of the tube, with its thin musculature and voluminous rugae, results in some of the lumen's rolling out of the clip, with resultant patency and pregnancy.

Clips that are dislodged from the applicator or tube and cannot be retrieved pose a clinical concern. Animal studies have shown that closed clips are peritonealized free in the abdominal cavity or attach themselves harmlessly to a peritoneal surface for a vascular supply. Open clips or loose springs in humans have invariably been taken up and surrounded by the omentum. We are unaware of any medical complication resulting from clips, open or closed, left free in the abdomen. For this reason, we do not recommend laparotomy for exploration and retrieval, since the cure would have more complications than the disease.

HEALING AFTER BAND PROCEDURE

As the Silastic band constricts the knuckle of the tube within it (Fig. 6–11), the tube undergoes gradual necrosis from anoxia over a period of 2 to 3 days. The nerves caught within the anoxic process die slowly from crushing, resulting in cramps that are most severe with the band (because of the relatively large volume of tissue dying), less severe with the clip (smaller volume of crushed tissue), and absent with coagulation techniques (nerves are instantly destroyed).

As with electrocoagulation, necrotic tissues stimulate a hyperemic reaction within the broad ligament to absorb anoxic cells within the loop and adjacent to it. This absorption process also takes 3 to 6 months. The end result at 6 months is usually complete separation of the proximal and distal stump of the tube with the Silastic band in its original, unstretched form being covered by peritoneum at one stump.

Although Silastic is biologically inert, the bands contain barium sulfate to make them visible in subsequent x-rays as required by the Federal Drug Administration (FDA). Some patients may react to this barium sulfate. For reasons that are unclear but may be attributed to brittleness of the Silastic caused by the admixture of barium sulfate, occasional defects in the band are induced when stretching it around the 5-mm applicator tube. Absorption of the knuckle of tube is not always complete, and viable cells within this knuckle can be seen.

As with the clip, improper application of the band on the ampulla may not completely occlude the tube (Fig. 6–12). The luminal rugae at this point may allow patency and also pregnancy.

FIGURE 6–11 Healing after band application

At surgery

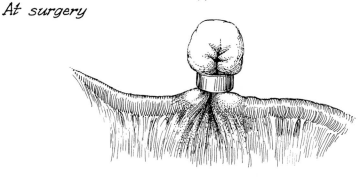

3 months

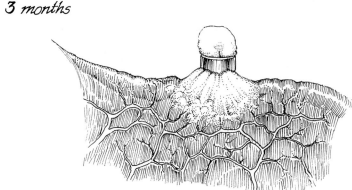

6 months

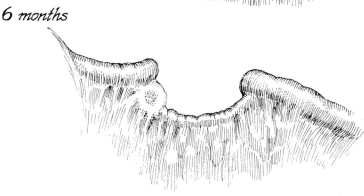

FIGURE 6–12 Improper application of the band *on ampulla*

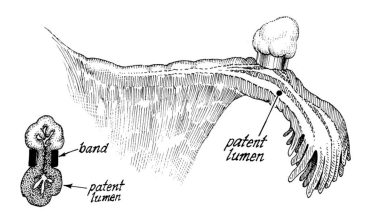

band

patent lumen

patent lumen

FIGURE 6–13 Uteroperitoneal fistula

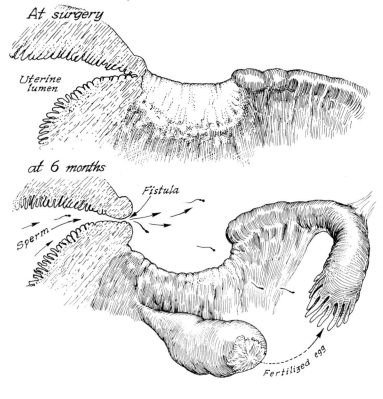

UTEROPERITONEAL FISTULA FORMATION

In situations in which the tube is destroyed very close to the uterus (Fig. 6–13), utero-peritoneal fistulas containing endometrial tissue have been seen. In an early series of patients undergoing hysterosalpingography after electrocoagulation, Courey and associates (1973) demonstrated peritoneal spillage in more than 10% of the patients studied for 3 months or more after surgery. This fistula formation is believed to be created by the continuing contractility of the uterus, forcing its small volume of fluid through the healing portions of the coagulated tube and resulting in a fistula to the peritoneum. These fistulas may be important in the cause of subsequent ectopic pregnancy, since spermatozoa could reach the peritoneal cavity, enter the distal stump of the fallopian tube, await the ruptured follicle, and fertilize an egg in the distal stump. The ratio of intrauterine to ectopic pregnancies after extensive electrocoagulation techniques has been about 1:2. Because of this theoretical possibility, it is currently recommended that a stump of approximately 1 to 2 cm of isthmus remain after all techniques of sterilization (Fig. 6–14), so that this muscular lumen can accommodate the small amounts of fluid coming from the uterus during its peristaltic contractions and not lead to fistula formation.

FIGURE 6–14 Prevention of a fistula

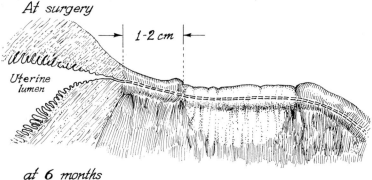

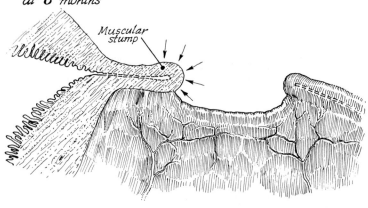

UNIPOLAR VERSUS BIPOLAR BOWEL BURNS

Unipolar circuits require passage of electrons through the body to the ground or return plate. Heat caused by high electron density sufficient to generate a bowel perforation (Fig. 6–15) is accompanied by less obvious but equally devitalizing heat caused by the electrons leaving an intense burn area along the bowel wall for 4 to 5 cm surrounding the perforated area. The management of a unipolar bowel perforation thus requires the resection of a 5- to 6-cm margin of bowel on either side of the crater (Thompson and Wheeless, 1973).

In contrast, a burn induced by picking up bowel with a bipolar forceps is caused by electrons flowing between the closely placed prongs or electrodes of the forceps and not any distance into tissue beyond them (Fig. 6–16). A resection adequate to reach healthy, viable tissue, depending on the degree of necrosis from infection present, needs to be much less extensive after a bipolar burn than after a unipolar burn. If the burns are recognized immediately, for example, a simple excision of the coagulated bipolar injury may suffice, whereas a segmental resection and anastomosis may be necessary with a unipolar burn.

FIGURE 6–15 Unipolar bowel injury

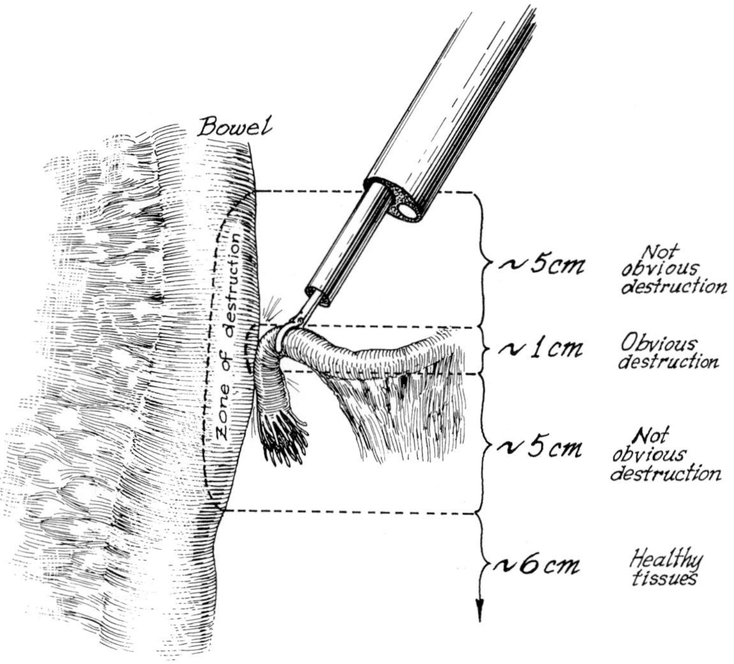

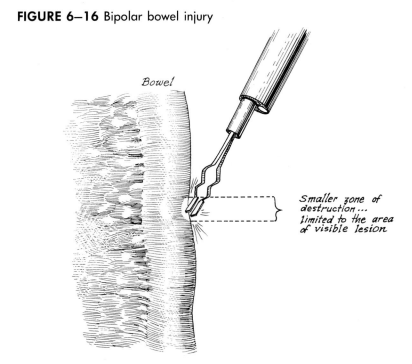

FIGURE 6–16 Bipolar bowel injury

REFERENCES

MICROBIOLOGY

Corson SL, Block S, Mintz C, et al: Sterilization of laparoscopes: Is soaking sufficient? J Reprod Med 23:49–56, 1979a.

Corson SL, Dole M, Kraus R, et al: Studies in sterilization of the laparoscope: II. J Reprod Med 23:57–59, 1979b.

ADHESIONS

Brumsted JR, Deaton J, Lavigne E, and Riddick DH: Postoperative adhesion formation after ovarian wedge resection with and without ovarian reconstruction in the rabbit. Fertil Steril 53:723–726, 1990.

Buckman RF Jr, Buckman PD, Hufnagel HV, and Gervin AS: A physiologic basis for the adhesion-free healing of deperitonealized surfaces. J Surg Res 21:67–76, 1976.

diZerega GS: The peritoneum and its response to surgical injury. In diZerega GS, Malinak LR, Diamond MP, and Linsky CB (eds): Treatment of Post Surgical Adhesions: Proceedings of the First International Symposium for the Treatment of Post Surgical Adhesions, Phoenix, AZ, September 15 to 17, 1989. New York, Wiley-Liss, 1990.

Drollette CM and Badawy SZ: A pathophysiology of pelvic adhesions: Modern trends in preventing infertility. J Reprod Med 37:107–121, 1992.

Ellis H: The cause and prevention of postoperative intraperitoneal adhesions. Surg Gynecol Obstet 133:497–511, 1971.

Ellis H: Internal overhealing: The problem of intraperitoneal adhesions. World J Surg 4:303–306, 1980.

Gervin AS, Puckett CL, and Silver D: Serosal hypofibrinolysis: A cause of postoperative adhesions. Am J Surg 125:80–88, 1973.

Hulka JF: Adnexal adhesions: A prognostic staging and classification system based on a five-year survey of fertility surgery results at Chapel Hill, North Carolina. Am J Obstet Gynecol 144:141–148, 1982.

Luciano AA, Maier DB, Koch EI, et al: A comparative study of postoperative adhesions following laser surgery by laparoscopy versus laparotomy in the rabbit model. Obstet Gynecol 74:220–224, 1989.

Lundorff P, Hahlin M, Källfelt B, et al: Adhesion formation after laparoscopic surgery in tubal pregnancy: A randomized trial versus laparotomy. Fertil Steril 55:911–915, 1991.

Nisell H and Larsson B: Role of blood and fibrinogen in development of intraperitoneal adhesions in rats. Fertil Steril 30:470–473, 1978.

Operative Laparoscopy Study Group: Postoperative adhesion development after operative laparoscopy: Evaluation at early second-look procedures. Fertil Steril 55:700–704, 1991.

Pagidas K and Tulandi T: Effects of Ringer's lactate, Interceed (TC7) and Gore-Tex Surgical Membrane on postsurgical adhesion formation. Fertil Steril 57:199–201, 1992.

Robbins GF, Brunschwig A, and Foote FW: Deperitonealization: Clinical and experimental observations. Ann Surg 130:466–479, 1949.

Ryan GB, Groberty J, and Majno G: Postoperative peritoneal adhesions: A study of the mechanisms. Am J Pathol 65:117–148, 1971.

Thompson JN, Paterson-Brown S, Harbourne T, et al: Reduced human peritoneal plasminogen activating activity: Possible mechanism of adhesion formation. Br J Surg 76:382–384, 1989.

Trimbos-Kemper TCM, Trimbos JB, and van Hall EV: Adhesion formation after tubal surgery: Results of the eighth day laparoscopy in 188 patients. Fertil Steril 43:395–400, 1985.

Tulandi T, Hum HS, and Gelfand MM: Closure of laparotomy incisions with or without peritoneal suturing and second-look laparoscopy. Am J Obstet Gynecol 158:536–537, 1988.

Wiskind AK, Toledo AA, Dudley AG, and Zusmanis K: Adhesion formation after ovarian wound repair in New Zealand white rabbits: A comparison of ovarian microsurgical closure with ovarian nonclosure. Am J Obstet Gynecol 163:1674–1678, 1990.

STERILIZATION

Courey NG, Cunanan RG Jr, and Taefi P: Sterilization via laparoscope. N Y State J Med 73:559–561, 1973.

Fishburne JI Jr and Hulka JF: Tubal healing following laparoscopic electrocoagulation. J Reprod Med 16:129–134, 1976.

Hulka JF: Studies in simpler tubocclusion methods. Am J Obstet Gynecol 122:337–348, 1975.

Thompson BH and Wheeless CR Jr: Gastrointestinal complications of laparoscopy sterilization. Obstet Gynecol 41:669–676, 1973.

7

Anesthesia

The special needs of anesthesia for laparoscopy have been thoroughly studied and reduced to essentials by Fishburne, who pioneered in the establishment of general and local anesthesia on an outpatient basis (Fishburne, 1983). Several features are unique to laparoscopy with which the anesthesiologist should be familiar.

PREOPERATIVE MEDICATION

Preoperative sedation should be chosen to be relatively short acting so that the patient can recover sufficiently to go home on the day of surgery. Intravenous diazepam can cause phlebitis at the point of entry, which the patient may complain of long after the rest of the laparoscopy has gone well. Midazolam (Versed) has proved to be useful for both general and local anesthesia but is three to four times as potent a respiratory depressant as diazepam, as can be seen on pulse oximetry monitoring. Depressed oxygenation can be countered with nasal oxygen under local anesthesia. Use of intravenous fentanyl (Sublimaze) or alfentanil (Alfenta) has been quite satisfactory for the short duration for general and local anesthesia.

Manipulation of the uterus or tubes can result in stimulating a *vagal reflex*, which may lead to bradycardia, hypotension, and cardiac arrhythmias and arrest. This reflex is seen under local and general anesthesia and can be treated with atropine. Similarly,

high-pressure CO_2 insufflation may cause bradycardia secondary to inferior vena cava compression, which can also be treated with atropine. Antihistamines dampen the vagal reflex and discomfort from the use of CO_2 but have a relatively long duration of action and prolong postoperative stays in an outpatient service.

If general anesthesia is planned, the patient should breathe 100% oxygen for at least 2 to 3 minutes before induction. This procedure is preferable to paralyzing the patient and using positive pressure for ventilating before endotracheal intubation. Mask hyperventilation can inflate the stomach and lead to a Veress needle or trocar injury. If masked hyperventilation is used, an oral gastric tube should be placed prior to establishing a pneumoperitoneum.

GENERAL ANESTHESIA

Approximately 10 minutes prior to induction, an antiemetic (e.g., droperidol [Inapsine] 1.25 mg) or a sedative (midazolam [Versed] 0.5 to 1.0 mg) is given intravenously. General anesthesia is induced after 2 minutes of 100% oxygen, followed by a bolus of short-acting narcotic (alfentanil, 25 to 75 µg/kg). Thirty seconds later a bolus of a barbiturate (thiopental [Pentothal], 1 to 2 mg/kg) is given intravenously. Within 30 seconds, a muscle relaxant (mivacurium [Mivacron], 150 to 200 µg/kg) is administered as a bolus. Intubation is achieved with a 7-mm endotracheal tube, and controlled respiration is established. At this point an end-tidal CO_2 monitor is placed.

General anesthesia is maintained with 40 to 50% oxygen, with 50 to 60% nitrous oxide (N_2O) inhalational anesthetic, isoflurane (Forane), alfentanil infused at a rate of 1 μg/kg/min, and mivacurium infused at a rate of 6 to 8 μg/kg/min. The patient usually wakes 5 to 10 minutes following completion of the operation.

CONCERNS DURING ANESTHESIA

Under general anesthesia (as well as under local anesthesia), it is helpful if the patient is relaxed. Failure to do so will result in the patient's expelling the gas from the peritoneal cavity during a bucking period when intra-abdominal pressure far exceeds the capacity of the valves and gaskets of the laparoscopes to contain it. Diagnostic and operative maneuvers become hazardous if the patient's abdominal muscles contract in response to pain, because grasped organs may be torn or bowel may rise into the operative field and possibly touch a live coagulation tip. Because of these factors, endotracheal intubation, pharmacologic neuromuscular blockade, and positive-pressure respiration are recommended for general anesthesia in laparoscopy.

The anesthesiologist should share with the surgeon the responsibility for monitoring the intra-abdominal gas pressure indicator, ensuring that the pressure is not excessive. Pressure should be maintained at no more than 15 to 20 mm Hg. At these levels, under local anesthesia, the patient is quite comfortable and may describe the sensation of her abdomen's being like that after having eaten a big Thanksgiving dinner. At pressures exceeding this level, the abdomen becomes distended, ventilation difficulties occur, and acute anxiety can begin under local anesthesia.

Under general anesthesia hypoventilation may lead to hypercarbic cardiac problems. Since the surgeon is often distracted by the technical problems of laparoscopy itself, it helps to have the anesthesiologist share the important gas pressure-monitoring function (see also Chapter 4).

At the end of the laparoscopic procedure, the Trendelenburg position should be maintained until all peritoneal gas is removed. Continuing this position allows the gas to escape from under the diaphragm and upward into the lower part of the abdomen and out the sleeve (see Fig. 4–5). The anesthesiologist's usual reflex is to get the patient out of the Trendelenburg position as soon as the surgeon is finished, often before the sleeve is removed. Doing so often leads to severe complaints of chest or shoulder pain accompanied by lower blood pressure in the recovery room caused by a residue of gas under the diaphragm.

Oversedation

Reviews of deaths during sterilization have indicated that anesthesia appears to be a major and preventable cause of death (Peterson et al, 1983). Local anesthesia, combined with sedation to the point of overmedication and unconsciousness, has led to deaths from anoxia during minilaparotomy overseas; in the United States, laparoscopic sterilization with general anesthesia and no intubation has led to deaths from hypoventilation or gastric aspiration causing cardiac arrest. As in using obstetric anesthesia, gynecologists performing laparoscopic surgery should be as familiar with the demands that they are placing on their anesthesiologists and their patients as the anesthesiologists are.

Explosions

There has been at least one overseas report of an explosion during laparoscopy using electrocoagulation in the presence of nitrous oxide. The incident was probably inaccurately reported with regard to the anesthetic technique used at the time. It is plausible to explain this situation as having occurred in the presence of explosive inhalation anesthesia. In my (J. F. H.) experience overseas, I have had to cancel operations on patients who had been successfully induced with thiopental sodium according to instructions but were then maintained with ether anesthesia because of its low cost.

Nitrous oxide in American operating rooms has created no documented hazard, although at least one surgeon has lost consciousness because his nose was next to an open operating channel during laparoscopy.

Air Embolism

Because of the fatal nature of air embolism, the anesthesiologist is well advised to have a stethoscope on the patient's chest or in the esophagus and to listen to it carefully during induction of pneumoperitoneum as well as throughout the procedure. During a difficult pneumoperitoneum attempt, or after a period of violent bucking after pneumoperitoneum is established, the anesthesiologist should be especially alert for the "mill-wheel murmur" characteristic of an air embolism in the right atrium and ventricle. The murmur is fortunately a loud, clear, and early signal of this lethal complication, and the embolism can be managed promptly with direct intracardiac insertion of a needle to aspirate the frothy blood from the right ventricle, or rapid insertion of a central venous catheter monitor through the superior vena cava, right atrium, and ventricle to aspirate the froth. During these efforts, the patient should be placed on her left side and with her head down to minimize the propulsion of gas into the pulmonary artery, where aspiration would no longer be possible.

LOCAL ANESTHESIA

As in obstetrics, local anesthesia with the maintenance of consciousness is safer than general anesthesia in laparoscopy. The patient's own reflexes are superior to the best anesthesiologist for maintaining pulse and blood pressure stability (Peterson et al, 1987), and postoperative recovery is shorter and less morbid. Most sterilization procedures can be done under local anesthesia conditions, since these patients have had deliveries and are familiar with surgical manipulations, as well as having relaxed abdominal walls. Although most patients in chronic pelvic pain do not tolerate the discomfort of laparoscopy under local anesthe-

sia, some benefit from "mapping" the pelvis for pain localization. The gentle techniques required for trocar insertion should be consciously learned in no less a deliberate manner than those we have learned for gentle delivery of the conscious patient.

When performing laparoscopy under local anesthesia, it is important that the patient be psychologically relaxed and as confident as possible. This is accomplished by close personal communication between the physician and the patient before and during surgery. Medication should be used as a supplement, not as a substitute for this communication. It is helpful to explain the sensations that the patient is experiencing during each step of the procedure (see "Vocal Local" later).

Positioning and Prepping

The patient should void just prior to entering the operating room, thus relieving the necessity for catheterization.

After being transferred to the operating table and connected to all monitoring devices, the patient should be premedicated with intravenous sedation (midazolam). The important positioning of the legs is done when medication has had a sedative effect to minimize the embarrassment of the lithotomy position. Each leg should be wrapped, including the foot, with a blanket to avoid uncomfortable chilling during surgery. The lateral aspect of the knee-supporting stirrups should be well padded to prevent postoperative "foot-drop" from peroneal nerve compression or hypoxia during surgery. The operation should not proceed until the patient states that her legs are comfortably positioned.

The patient is prepped with warm solution from above the umbilicus in a 6-in.–wide stripe down through the symphysis and to the bottom of the buttocks. No shaving is necessary. The vagina is prepped gently with antiseptic solution, and the Graves vaginal speculum is then inserted. When the cervix is visualized, the controlling tenaculum is inserted into the cervix and uterus. This may cause discomfort in some patients. If it is uncomfortable, pelvic adhesions may be suspected, and additional

FIGURE 7–1 Field block technique

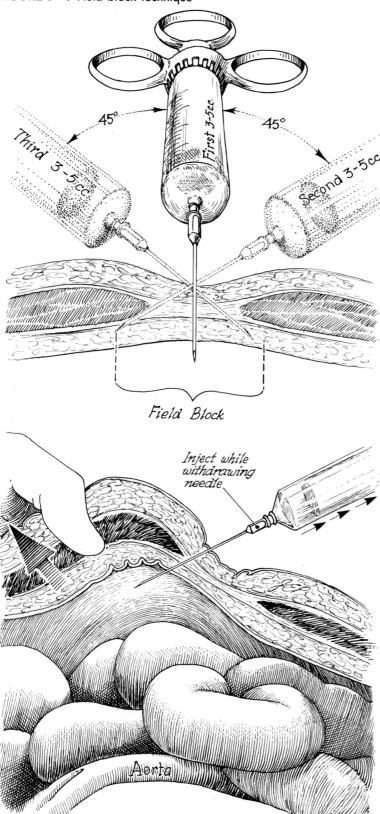

Field Block

Inject while withdrawing needle

Aorta

analgesia with alfentanil may be required. The patient is then draped appropriately to prevent her feet from contaminating the instruments during surgery.

Abdominal Wall Block

One per cent lidocaine hydrochloride solution is then used to raise a bleb in the skin just beneath the umbilicus. A 1-in. sharp small-gauge needle should be used to infiltrate the skin. The needle should then be changed to allow a longer 19- to 20-gauge 2-in. needle to be used to infiltrate the hand-elevated abdominal wall. The infiltration should begin at an angle of 45 degrees with respect to the umbilicus and should be aimed toward the uterus. Experience will allow the physician to gauge how deep the needle should go and how much anesthetic should be left at each level. On very thin patients, the aorta feels almost subcutaneous at this point, and it may be advisable to stretch the abdominal wall away from the aorta (Fig. 7–1). Then the surgeon injects 10 ml of anesthetic along the anticipated track of the Veress needle and trocar as the needle is withdrawn to the subcutaneous area. A "field block" anesthetic technique (see Fig. 7–1) of infiltrating 3 to 5 ml of anesthetic directly along the future track, 3 to 5 ml at an angle of 45 degrees to the left of the track, and an additional 3 to 5 ml to the right of the track will block most nerves coming to the abdominal wall at the site of trocar insertion and will ensure greatest comfort. If the patient is obese, in all probability the entire length of a 4-in. needle is necessary to penetrate the abdominal wall.

Gas for Insufflation

N_2O is the indicated insufflation agent under local anesthesia. CO_2 turns to carbonic acid on moist peritoneal surfaces and causes discomfort, ranging from mild to intolerable. This rapidly destroys any rapport and comfort that the patient may have achieved. CO_2 is indicated only when laser surgery is anticipated; all other laparoscopic procedures, including electrocoagulation, can be safely performed with N_2O.

Intra-Abdominal Topical Anesthesia

For laparoscopic sterilization 5 ml of rapidly absorbed 0.5% bupivacaine hydrochloride should be applied by flowing onto the surface of each fallopian tube, starting from the cornu and flowing well past the area of coagulation or clipping on both the upper and lower surface of each tube. Approximately 2 ml for each of these four surfaces will allow rapid peritoneal absorption and anesthetizing of the tubal nerve supply adequate for coagulation. These agents are effective within 30 seconds of peritoneal application, thus the sterilization procedure can proceed directly after local application. For occasional lysis of adhesions under local anesthesia, these agents can be flowed onto the adhesion surfaces with a surprising level of comfort achieved for this surgery. Blood level studies by Spielman (1989) have revealed that these dosages applied to the abdominal wall and peritoneal surfaces will lead to levels well below minimal toxic levels for these anesthetic agents.

"Vocal Local"

If local anesthesia is used, most hospitals require the presence of a "sitter" who can perform a valuable service by providing "vocal local"—constantly talking to the patient and assuring her that everything is going well, as well as assuring that general anesthesia can be resorted to if necessary. This role can often be assumed by the surgeon who converses with the patient during the procedure. One of the most difficult aspects of local anesthesia for most surgeons is that the patient, rather than the surgeon, becomes the center of attention for all noises and comments made in the room during surgery. The awareness of the impact that casual comments or normal noises can make on the patient's psyche and appropriate deference to the patient by everyone in the operating room contribute to the successful and relaxed completion of surgery.

REFERENCES

Fishburne JI Jr: Anesthesia for laparoscopy: Considerations, complications and techniques. J Reprod Med 21:37–40, 1978.

Fishburne JI Jr: Anesthesia for the outpatient: Sterilization and other procedures. AVS Biomed Bull 4(1):1–6, 1983.

Peterson HB, DeStefano F, and Rubin GL: Deaths attributable to tubal sterilization in the United States, 1977 to 1981. Am J Obstet Gynecol 146:131–136, 1983.

Peterson HB, Hulka JF, Spielman FJ, et al: Local versus general anesthesia for laparoscopic sterilization: A randomized study. Obstet Gynecol 70:903–908, 1987.

Spielman FJ: Laparoscopic surgery. Probl Anesth 3:151–159, 1989.

FURTHER READINGS

Lim HS: Preventing and managing the complications of local and general anesthesia. In Phillips JM (ed): Endoscopy in Gynecology. The Proceedings of the Third International Congress on Gynecologic Endoscopy, San Francisco. Downey, CA, American Association of Gynecologic Laparoscopists, 1978, pp 296–298.

Abdominal Entry

Entering the abdomen is the most dangerous part of the laparoscopic procedure. Most physicians use a Veress needle or similar large-bore needle for introduction of gas. An intra- or subumbilical incision is usually made, and the needle is inserted into the abdomen. It is at this point that approximately half of vessel lacerations occur. For this reason, meticulous attention to detail is necessary. In this chapter we review the important anatomic relationships of the abdominal wall and underlying blood vessels in detail to explain the surgical maneuvers necessary to enter the abdominal cavity safely.

FIGURE 8–1 Umbilical incisions

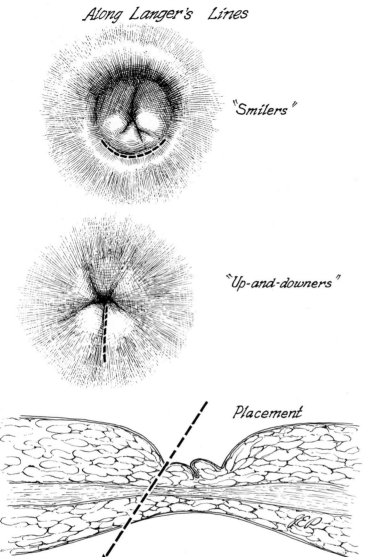

Along Langer's Lines

"Smilers"

"Up-and-downers"

Placement

SKIN INCISION

Location

The choice of location for the skin incision is important. Cosmetically, it should be made along Langer's lines indicated by pre-existing folds or creases in the umbilicus (Fig. 8–1), either horizontal or vertical, so that the skin falls back naturally to these lines and may not even require a suture. Most practitioners agree that the lower edge of the umbilical depression is the area of choice. It is particularly important to stay close to this edge in obese patients, since the peritoneum joins the umbilical plate at this point, making the distance necessary to traverse the preperitoneal fat minimal. Making this incision more surgically convenient below the umbilical plate in the obese may make peritoneal entrance difficult as the trocar may only stretch the peritoneum because of its loose connection to preperitoneal fat (Hurd et al, 1991).

Size

The skin incision for the trocar and sleeve must be adequate in size. The incision can be tested with the back of a standard scalpel holder (about 1 cm in width) or more directly by inserting the surgeon's small finger into the incision to feel for adequacy of length and freedom from bands of connective tissue remaining if the skin is not cut deeply enough.

VERESS NEEDLE

Insertion Technique

Figure 8–2 shows the principles that we have found to be most useful in the safe introduction of a Veress needle. The lower abdomen between the symphysis and umbilicus is divided into halves, and the lower half of this area (just above the pubic hairline approximately in the area of the bladder) is grasped by the surgeon's left hand and elevated. The elevation is at a 45-degree angle upward and caudad. This elevation slightly raises the umbilicus with its underlying peritoneum and puts that peritoneum on a stretch in a plane roughly perpendicular to the axis of the true pelvis. The Veress needle can then be inserted smartly at the umbilical level at right angles to this plane (45 degrees caudad off the vertical) straight into the axis of the true pelvis. During this two-handed maneuver, the surgeon should remember (and in training say out loud) three cardinal rules:

1. Aim toward the uterus. (If punctured, it forgives.)
2. Aim away from the pelvic blood vessels. (If punctured, they do not forgive.)
3. Aim at right angles to the skin (shortest distance to the peritoneum).

With this maneuver, the amount of preperitoneal fat to be traversed will be minimized in normal and moderately obese women.

FIGURE 8–2 Elevating the abdomen

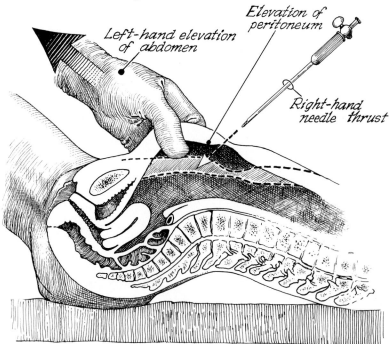

Left-hand elevation of abdomen

Elevation of peritoneum

Right-hand needle thrust

FIGURE 8–3 Lateral needle swing

CHECKS FOR ABDOMINAL ENTRY

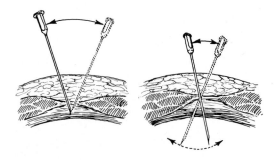

Large arc indicates tip is fixed

Small arc indicates tip is free

FIGURE 8–4 Epidural space test

Drop of saline in needle hub disappears in the low pressure of the peritoneal space

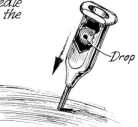

Drop

FIGURE 8–5 Syringe barrel flow test

Easy flow of saline or anesthetic into peritoneal cavity

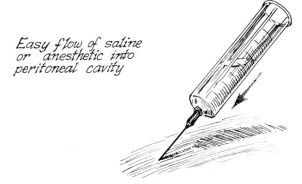

FIGURE 8–6 Syringe aspiration

Inject 2 cc. saline . . . aspirate and look for:
Blood, Bowel, Bladder, Bile

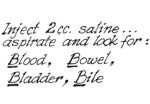

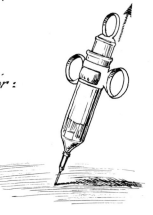

Tests for Peritoneal Entry

When the needle is inserted, a number of quick tests can be done to ensure that the entry is proper:

1. Swing the needle in an arc and visualize whether the tip of the needle is swinging in a counterarc with the pivot point at the rectus fascia midway down the needle (Fig. 8–3). If the needle is swinging with the tip as the pivot point, the needle is probably incompletely through the peritoneum. Elevate the abdominal wall again and redirect the needle more deeply. This time it should pass through the peritoneum and allow the tip to swing free.

2. A "hanging drop" or "epidural space" test (Fig. 8–4) observes a hanging drop of fluid in the Veress needle that flows downward freely if the needle is in the peritoneal cavity. Lifting the lower abdominal wall manually decreases intra-abdominal pressure and enhances free flow. The drop remains hanging if the needle tip is still preperitoneal.

3. Attach a syringe barrel and pour 1 to 2 ml of fluid (local anesthetic, saline) into it (Fig. 8–5). If the needle is in the abdominal cavity, the fluid will flow into the peritoneum. If it is preperitoneal, the flow will be much slower, although it can also dissect its way into the preperitoneal fat.

4. Aspirate with a syringe (Fig. 8–6) to make sure that the "four Bs" are absent—blood, bile, bladder, and bowel.

5. Attach the gas flow and inflate at no more than 1 l/min (Fig. 8–7), making sure that the pressure does not exceed 10 mm Hg at this rate of flow. If slight elevations in pressure coincide with the patient's expiratory efforts, the needle is probably in the peritoneal space.

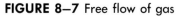

FIGURE 8–7 Free flow of gas

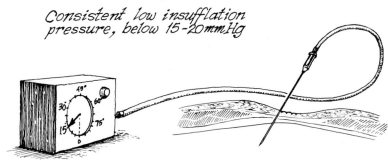

Consistent low insufflation pressure, below 15–20mmHg

FIGURE 8—8 Peritoneum blocking needle hole

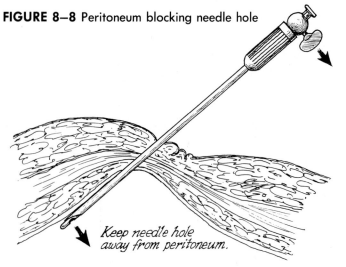

Keep needle hole away from peritoneum.

FIGURE 8—9 Tissue blocking the needle channel

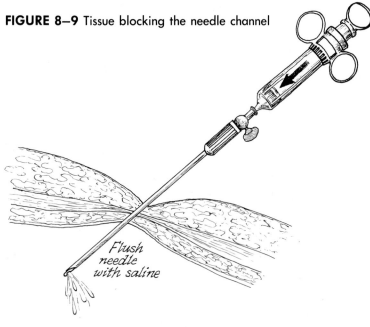

Flush needle with saline

FIGURE 8—10 Water in the line

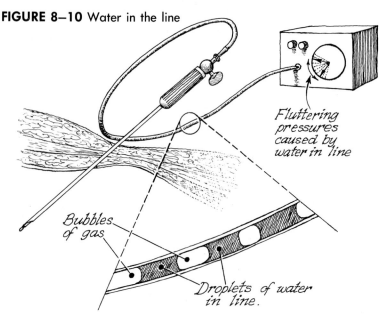

Fluttering pressures caused by water in line

Bubbles of gas

Droplets of water in line.

Troubleshooting Insufflation Problems

HIGH PRESSURE. With the Veress needle, the lateral opening at the tip (always on the same side as the valve lever) should always be directed downward to avoid the possibility that peritoneum is pressing against the opening (Fig. 8–8).

High pressures may also be caused by a piece of tissue blocking the needle opening. Flushing vigorously with 2 to 3 ml of fluid ensures that the needle lumen is clear (Fig. 8–9).

Fluttering seen on the pressure meter may be caused by intra-abdominal segments of water remaining in the insufflation tubing because of incomplete rinsing (Fig. 8–10).

If the pressure rises initially, or if it continues to be elevated irregularly, preperitoneal dissection should be suspected. In this case, the gas should be discontinued, the gas pocket should be evacuated, and a second effort should be made at reaching the peritoneum.

RE-ENTRY. Repeated unsuccessful attempts to enter the peritoneum can leave the preperitoneal tissue dissected away from the intact peritoneum (Fig. 8–11). A useful solution is to make a small incision for the Veress needle at the left upper edge of the umbilicus (to avoid the ligamentum teres) and insert the needle toward the pelvis (Fig. 8–12). This maximizes the chance of penetrating the peritoneum, since the needle will be traversing the peritoneum at a right angle and next to the area where it is fixed to the skin and fascia via the umbilical plate. When the peritoneum is finally positively reached after such multiple preperitoneal attempts, it is advisable to inflate the abdomen beyond the normal 15 to 20 mm Hg (Fig. 8–13). The surgeon should maintain careful communication with the anesthesiologist or the awake patient to detect respiratory difficulties caused by diaphragmatic pressure. This elevated intra-abdominal pressure (20 to 25 mm Hg) will hold the peritoneum against the preperitoneal and the skin fat like a distended balloon and will allow the trocar to enter (through the incision below the umbilicus) more easily. Another method uses the view created by the gas in the preperitoneal space to place the Veress needle into the peritoneum under direct laparoscopic vision (Kabukoba and Skillern, 1992).

COMPLETELY FAILED ENTRY. Since laparoscopy is an elective procedure in most cases, we allow ourselves three strikes before we call ourselves out in attempting to enter the abdominal cavity. After three attempts, the abdominal wall has been traversed repeatedly, and the surgeon is usually quite disconcerted and in no mental condition to continue an elective procedure. If a colleague is available to have an additional three tries, that surgeon should be given the opportunity to do so. Open laparoscopy or minilaparotomy may be elected. Otherwise, the procedure can be canceled at this point and rescheduled.

FIGURE 8–11 "Tenting" of the preperitoneum

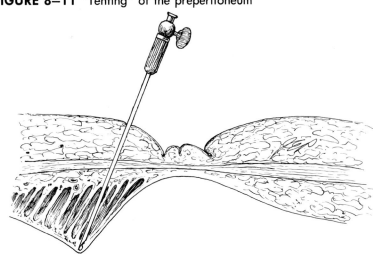

FIGURE 8–12 Re-entry above the umbilicus

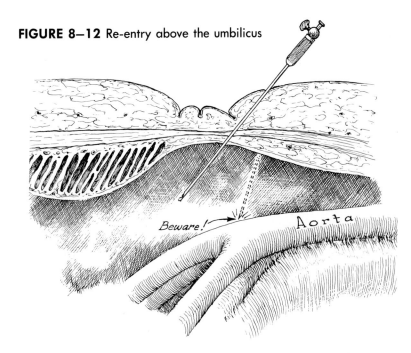

FIGURE 8–13 Extra inflation of the abdomen

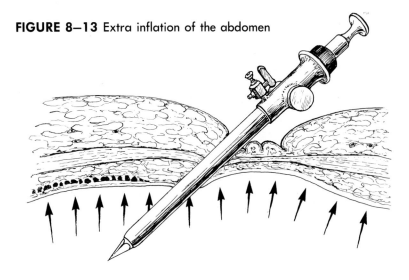

TROCAR

Trocar entry is the most dangerous part of the procedure. The principles outlined earlier concerning the technique of inserting the Veress needle pertain even more strongly to trocar entry (Fig. 8–14). Sharp trocars allow for less force to be exerted by the laparoscopist's right hand, causing minimal collapse of the abdominal wall against the underlying vessels under this pressure. The laparoscopist should again keep the three cardinal points in mind:

1. Aim toward the uterus.
2. Aim away from the pelvic blood vessels.
3. Aim at right angles to the skin.

The surgeon's concentration should focus equally on both right and left hands during entry (see Fig. 8–14). The left hand is the "guardian of the vessels" and should constantly elevate the abdomen upward. The laparoscopist should not rely on the pneumoperitoneum to do this, because in some cases the trocar is not sharp enough or the abdominal fascia is too resistant to keep the trocar away from the pelvic blood vessels.

FIGURE 8–14 Elevating the abdomen

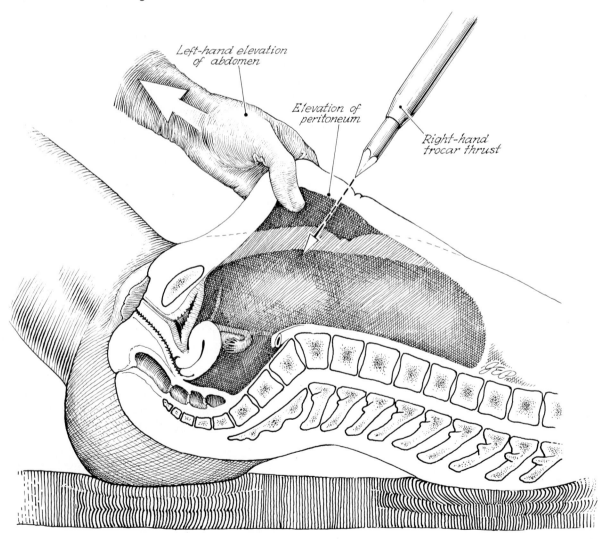

Left-hand elevation of abdomen

Elevation of peritoneum

Right-hand trocar thrust

Keeping the Sleeve In

As the trocar and sleeve pass through the fascia and peritoneum, the alert surgeon should feel these two distinct "gives" and should assume that he or she is in the peritoneum. At this point, especially with obese women, it is advisable to hold the trocar under very slight forward pressure and advance the sleeve over the trocar about 5 cm (Fig. 8–15), or in obese women until the trumpet valve touches the skin. This ensures that the sleeve is well within the peritoneum and is not pulled back pre-peritoneally when the trocar is removed. While holding the sleeve against the abdominal wall with the trumpet valve held down (Fig. 8–16), an audible rush of gas out of the abdomen as the trocar is removed is the most comforting signal that pneumoperitoneum has been established.

FIGURE 8–15 Advancing the sleeve over the trocar

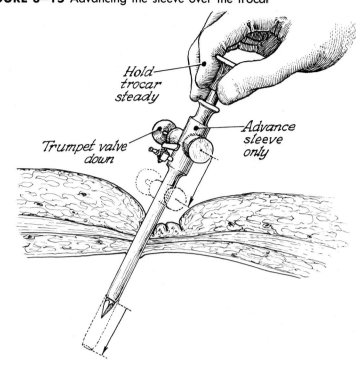

FIGURE 8–16 Confirming the pneumoperitoneum

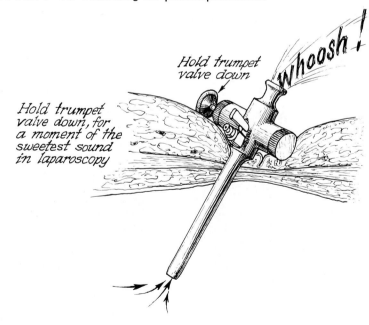

FIGURE 8–17 Inserting the optics

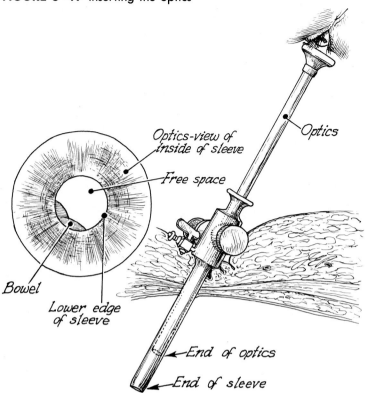

Optics-view of inside of sleeve

Free space

Optics

Bowel

Lower edge of sleeve

End of optics

End of sleeve

The laparoscope should then be inserted beyond the trumpet valve but within the sleeve (Fig. 8–17) and advanced under vision to the end of the sleeve to identify the abdominal contents. Free abdominal space should be positively identified. If adhesions are present, the scope should be advanced slowly to "spelunk" one's way into the abdominal cavity. If, after all this, the surgeon is still preperitoneal, the day's efforts should probably be abandoned.

Correct Angle of Insertion

In learning how to enter the abdomen correctly, it is helpful to have a colleague stand at the foot of the table along the axis at the patient's midline (Fig. 8–18). Many surgeons inadvertently aim the Veress needle and trocar to the left or the right of the midline, which can lead to accidental laceration of the left or right common iliac artery or vein on deep penetration. This accident can be eliminated by the colleague's directing the physician to a proper direction along this axis.

FIGURE 8–18 Checking vertical entry

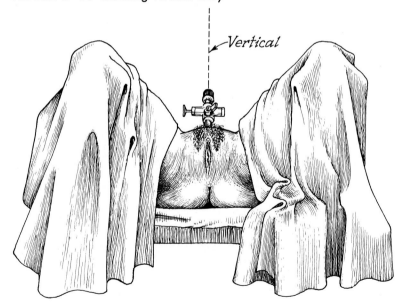

Vertical

Disposable Trocars and Sleeves

Trocars and sleeves were initially manufactured to be permanent, reusable instruments. In practice, the processing between patients (e.g., gathering, cleaning, and resterilizing) by most services treats trocars like clamps without regard to protecting their sharp tips. This results in dulling the tip of the trocar after about a dozen cycles. Dull trocars are actually more dangerous than sharp ones, since the increased force required to enter the abdomen lowers the surgeon's fine control and may make the surgeon press the umbilical area down onto the underlying large vessels, despite pneumoperitoneum. Resharpening trocars is difficult for the operating room personnel to do and is expensive and time consuming when done by the manufacturer.

Disposable trocars offer the advantage of a sharp tip for entry, with documented diminution of complications and force required (Corson et al, 1989). Trocars with stainless steel tips and plastic shanks (Rocket) are "resposable," good for use about a dozen times until operating room processing wears them down.

Disposable trocar-and-sleeve units (SURGIPORT; U.S. Surgical) as well as Veress needles (SURGINEEDLE; U.S. Surgical) are designed to be discarded after one use. The advantage of ensured sterility and sharpness is offset by their increased cost. For services with infrequent laparoscopic procedures, the cumulative cost of processing, sterilizing, and correctly assembling (often in the operating room by the surgeon during anesthesia time) standard Veress needles and sleeves may exceed the cost of using disposable ones. Disposable trocars and sleeves have a plastic sheath that in theory snaps forward to protect the abdominal contents from trocar injury, but in practice vascular and bowel injuries have occurred if full surgical precautions and skills described earlier are not used in insertion (the magic is not in the wand).

SECOND PUNCTURE

Entry Technique

The technique of entry of secondary trocars deserves similar careful attention. The incision site should be off the midline to avoid the fascial aponeurosis, to the left for convenience if the surgeon is standing at the patient's left and above the pubic hairline to avoid the bladder, which should be empty.

Laparoscopy has already been performed, and pneumoperitoneum is present. The inferior epigastric vessels can usually be seen through the laparoscope, and the abdominal wall should be indented at the proposed point of entry to ensure that the second puncture avoids these vessels.

Placement of the lower quadrant trocar sleeves just above the pubic hairline and lateral to the deep epigastric vessels (and thus, the rectus abdominis muscle) is preferred for operative procedures. These vessels, an artery flanked by two veins (venae comitantes), are found lateral to the umbilical ligaments (obliterated umbilical artery) by direct laparoscopic inspection of the anterior abdominal wall. They cannot be consistently found by traditional transillumination. The deep epigastric vessels arise near the junction of the external iliac vessels with the femoral vessels and make up the medial border of the internal inguinal ring. The round ligament curls around these vessels to enter the inguinal canal. When the anterior abdominal wall parietal peritoneum is thickened from previous surgery or obesity, the position of these vessels is judged by palpating and depressing the anterior abdominal wall with the back of the scalpel; the wall appears thicker where rectus muscle is enclosed, and the incision site should be chosen lateral to this area near the anterior superior iliac spine.

FIGURE 8–19 Second-puncture entry

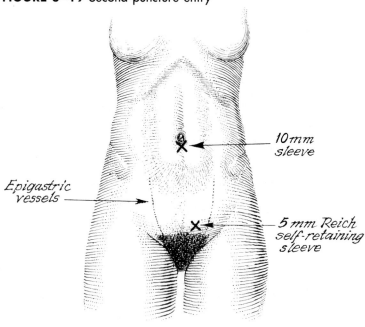

10 mm sleeve

Epigastric vessels

5 mm Reich self-retaining sleeve

FIGURE 8–20 Laparoscopic view of the second trocar

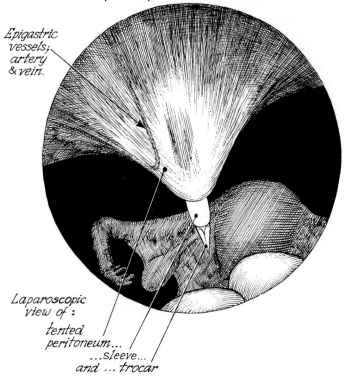

Epigastric vessels; artery & vein.

Laparoscopic view of:
tented peritoneum...
...sleeve...
and ...trocar

The surgeon should not look through the laparoscope during the initial stages of second-puncture entry. Rather, the surgeon should look at the trocar directly from outside (Fig. 8–19), again aiming the trocar toward the uterus and away from the common iliac vessels. Keeping a forefinger extended on the sleeve to stop the trocar at the estimated thickness of the abdominal wall helps. A 5-mm skin incision for a 5-mm second trocar should be checked directly by inserting the trocar and sleeve to ensure that the skin incision does not hold the sleeve back and cause excessive abdominal wall depression as the surgeon pushes the trocar and sleeve in.

Once the skin and fascia have been penetrated, the peritoneum in the suprapubic area is often quite loose and requires a very deep thrust to penetrate. This is most safely performed under direct laparoscopic visualization (Fig. 8–20). The tip of the trocar should be visible at all times; it should be directed into the cul-de-sac away from fixed structures and should avoid the epigastric vessels. The trocar should be thrust sufficiently deeply through the peritoneum so that the sleeve also penetrates this loose peritoneum. Failure to do this may lead to excessive peritoneal trauma and hematoma formation.

Crossed Swords to Chopsticks

Occasionally the second-puncture sleeve or instruments cannot be seen through the laparoscope. This is usually because the surgeon has "crossed swords" so that the second trocar is behind the field of view of the optics (Fig. 8–21). To check for this, the surgeon looks from *outside* the abdomen at the angle that the two sleeves and instruments are making. It is necessary to change the relationship to "chopsticks" so that the two instruments are nearly parallel and very slightly converging. The second-puncture instrument should then be easily seen in the optic's field of view.

WOUND CLOSURE

Withdrawing the Trocar to Check for Possible Bowel Injury

If the patient has a history of previous abdominal surgery suggesting adherent bowel, the track of the trocar and sleeve should be inspected with the laparoscope within the sleeve as the sleeve is slowly withdrawn to look for bowel injury. After the "vocal cords" of the peritoneum are seen, the trocar should be advanced back into the abdominal cavity to allow the gas to escape. The patient should be advised concerning increasing abdominal pain that may possibly indicate bowel injury and that may require further surgery. Bowel injury may be difficult to diagnose at laparoscopy in these situations, and immediate exploratory laparotomy may also be considered appropriate under some circumstances.

FIGURE 8–21 "Crossed swords" to "chopsticks"

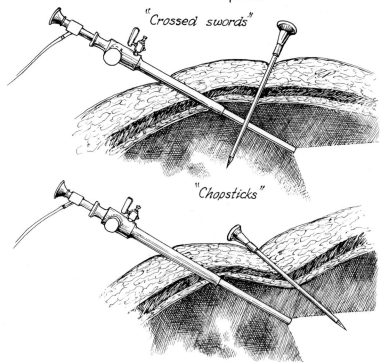

"Crossed swords"

"Chopsticks"

FIGURE 8–22 Closing an umbilical incision

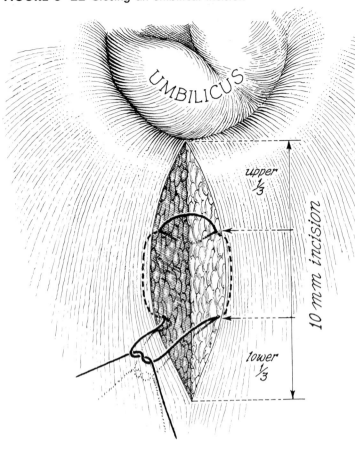

Suturing

The peritoneum and fascia close after a puncture wound without need for suturing. Furthermore, if the skin incision is along Langer's lines, no suture may be required for approximation. If a suture is required to approximate the skin, for 10-mm trocars a 3–0 absorbable subcuticular suture will make it unnecessary for the patient to return for suture removal. A subcuticular suture in the middle third of a 10-mm incision (Fig. 8–22) will approximate skin rapidly, if the suture is not pulled too tightly on the first two knots. Alternately, the umbilical incision can be closed with a 4–0 Vicryl suture opposing deep fascia and skin dermis. The knot is buried beneath the fascia.

A 5-mm second puncture can be closed with a buried knot if the needle starts deep and exits at the skin edge (Fig. 8–23). This procedure minimizes postoperative healing complaints. All lower quadrant incisions over 7 mm require precise identification and closure of the deep fascia to prevent incisional hernias. Alternately, suture material can be avoided in 5-mm lower quadrant incisions as their prolonged dissolution results in scarring. The lower quadrant 5-mm and 3-mm incisions are loosely approximated with Javid vascular clamps (V. Mueller) and are covered with collodion (AMEND) to allow drainage of excess lactated Ringer's solution if increased intra-abdominal pressure is present. Patients are instructed to expect incision leakage for 24 hours and to wait for 1 week for the collodion to slough off. These wounds heal by secondary intention because they are clean, free from pressure, surrounded by mobile tissue, and have good blood supply. Minimal scarring results.

FIGURE 8–23 Closing a second incision

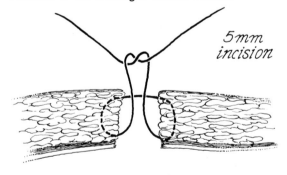

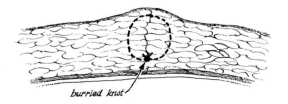

ALTERNATE ENTRY METHODS

The aforementioned description is my (J. F. H.) preferred method, formulated after numerous experiences in teaching residents and physicians overseas. These methods all have a low level of what I call *teacher's coronary index*, defined as the amount of spasm that the teacher's coronary arteries experience while watching a trainee perform a certain maneuver. All the techniques described earlier can be monitored by an instructor and certainly by the surgeon. Surprisingly, direct entry of the abdomen with trocar and sleeve without pneumoperitoneum (see later) carries with it a low teacher's coronary index after the initial experiences are survived. Nevertheless, other techniques of entry should be acknowledged as working very satisfactorily in other hands. We now discuss them in order of frequency of use.

Open Laparoscopy

Through a 2- to 3-cm vertical skin incision at the edge of the umbilical plate, Baby Deaver retractors (Eder Instrument Corp.) are used for exposure and sharp dissection and entry of the fascia. Two strong sutures are placed on both edges of the fascial entry, and these sutures are used to elevate the abdominal wall for sharp or blunt entry into the peritoneum (Fig. 8–24). A smooth-tipped Hasson trocar and sleeve are then inserted with an acorn-shaped metal obturator on the sleeve that maintains an air seal when the fascial sutures are tied to the sleeve. At the end of the procedure, the abdominal wall can be closed in layers using the elevating sutures for fascia. Closure of the peritoneum is not essential. This technique was developed by Hasson (1974) to minimize risk of large vessel injury during entry. It is particularly appropriate for patients with suspected abdominal wall adhesions and for muscular males or children with strong abdominal walls. Physicians lacking sufficient upper arm strength for abdominal wall elevation and trocar entry may prefer this routinely. General surgeons doing occasional emergency laparoscopies

FIGURE 8–24 Hasson cannula for "open laparoscopy"

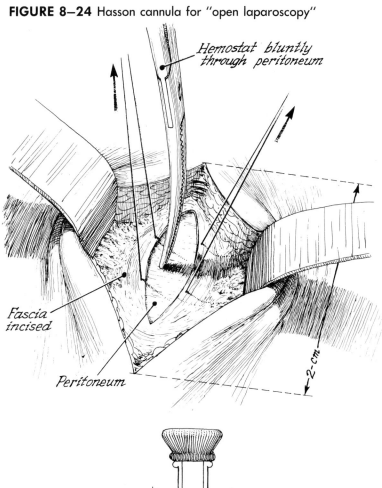

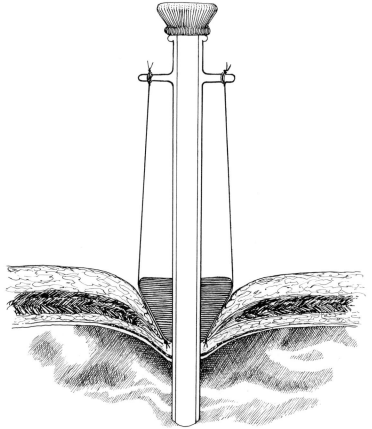

will find the method secure because it uses the technique and instincts of standard laparotomy on a small scale for abdominal entry.

Direct Trocar Entry

The abdominal wall is elevated as has been shown earlier (see Fig. 8–14), and the trocar is inserted without pneumoperitoneum. Strict attention is paid to the standard surgical principles of good relaxation, adequate skin incision, sharp instruments, and anatomy. Immediately after trocar entry, air is let into the trocar by elevating the abdomen, and the laparoscope is inserted into the sleeve to look at the end of the sleeve. Omentum and bowel move freely under the trocar end; preperitoneal fat does not. When proper entry is ensured, both insufflation and inspection can begin immediately, saving several minutes of blind insufflation and testing. This method has proved to be suitable for the majority of elective sterilizations. Most women seek sterilization after having had one or two children. Pregnancy has distended these abdominal walls, making the fascia thinner for easy trocar entry and the wall more relaxed for easy elevation by hand. Also, most women have not had previous abdominal surgery that may leave adherent bowel. With such patient selection, the technique can reduce operating time, and therefore anesthesia time significantly in busy outpatient laparoscopy programs (Byron et al, 1991; Copeland et al, 1983; Jarrett, 1990; Poindexter et al, 1990).

Towel Clip Elevation

For years the Johns Hopkins University school of laparoscopy has advocated the use of towel clips to elevate the skin around the umbilicus for needle and trocar entry. This requires the assistance of another hand while the surgeon is holding one towel clip and inserting the instrument with another (the third hand holds the second towel clip).

No Elevation

Others rely instead on a more gentle and cautious insertion of the Veress needle and creation of a well-distended abdomen against which a trocar and sleeve can be inserted with little risk of depressing the pneumoperitoneum if the trocar is sharp. Very skilled and experienced internists ask the patient to bear down under local anesthesia during trocar entry, thus in effect elevating the abdomen above the pneumoperitoneum and creating a rigid structure through which the trocar can be inserted rather than the relaxed wall preferred by gynecologic laparoscopists.

Gastroenterologists prefer a left upper quadrant point of entry to avoid the impressively dilated paraumbilical veins that can occur with advanced cirrhosis of the liver.

Reich Entry Technique

With the surgeon standing on the patient's left side and the patient supine, the left thumb (with or without sponge) is inserted into the umbilicus as deep as possible, after which the thumb and surrounding umbilicus are rolled over the lower left forefinger, stretching and widening the umbilical fossa, which is further enlarged with the blunt back end of the scalpel. A No. 15 blade (never a No. 11 blade) should be used to make a vertical midline incision on the inferior wall of the umbilical fossa, extending to and just beyond its lowest point. In thin patients, this incision frequently traverses the deep fascia, but intraperitoneal injury is avoided by the pulling of the umbilicus onto the surgeon's forefinger, a maneuver that controls the incision's depth.

A disposable Veress needle is grasped near its tip, like a dart, between the thumb and forefinger. The lower anterior abdominal wall is stabilized, not elevated, by grasping its full thickness in the operator's fist and by pulling it downward to bring the umbilicus to below the aortic bifurcation. The Veress needle tip is then inserted at right angles to the anterior abdominal wall for a distance of 1 cm. Insertion of the Veress needle should be an anatomic exercise with the surgeon cognizant of the anatomic structures traversed. Individual layers can be felt—deep fascia and peritoneum, or occasionally, peritoneum alone. If the Veress needle is inserted according to these principles, little need exists for testing to ensure proper positioning of the needle. After complete insertion, the needle is connected to a CO_2 insufflator flowing at 1 l/min with a pressure of less than 10 mm Hg. Insufflation is continued until a pressure of 20 to 25 mm Hg is obtained, usually after 4 to 6 liters.

The umbilical or "first-puncture" trocar, with its surrounding trumpet-valve trocar sleeve, is placed within the umbilicus. It is not necessary to lift the anterior abdominal wall during insertion of the trocar after establishment of a 4- to 6-liter pneumoperitoneum at 20 to 25 mm Hg, as the parietal peritoneum and skin move as one unit. The trocar should be "palmed" so that only 1 cm of the sharp tip protrudes beyond the operator's fingers. Holding the trocar sleeve higher unsheathes a "lethal weapon." Following shallow penetration to seat the trocar in the peritoneum at a 60- to 90-degree angle, the trocar is upturned to approximately 60 degrees. This continuous motion is "almost straight down" at first and then becomes "almost horizontal," with the wrist rotating nearly 90 degrees. Twisting of the trocar while under pressure is minimal. The result is a parietal peritoneal puncture directly beneath the umbilicus.

When this intraumbilical approach is used, the trocar exits the undersurface of the umbilicus closer to the aortic bifurcation than is encountered with the more common transverse infraumbilical incision with the trocar inserted at a 30-degree angle. Accordingly, an important prerequisite to performing an intraumbilical puncture is the surgeon's ability to palm the trocar. Some trocars are too long, and some hands are too small. (The long length of the Auto Suture SURGIPORT with safety shield makes it unsuitable for this palming technique.) If palming is neither feasible nor possible, the trocar should be "aimed" at the hollow of the sacrum to avoid the aortic bifurcation, or because elevation of the lower abdominal wall is not necessary with

adequate pneumoperitoneum, the trocar can be controlled with two hands to avoid a sudden thrust—the thumb and forefinger of one hand provide resistance to the insertional pressure exerted by the other. The high pressure settings used during initial insertion of the trocar are lowered thereafter to diminish the development of vena caval compression and subcutaneous emphysema. A relatively constant intra-abdominal pressure between 10 and 15 mm Hg is maintained during long laparoscopic procedures (Reich, 1989).

Ninth Intercostal Space

Special entry techniques are necessary in patients who have undergone multiple laparotomies or who may have extensive adhesions either discerned clinically or from another doctor's operative record. If CO_2 insufflation is not obtainable through the umbilicus, Veress needle puncture is done in the left ninth intercostal space, anterior axillary line (Reich, 1992). The trocar is then inserted at the left costal margin in the midclavicular line, giving a panoramic view of the entire peritoneal cavity. Likewise when extensive adhesions are encountered initially surrounding the umbilical puncture, the surgeon should immediately seek a higher site. Thereafter, the adhesions can be freed down to and just beneath the umbilicus, at which time it becomes possible to establish the umbilical portal for further work.

Which Technique to Choose

These variations in techniques of abdominal entry among skilled and experienced clinicians are mentioned to disclaim any absolute dictum implied by the detailed description of the technique discussed earlier in this chapter. As in the choice of which sterilization technique to use, the concluding recommendation is for physicians to continue using that technique with which they are the most comfortable (which has the lowest coronary index for them) until they are persuaded by colleagues, publications such as this one, or surgical misadventure to change their technique.

FURTHER READINGS

Byron JW, Markenson G, and Miyazawa K: A prospective evaluation comparing Veress needle and direct insertion techniques for laparoscopy (Abstract). Presented at the annual meeting of the American College of Gynecologists, New Orleans, May 1991.

Copeland C, Wing RR, and Hulka JF: Direct trocar insertion at laparoscopy: An evaluation. Obstet Gynecol 62:655–659, 1983.

Corson SL, Batzer FR, Gocial B, and Maislin G: Measurement of the force necessary for laparoscopic trocar entry. J Reprod Med 34:282–284, 1989.

Hasson HM: Open laparoscopy: A report of 150 cases. J Reprod Med 12:234–238, 1974.

Hurd WH, Bude RO, Delancey JOL, et al: Abdominal wall characterization with magnetic resonance imaging and computed tomography: The effect of obesity on the laparoscopic approach. J Reprod Med 36:473–476, 1991.

Jarrett JC: Laparoscopy: Direct trocar insertion without pneumoperitoneum. Obstet Gynecol 75:725–727, 1990.

Kabukoba JJ and Skillern LH: Coping with extraperitoneal insufflation during laparoscopy: A new technique. Obstet Gynecol 80:144–145, 1992.

Reich H: Laparoscopic bowel injury. Surg Laparosc Endosc 2:74–78, 1992.

Reich H: New techniques in advanced laparoscopic surgery. In Sutton C (ed): Bailliere's Clinical Obstetrics and Gynecology, Vol 3. New York, Harcourt Brace Jovanovich, 1989, pp 655–681.

STANDARD GYNECOLOGIC TECHNIQUES

Laparoscopy requires a unique combination of knowledge of basic physics and anatomy to enable the surgeon to perform the technique necessary, solve problems as they arise, and understand both normal and abnormal findings. We have chosen as "standard" those procedures that most residency training programs now include, and we have reserved the more extensive surgical procedures for the next section, Advanced Laparoscopic Surgery. The material has been chosen based on the technical and diagnostic problems that occur most frequently in the learning process of laparoscopy.

Description of Findings, Indications, and Timing of Surgery

*We see only what
we look for—we
look for only what
we know.*

In this era of video recordings of laparoscopic findings and surgery, it has become even more important for the surgeon to make more accurate observations. We are learning that the selection of the most appropriate method of treatment (laparoscopic surgery versus laparotomy versus in vitro fertilization [IVF]) depends a good deal on the nature and extent of the disease present. In this chapter we review the current methods used to describe surgery and findings, and we discuss prognostic implications of these findings.

TABLE 9–1. CLASSIFICATION OF OPERATION PERFORMED (CURRENT PROCEDURAL TERMINOLOGY [CPT] CODE)*

Code	Terminology	Description
Laparoscopy		
56300	Diagnostic only	Separate procedure
Operative Laparoscopy		
56301	Fulguration of oviducts	Sterilization
56302	Occlusion of oviducts by device	Clip, band, ring
56303	Fulguration or excision of lesions by any method	Ovary, pelvic viscera, peritoneal surface
56304	Lysis of adhesions	
56305	Biopsy	Single or multiple
56306	Aspiration	Single or multiple
56307	Removal of adnexal structures	Partial or total oophorectomy and/or salpingectomy
56308	Laparoscopic assisted vaginal hysterectomy	With or without removal of tube(s) and/or ovary(s)
56309	Subserosal myomectomy	Single or multiple
Adhesions by Laparotomy		
58740	Lysis of adhesions	No fimbrial surgery
58740–20	With microsurgery	
Tubal Surgery by Laparoscopy or Laparotomy		
56304	Salpingostomy	Permanent opening of blocked tube
59150	Ectopic salpingotomy	Incision into tube
59151	Ectopic salpingectomy	Removal of tube
Sterilization Reversal by Laparotomy		
58750–20	Microsurgical anastomosis	Connecting segments of tube (after sterilization)
	Cornual-isthmic	
	Cornual-ampullary	
	Isthmic-isthmic	
	Isthmic-ampullary	
	Ampullary-ampullary	

*Based on annual versions of American Medical Association: CPT. Physician's Current Procedure Terminology. Chicago, AMA; 1993 revisions from Rizzo J and Marinelli T: CPT corner. The AMGO News (Association of Managers of Gynecology and Obstetrics) 14:4–5, 1993.

CLASSIFICATION SYSTEMS

Three ways of describing adnexal disease are by *operation performed*, by *disease found*, and by *prognostic factors*.

Operation Performed

In Table 9–1 we present the 1993 American Medical Association codes and nomenclature for inclusion in the *Physicians' Current Procedural Terminology* (CPT) code. Extensive procedures, such as a difficult lysis of adhesions, can be changed with a -20 modifier.

Disease Found

The American Fertility Society (AFS) is in the process of developing classifications for disease found, and we present the current version of these classifications in this chapter (1985 to 1988 Committee on Classification of the American Fertility Society). Ultimately, these classifications will be based on the prognostic factors that significantly influence success. At the moment, the AFS classifications are descriptive and anatomic rather than prognostic (Fig. 9–1).

Figure 9–1. From The American Fertility Society classifications of adnexal adhesions, distal tubal occlusion, tubal occlusion second to tubal ligation, tubal pregnancies, mullerian anomalies and intrauterine adhesions. Fertil Steril 49:945, 1988. Reproduced with permission of the publisher, The American Fertility Society.

FIGURE 9–1 The American Fertility Society Classification of Adnexal Adhesions

Patient's Name _____ Date _____ Chart # _____

Age _____ G _____ P _____ Sp Ab _____ VTP _____ Ectopic _____ Infertile Yes _____ No _____

Other Significant History (i.e. surgery, infection, etc.) _____

_____

HSG _____ Sonography _____ Photography _____ Laparoscopy _____ Laparotomy _____

	ADHESIONS		<1/3 Enclosure	1/3 - 2/3 Enclosure	>2/3 Enclosure
OVARY	R	Filmy	1	2	4
		Dense	4	8	16
	L	Filmy	1	2	4
		Dense	4	8	16
TUBE	R	Filmy	1	2	4
		Dense	4·	8·	16
	L	Filmy	1	2	4
		Dense	4·	8·	16

· If the fimbriated end of the fallopian tube is completely enclosed, change the point assignment to 16.

Prognostic Classification for Adnexal Adhesions

	LEFT		RIGHT
A. Minimal	_____	0-5	_____
B. Mild	_____	6-10	_____
C. Moderate	_____	11-20	_____
D. Severe	_____	21-32	_____

Treatment (Surgical Procedures): _____

_____

_____

_____

_____

Prognosis for Conception & Subsequent Viable Infant**

_____ Excellent (> 75%)

_____ Good (50-75%)

_____ Fair (25%-50%)

_____ Poor (< 25%)

**Physician's judgment based upon adnexa with least amount of pathology.

Recommended Followup Treatment: _____

_____

_____

Additional Findings: _____

_____

_____

_____

_____

_____

```
                    DRAWING
   L                                        R
```

Property of
The American Fertility Society

For additional supply write to:
The American Fertility Society
2140 11th Avenue, South
Suite 200
Birmingham, Alabama 35205

FIGURE 9–2 Adnexal adhesion staging: ovarian involvement

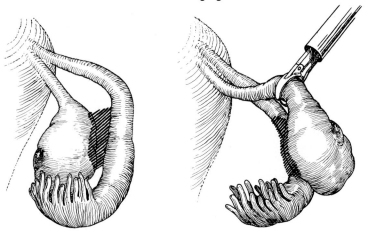

*Over **50%** of ovary visible*

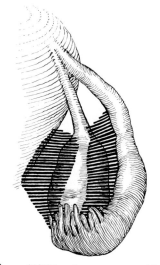

*Less than **50%** of ovary visible*

Prognostic Factors

In this chapter we present our current approaches to prognostic classifications. We have analyzed our own patients and those reported by others to identify prognostic features in the diseases treated (Hulka, 1982). We have strictly defined success in infertility surgery as involving patients who had "take-home babies" (THB) rather than pregnancies. When findings predict an increase in pathologic pregnancies (abortions and ectopic pregnancies), they are identified. To simplify prognosis, we divide patients into three categories:

- Stage I. Patients with a good prognosis for whom surgery is clearly indicated (mild)
- Stage II. Patients for whom surgery may result in a THB rate better than with IVF or gamete fallopian transfer (GIFT) (moderate)
- Stage III. Patients who will not benefit from surgery and who should proceed directly to IVF or GIFT (severe)

ADNEXAL ADHESIONS

The success of lysis of adhesions depends in large part on their extensiveness and cause. The AFS has recommended a system of describing adnexal adhesions (see Fig. 9–1) in which a numeric value is assigned to each adnexum based on accurate observations concerning the nature of the adhesions and the extent of tubal and ovarian involvement. These observations are presented in detail:

1. *Extent of ovarian surface visible* (Fig. 9–2). Since the egg must leave the ovary to get into the tube, the amount of free surface becomes critically important. We have found that an adnexum with more than half of the ovary free of adhesions has a good prognosis for pregnancy. Patients with less than half of an ovary visible have a poor prognosis.

2. *Nature of adhesions* (Fig. 9–3). Thin, avascular adhesions are easily lysed and tend not to recur. In contrast, thick or vascular adhesions that require separation result in damaged surfaces on which adhesions rapidly reform.

For prognostic purposes, our thinking has reduced the varieties of conditions found in adnexal adhesions into three categories. These have practical value since they tell us what to offer the patient in terms of further management (Table 9–2; see also Atlas, Plates 11 and 12).

FIGURE 9–3 Stretching adhesions for staging

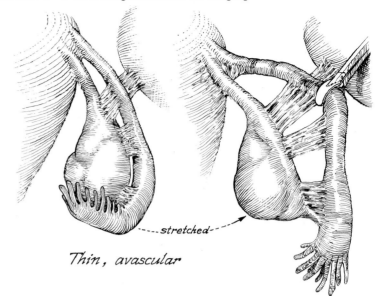

Thin, avascular

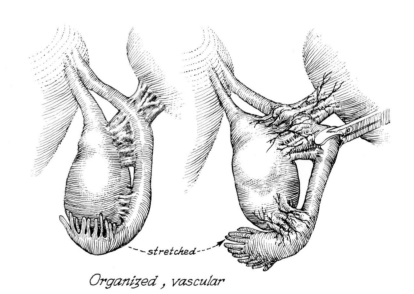

Organized, vascular

TABLE 9–2.	PROGNOSTIC CLASSIFICATION OF ADHESIONS
Stage I:	Thin adhesions involving less than half the ovary Prognosis: more than 50% THB* Plan: laparoscopic lysis
Stage II:	(Any combination of findings between I and III) Prognosis: 10–50% THB Plan: laparoscopic lysis
Stage III:	Thick adhesions covering more than half the ovary Prognosis: less than 10% THB Plan: In vitro fertilization

*THB = take-home babies.

DISTAL OCCLUSION

Although hysterosalpingography (HSG) first raises the possibility of distal tubal occlusion, laparoscopy is the final method of diagnosis. There is a 15 to 30% discrepancy rate in diagnosing distal tubal occlusion between HSG and surgery.

Modern diagnostic laparoscopy often requires fairly extensive lysis of adhesions to get to the distal end of the tube to make important diagnostic observations. True hydrosalpinx must be distinguished from a patent tube bound to an ovary by adhesions causing intratubal loculation. The prognosis for a patent but adherent tube is much better than for a true hydrosalpinx where fimbriae have been destroyed.

The AFS recommendations give numeric weights to the diameter of the tube and its estimated thickness (Fig. 9–4).

Studies evaluating the internal tubal epithelium at microsurgery, laparoscopy, or salpingoscopy have suggested that the gross appearance of the epithelium is a significant factor for subsequent pregnancy, with the following prognostic values:

1. Normal rugae (a rare finding): about 70% chance of pregnancy
2. Agglutinated or damaged: 10 to 30% chance of pregnancy
3. Patchy or complete absence: less than 10% chance of pregnancy

Opening the tube at laparoscopy and performing a *diagnostic salpingotomy* with a 5- or 10-mm optic can give valuable information concerning the state of the mucosa on the rugae in the ampulla.

(From Revised American Fertility Society Classification of Endometriosis: 1985. Fertil Steril 43:351, 1985. Reproduced with permission of the publisher, The American Fertility Society.)

FIGURE 9–4 The American Fertility Society Classification of Distal Tubal Occlusion

Patient's Name _____ Date _____ Chart # _____

Age _____ G _____ P _____ Sp Ab _____ VTP _____ Ectopic _____ Infertile Yes _____ No _____

Other Significant History (i.e. surgery, infection, etc) _____

HSG _____ Sonography _____ Photography _____ Laparoscopy _____ Laparotomy _____

		<3 cm	3-5 cm	>5 cm
Distal ampullary diameter	L	1	4	6
	R	1	4	6
Tubal wall thickness		Normal/Thin	Moderately Thickened or Edematous	Thick & Rigid
	L	1	4	6
	R	1	4	6
Mucosal folds at neostomy site		Normal/ > 75% Preserved	35% to 75% Preserved	<35% Preserved Adherent Mucosal Fold
	L	1	4	6
	R	1	4	6
Extent of adhesions		None/Minimal/Mild	Moderate	Extensive
	L	1	3	6
	R	1	3	6
Type of adhesions		None/Filmy	Moderately Dense (or Vascular)	Dense
	L	1	2	4
	R	1	2	4

Prognostic Classification for Terminal Salpingostomy (Salpingoneostomy)

	LEFT		RIGHT
A. Mild	_____	1-3	_____
B. Moderate	_____	9-10	_____
C. Severe	_____	>10	_____

Treatment (Surgical Procedures):

Salpingostomy	L	R
A. Terminal	_____	_____
B. Ampullary	_____	_____

Other: _____

_____

_____

_____

_____

Prognosis for Conception & Subsequent Viable Infant*

_____ Excellent (> 75%)

_____ Good (50 - 75%)

_____ Fair (25%-50%)

_____ Poor (< 25%)

*Physician's judgment based upon adnexa with least amount of pathology.

Recommended Followup Treatment: _____

Additional Findings: _____

_____

_____

_____

_____

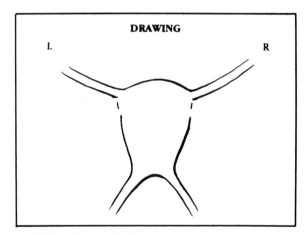

For additional supply write to:
The American Fertility Society
2140 11th Avenue, South
Suite 200
Birmingham, Alabama 35205

Property of
The American Fertility Society

TABLE 9–3. **PROGNOSTIC CLASSIFICATION OF DISTAL OCCLUSION**

Stage I:	External adhesions blocking tube, normal rugae, "pure" hydrosalpinx
	Prognosis: 30–70% THB*
	Plan: microsurgery
Stage II:	Ovarian adhesions, damaged rugae
	Prognosis: 0–30% THB, increased risk of ectopic pregnancy
	Plan: laparoscopic therapeutic salpingostomy
Stage III:	Denuded and agglutinated rugae, or adhesions covering ovary
	Prognosis: 0% THB, increased risk of ectopic pregnancy
	Plan: In vitro fertilization

*THB = take-home babies.

Surgery on closed tubes with more than half the ovary covered with adhesions has not resulted in any subsequent live births in our institution (see Atlas, Plate 10). As with adhesions, we have reduced the findings of distal occlusion into three categories with distinct practical implications for further management. These prognostic factors and therapeutic implications are summarized in Table 9–3. As Table 9–3 indicates, a diagnostic laparoscopy in which tubal occlusion is suspected should anticipate and be prepared for possible lysis of adhesions and salpingostomy by laparoscopy.

The management of occlusion has vacillated between microsurgery and laparoscopic salpingostomy. It is our current belief that if at diagnostic salpingotomy (during laparoscopy) the tubal damage is minimal and rugae are present, the patient will have her best chance for subsequent pregnancy if a microsurgical approach is planned. The tubes can be handled delicately, with minimal trauma and scar formation, and continuing patency and function are more assured than with the less delicate techniques of laparoscopic salpingostomy. *Therapeutic salpingostomy by laparoscopy* is appropriate in the presence of adhesive disease and damaged rugae. Under these conditions, the prognosis for subsequent pregnancy is low (approximately 20% or less) and a separate microsurgical operation is not justified by the prognosis.

Ancillary procedures to improve the outcome of salpingostomy have included postoperative hydrotubation and second-look laparoscopy, including reopening of the tube. None of these procedures has been documented as improving subsequent fertility rates.

PROXIMAL OCCLUSION

Patency of the isthmic-uterine junction can be compromised either by obstruction or by the presence of salpingitis isthmica nodosa (SIN). SIN can be suspected at laparoscopy by a funnel-like or nodular connection of the uterus and isthmic portion of the tube. However, diagnosis of true uterotubal obstruction is difficult and currently includes selective salpingography and cannulation with roentgenogram or ultrasound guidance as well as hysteroscopic cannulation. Hysteroscopic cannulation is often planned together with diagnostic laparoscopy for a definitive evaluation of the extent of tubal disease. Proximal occlusion must be taken into account in anticipating success of adnexal surgery. Repair of the combination of a true proximal and distal blockage has resulted in rare pregnancies.

These descriptive details can be best remembered by looking at the adnexa from the egg's point of view. It must (1) get out of the *ovarian surface*, (2) through the *adhesions*, (3) into the *distal tube*, and (4) past the *isthmic-uterine junction* to result in an intrauterine pregnancy.

TABLE 9–4. ACOSTA CLASSIFICATION OF PELVIC ENDOMETRIOSIS*

Mild
1. Scattered, fresh lesions (i.e., implants not associated with scarring or retraction of the peritoneum) in the anterior or posterior cul-de-sac or pelvic peritoneum
2. Rare surface implant on ovary, with no endometrioma, without surface scarring and retraction, and without periovarian adhesions
3. No peritubular adhesions

Moderate
1. Endometriosis involving one or both ovaries, with several surface lesions, with scarring and retraction, or small endometriomata
2. Minimal periovarian adhesions associated with ovarian lesions described
3. Minimal peritubular adhesions associated with ovarian lesions described
4. Superficial implants in the anterior or posterior cul-de-sac with scarring and retraction; some adhesions, but not sigmoid invasion

Severe
1. Endometriosis involving one or both ovaries with endometrioma >2 × 2 cm (usually both)
2. One or both ovaries bound down by adhesions associated with endometriosis, with or without tubal adhesions to ovaries
3. One or both tubes bound down or obstructed by endometriosis; associated adhesions or lesions
4. Obliteration of the cul-de-sac from adhesions or lesions associated with endometriosis
5. Thickening of the uterosacral ligaments and cul-de-sac lesions from invasive endometriosis with obliteration of the cul-de-sac
6. Significant bowel or urinary tract involvement

*From Acosta AA, Buttram VC Jr, Besch PK, et al: A proposed classification of pelvic endometriosis. Obstet Gynecol 42:19–25, 1973. Reprinted with permission from The American College of Obstetricians and Gynecologists.

EVALUATION PRIOR TO ANASTOMOSIS

Patients seeking reversal of sterilization should have documentation of the sterilization procedure performed, preferably the dictated operative note. Fimbriectomies are seldom successfully reversed, and IVF is recommended. Electrocoagulating techniques may need a laparoscopy to determine the amount of useful tube left. This situation holds true for unipolar and bipolar coagulation techniques, since there is great individual variation in the techniques used as well as resultant tissue destruction. If less than 4 cm of tube (proximal plus distal stump) remains bilaterally, the prognosis is poor for a successful THB, and risk of abortion and ectopic pregnancy is increased. Currently, IVF is recommended.

On the other hand, mechanical occlusion techniques (e.g., Pomeroy, band, clip) seldom destroy sufficient tube to justify such a prognostic laparoscopy prior to microsurgical reversal. With documentation of a mechanical occlusive procedure, microsurgery can be scheduled directly with a prognosis for a successful pregnancy higher than IVF currently offers. Surgery not involving the ampulla, such as an isthmic-isthmic anastomosis, has a much lower chance of ectopic pregnancy than if the ampulla were involved. Reversal of sterilization is discussed in more detail in Chapter 11.

ENDOMETRIOSIS

Several classification systems for the numerous findings in endometriosis have been proposed. We present here the simple classification system that was proposed by Acosta and colleagues (Acosta et al, 1973) and that was used in reports of many medical and surgical therapeutic efforts (Table 9–4).

The description and classification recommended by the AFS assigns a numeric weight to the severity of findings to arrive at a total score (Fig. 9–5). Although each adnexum is described separately, the final score includes findings of both adnexa. The extent of ovarian enclosure by adhesions is described, and the adhesions are described throughout as "filmy" or "dense." The AFS classification includes very important observations on the size of ovarian endometriomata but does not describe depth of infiltrating lesions.

Pregnancy rates following medical or surgical treatment for minimal or mild endometriosis appear to be in the 60 to 70% range, with no advantage detectable concerning surgery (including laser) versus medical or combined therapy. More extensive endometriosis has subsequent pregnancy rates ranging downward from this figure.

RECORDING OF FINDINGS

Many aids have been devised for description of abnormal findings. The AFS forms for endometriosis, adnexal adhesions, tubal occlusion, and anastomosis (see Figs. 9–1, 9–4, and 9–5) are useful for disciplining the laparoscopist to make the specific observations required, as well as being useful as permanent records. Video tapes and selected color prints are being used as additional records and help in research to allow independent staging of adnexal disease. They are also useful as medicolegal documents, since judges and juries appreciate the honesty of the surgeon's presenting exactly what was found and what happened. Finally, it is very helpful for records of tubo-occlusion for sterilization to include confirmation by a named colleague that the proper structure was occluded properly. Two doctors on record is a deterrent to subsequent malpractice accusations.

FIGURE 9–5 The American Fertility Society Revised Classification of Endometriosis. (From The American Fertility Society: The American Society Revised Classification of Endometriosis. Fertil Steril 43:351–352, 1985. Reproduced with permission of the publisher, The American Fertility Society.)

THE AMERICAN FERTILITY SOCIETY
REVISED CLASSIFICATION OF ENDOMETRIOSIS

Patient's Name _____ Date_____

Stage I   (Minimal) - 1-5
Stage II (Mild)   - 6-15
Stage III (Moderate) - 16-40
Stage IV (Severe)   - >40
Total_____

Laparoscopy_____ Laparotomy_____ Photography_____
Recommended Treatment_____
_____
Prognosis_____

PERITONEUM	**ENDOMETRIOSIS**	<1cm	1-3cm	>3cm
	Superficial	1	2	4
	Deep	2	4	6
OVARY	R Superficial	1	2	4
	Deep	4	16	20
	L Superficial	1	2	4
	Deep	4	16	20

	POSTERIOR CULDESAC OBLITERATION	Partial	Complete
		4	40

	ADHESIONS	<1/3 Enclosure	1/3-2/3 Enclosure	>2/3 Enclosure
OVARY	R Filmy	1	2	4
	Dense	4	8	16
	L Filmy	1	2	4
	Dense	4	8	16
TUBE	R Filmy	1	2	4
	Dense	4*	8*	16
	L Filmy	1	2	4
	Dense	4*	8*	16

*If the fimbriated end of the fallopian tube is completely enclosed, change the point assignment to 16.

Additional Endometriosis: _____ Associated Pathology: _____
_____ _____
_____ _____

To Be Used with Normal
Tubes and Ovaries

L   R

To Be Used with Abnormal
Tubes and/or Ovaries

L   R

For additional supply write to: The American Fertility Society, 2140 11th Avenue South,
Suite 200, Birmingham, Alabama 35205-2800

EXAMPLES & GUIDELINES

STAGE I (MINIMAL)	STAGE II (MILD)	STAGE III (MODERATE)

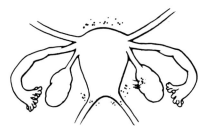 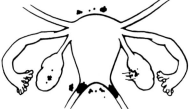 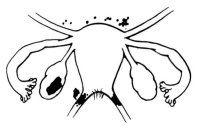

PERITONEUM	**PERITONEUM**	**PERITONEUM**
Superficial Endo – 1-3cm - 2	Deep Endo – >3cm - 6	Deep Endo – >3cm - 6
R. OVARY	**R. OVARY**	**CULDESAC**
Superficial Endo – < 1cm - 1	Superficial Endo – < 1cm - 1	Partial Obliteration - 4
Filmy Adhesions – < 1/3 - 1	Filmy Adhesions – < 1/3 - 1	**L. OVARY**
TOTAL POINTS 4	**L. OVARY**	Deep Endo – 1-3cm - 16
	Superficial Endo – <1cm - 1	TOTAL POINTS 26
	TOTAL POINTS 9	

STAGE III (MODERATE)	STAGE IV (SEVERE)	STAGE IV (SEVERE)

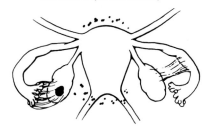 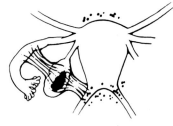 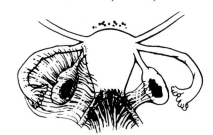

PERITONEUM	**PERITONEUM**	**PERITONEUM**
Superficial Endo – >3cm -4	Superficial Endo – >3cm -4	Deep Endo – >3cm - 6
R. TUBE	**L. OVARY**	**CULDESAC**
Filmy Adhesions – < 1/3 - 1	Deep Endo – 1-3cm - 32**	Complete Obliteration - 40
R. OVARY	Dense Adhesions – < 1/3 - 8**	**R. OVARY**
Filmy Adhesions – < 1/3 - 1	**L. TUBE**	Deep Endo – 1-3cm - 16
L. TUBE	Dense Adhesions – < 1/3 -8**	Dense Adhesions – < 1/3 - 4
Dense Adhesions – < 1/3 - 16*	TOTAL POINTS 52	**L. TUBE**
L. OVARY		Dense Adhesions – >2/3 - 16
Deep Endo – <1 cm -4	*Point assignment changed to 16	**L. OVARY**
Dense Adhesions – < 1/3 -4	**Point assignment doubled	Deep Endo – 1-3cm - 16
TOTAL POINTS 30		Dense Adhesions – >2/3 - 16
		TOTAL POINTS 114

Determination of the stage or degree of endometrial involvement is based on a weighted point system. Distribution of points has been arbitrarily determined and may require further revision or refinement as knowledge of the disease increases.

To ensure complete evaluation, inspection of the pelvis in a clockwise or counterclockwise fashion is encouraged. Number, size and location of endometrial implants, plaques, endometriomas and/or adhesions are noted. For example, five separate 0.5cm superficial implants on the peritoneum (2.5 cm total) would be assigned 2 points. (The surface of the uterus should be considered peritoneum.) The severity of the endometriosis or adhesions should be assigned the highest score only for peritoneum, ovary, tube or culdesac. For example, a 4cm superficial and a 2cm deep implant of the peritoneum should be given a score of 6 (not 8). A 4cm deep endometrioma of the ovary associated with more than 3cm of superficial disease should be scored 20 (not 24).

In those patients with only one adnexa, points applied to disease of the remaining tube and ovary should be multiplied by two. **Points assigned may be circled and totaled. Aggregation of points indicates stage of disease (minimal, mild, moderate, or severe).

The presence of endometriosis of the bowel, urinary tract, fallopian tube, vagina, cervix, skin etc., should be documented under "additional endometriosis." Other pathology such as tubal occlusion, leiomyomata, uterine anomaly, etc., should be documented under "associated pathology." All pathology should be depicted as specifically as possible on the sketch of pelvic organs, and means of observation (laparoscopy or laparotomy) should be noted.

FIGURE 9–6 Luteinized unruptured follicle (LUF) syndrome

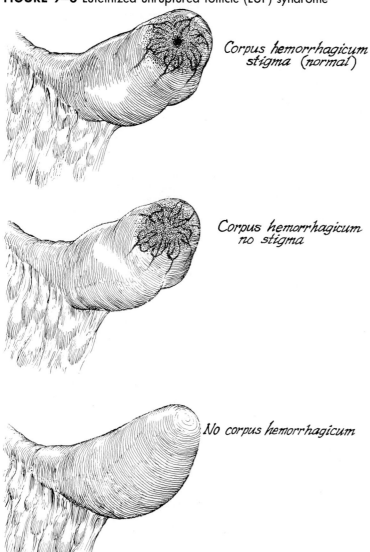

Corpus hemorrhagicum stigma (normal)

Corpus hemorrhagicum no stigma

No corpus hemorrhagicum

TIMING OF LAPAROSCOPY FOR INFERTILITY

For maximum information, timing of a laparoscopy for infertility is important. The more obvious problems of infertility should have already have been tested and evaluated: male factor, ovulation, and HSG to document normal internal uterine and tubal architecture as well as patent tubes.

Ovulation is most strictly defined by elevation of plasma progesterones to levels above 15 ng/ml in plasma obtained 5 to 10 days prior to the next menses. This may require administration of clomiphene citrate. Once ovulation has been documented by these criteria for three or four cycles, and pregnancy has not yet occurred, a laparoscopy is most appropriately done within 1 to 4 days after presumed ovulation. No particular precautions against pregnancy in that cycle are recommended, and the few pregnancies that we have had when laparoscopy was performed in the pregnancy cycle have been normal. This part of the cycle yields the most information concerning truly normal ovulation, as can be detected on gross inspection of the ovary: a fresh corpus hemorrhagicum with a fresh stigma or point of exit of the recently released ovum (Fig. 9–6; see also Atlas, Plate 5). These findings can be quite clearly seen in normal ovulation but are surprisingly absent in some patients (see Atlas, Plate 6). The condition of a luteinized unruptured follicle (LUF) (Marik and Hulka, 1978) has been well documented in humans with combined endocrine and ultrasound documentation and appears to occur in many women in an occasional cycle and in about 15% of infertile women consistently (Eissa et al, 1987; Hamilton et al, 1990). Treatment with clomiphene citrate or human chorionic gonadotrophin at the time of LH surge has been reported (Bateman et al, 1990). Ovulatory disturbances of this kind are often found in patients with endometriosis but are overlooked because the surgeon is distracted by endometriosis findings. Finally, in couples undergoing donor insemination, we perform laparoscopy after the sixth unsuccessful but well-timed insemination cycle.

With Possible Therapeutic Laparoscopic Surgery

All our diagnostic laparoscopies are done on an outpatient basis and are not scheduled as "laparoscopy, possible laparotomy." However, we try to schedule three or more 1-hour procedures during a session, anticipating that in at least one patient prolonged laparoscopic surgery will be required for endometriosis or adhesions. When endometriosis is found, electrocoagulation or laser ablation of implants is performed. Laser dissection of adhesions is usually required because of their density in active endometriosis. The differential diagnosis between an abnormal corpus hemorrhagicum or persistent corpus luteum and an endometrioma is extremely difficult to make at surgery. To avoid prolonged and unnecessary ovarian cystectomies for removal of functional cysts that would resolve with time, we prefer to open and drain unsuspected cysts discovered at diagnostic laparoscopy in women younger than 35 years of age, performing cystectomies only for the more obvious chocolate-filled endometriomas. Ovarian cystectomies are best managed by separate scheduling after ultrasonographic documentation of persistence for more than 3 months.

Adnexal adhesions are routinely lysed at diagnostic laparoscopy. We have been aggressive in our laparoscopic lysis, using techniques described in Chapter 15. Sharp scissor dissection, close to the surface of the ovary, is sufficient for most ovarian adhesions, with occasional laser or electrosurgery with cutting current for dense adhesions. Since these patients are undergoing diagnostic laparoscopy after normal patency at HSG, the tube usually has relatively few adhesions and can be well mobilized. If the HSG showed tubal occlusion, the patient is scheduled for a possible 3-hour laparoscopic lysis and salpingostomy, not just diagnostic laparoscopy.

With GIFT Procedure

GIFT involves placing freshly harvested eggs and washed sperm directly into a normal fallopian tube. Because of the high (> 25%) pregnancy rate obtained, services that provide GIFT can schedule an indicated diagnostic laparoscopy and GIFT procedure at the same time. The diagnostic part of this combined procedure is compromised only in that normal ovulation cannot be observed or documented in the hyperstimulated cycle necessary for multiple egg retrieval. Ablation of endometrial implants at the same time of GIFT does not appear to interfere with pregnancy results.

"SECOND-LOOK" LAPAROSCOPY

After Microsurgery

Since the introduction of the concept of a second-look laparoscopy after lysis of adhesions, its use has been controversial. The original recommendation of a 4- to 6-week delay (Raj and Hulka, 1982) has been reduced, since postoperative adhesion re-formation is rapid and collagen deposition begins on days 9 to 11 (diZerega, 1990). Semm recommends leaving a soft tubular rubber drain in the trocar wounds after laparoscopic conservative management of ectopic pregnancy and performing a second-look laparoscopy using these abdominal entries 3 days afterward to lyse the adhesions and maximize the patient's subsequent fertility (Semm, 1990). Although diminution of adhesions after second-look lysis has been observed, improvement of subsequent fertility has not (Trimbos-Kemper et al, 1985; Tulandi et al, 1989). The use of second-look laparoscopy has documented the efficacy of adhesion preventive agents or in endometriosis suppression. However, insurance companies in the United States are reluctant to pay for these procedures, citing lack of evidence that the patient's fertility is improved. The therapeutic benefit, in terms of live births, needs to be established by difficult large-scale prospective trials.

TABLE 9–5.	**DIFFERENTIAL DIAGNOSIS OF THE ACUTE ABDOMEN**
Normal pelvis	Acute suppurative salpingitis
Unruptured ovarian cyst	Pelvic abscess
Ruptured endometrioma	Diverticulitis
Ruptured corpus luteal cyst	Regional enteritis
Torsion of the abdomen	Acute appendicitis
Endometriosis	Perforated viscus
Ectopic pregnancy	

Waiting for longer than 6 weeks can result in dense adhesions, like those shown in the Atlas on Plate 13. We believe that the opportunity to evaluate our medical and surgical efforts, relyse adhesions, occasionally reopen fimbriae by opening a grasping forceps inside the ampulla, and inform the patient of her prognosis makes second-look laparoscopy useful to the patient and our field as we develop the management of endometriosis, ectopic pregnancy, and adhesions.

After Chemotherapy for Ovarian Cancer

After completion of chemotherapy, second-look laparoscopy can save about one in three patients from a second-look laparotomy. If at laparoscopy, persistent disease is documented and biopsied, no further laparotomy is indicated. If, however, no residual disease can be found, a laparotomy for a more thorough exploration by vision and palpation may be indicated to arrive at a diagnosis as to the presence or absence of tumor. The usefulness of ultrasound to document a recurrence and eliminate the need for exploration by laparoscopy or laparotomy is not established at this time.

ACUTE PAIN

The acute abdomen with an unclear cause is a good indication for laparoscopy, with the timing considerations that follow. The differential diagnosis of acute abdominal pain is given in Table 9–5, illustrating the usefulness of laparoscopy in diagnosis and therapy of this condition. See also Chapter 32 for a discussion of laparoscopy in the emergency situation.

IN CHILDREN. In a study of the use of laparoscopy to evaluate appendicitis in children, a 12-hour observation period in patients with an unclear diagnosis was incorporated to allow the signs and symptoms to clarify (Leape and Ramenofsky, 1977 and 1980). If at the end of this observation period the diagnosis was still obscure, a laparoscopy was found to avert the need for laparotomy in about one of three such unclear situations.

IN ACUTE SALPINGITIS. Laparoscopy can positively diagnose acute salpingitis after the patient is admitted to the hospital (see Atlas, Plate 16) and, more important, rule it out to avoid mislabeling the patient with the stigma and concern of pelvic inflammatory disease (PID). Routine laparoscopy for diagnosis of PID in Europe also provides the opportunity for drainage of tubo-ovarian abosses (see Atlas, Plate 17), leading to faster recovery. Based on clinical criteria alone, PID is incorrectly diagnosed in 30 to 50% of women (Jacobson, 1980; Sellors et al, 1991). Although laparoscopy has been used routinely for diagnosis in Lund, Sweden, in several thousand women with no detectable increase in complications from the procedure, cost factors in the United States cause laparoscopy to be used more sparingly in the diagnosis of this disease.

IN ACUTE APPENDICITIS. In the adult male or female, as in children, a more aggressive use of laparoscopy to rule out appendicitis may become more widespread as surgeons find this instrument useful. An acute appendix can be removed through the laparoscope. Finding a normal appendix with a laparoscope allows a thorough evaluation to be made of the abdomen in order to make a correct diagnosis, which is of great importance to the patient. The problem is discussed more extensively in Chapter 31.

IN UNRUPTURED ECTOPIC PREGNANCY. Sensitive β subunit pregnancy tests and vaginal ultrasonic detections of ectopic pregnancies, even prior to the onset of acute pelvic pain, have made the diagnosis and management of the unruptured ectopic pregnancy a semielective laparoscopic procedure. In Chapter 19 we present the current laparoscopic management of ectopic pregnancy. Once pelvic pain suggests a rupture of an ectopic pregnancy, in the presence of unstable vital signs with documented hemoperitoneum, it is preferable to do an immediate laparotomy to stop bleeding and save surgical time rather than do a laparoscopy.

TABLE 9–6. CHRONIC PAINS OF THE LOWER ABDOMEN (302 CASES—1956 TO 1973)*

Findings	No.	%
Normal findings	21	6.95
Endometriosis	33	27.46
Adhesions	30	9.93
Myoma	8	2.64
Ovarian tumors (dermoid, paraovarian cysts, strangulations)	33	10.92
Intestinal tumors, sigmoiditis, regional ileitis, diverticulitis	26	8.66
Inflammatory processes (appendicitis, adnexitis, old ectopic pregnancy, tuberculosis)	29	9.60
Conglomerous tumors	13	4.30
Spastic fibrotic ligaments, varicocele	37	12.25
Allan-Masters syndrome	14	4.63
Chronic peritonitis	4	1.32
Others (malplaced IUD, pregnancy and myoma, hydrops of the gallbladder)	4	1.32
Total	302	100

*Adapted from Frangenheim H and Kleindienst W: Chronic pelvic disease of unknown origin. In Phillips JM and Keith L (eds): Gynecological laparoscopy: Principles and Techniques. Selected papers and discussion from the First International Congress of the American Association of Gynecological Laparoscopists in New Orleans, Louisiana. New York, Stratton Intercontinental, 1974, pp 43–53.

CHRONIC PAIN

The patient with chronic pelvic pain may be a candidate for laparoscopy if at least 6 months have gone by during which more conservative forms of therapy (e.g., antibiotics, psychotherapy, endocrine suppression) have proved unsuccessful. Studies of pelvic findings in patients undergoing laparoscopy for chronic pain have revealed pathology in 70 to 80% of patients (Cunanan et al, 1983; Kresch et al, 1984). However, comparisons of findings in patients with chronic pain to patients with infertility and no complaints of pain have generally shown no statistical difference between the nature or distribution of adhesions or other pathology found (Peters et al, 1991; Rapkin, 1986; Stout et al, 1991; Walker et al, 1988). In pain associated with endometriosis, deep infiltrating lesions are causally related to the symptoms and may require difficult excision (Koninckx et al, 1991; Ripps and Martin, 1991). On the other hand, endometriosis does not consistently cause pain: it has been found in up to 45% of asymptomatic women (Rawson, 1991). The variety of findings that are possible appear in Table 9–6.

Chronic pain persisting over 1 year can alter the nerve pathways and the spinal pain "gate." In these patients, surgical management of lesions found may not cause permanent relief: The pain can be re-established through the "open gate" pathways after about 6 months (Steege and Stout, 1991). For example, hysterectomy for pain with documented pathology was found to result in recurrent pain in 23% of patients (Stovall et al, 1990). Although some form of psychiatric pain management therapy is indicated, most patients undergo repeated, temporarily successful surgery.

On the other hand, the therapeutic benefit of diagnostic laparoscopy alone (no surgical procedures) in women with normal findings has been reported (Baker and Symonds, 1992). In this study, women with no pelvic pathology were referred to their physicians with no psychiatric care and were free of pain 6 months postoperatively. Thus, we need to be intellectually cautious in the causal relationships between pathology and pain, as well as the causal relationships between surgery and cure.

REFERENCES

INFERTILITY

Acosta AA, Buttram VC Jr, Besch PK, et al: A proposed classification of pelvic endometriosis. Obstet Gynecol 42:19–25, 1973.

Bateman BG, Kolp LA, Nunley WC Jr, et al: Oocyte retention after follicle luteinization. Fertil Steril 54:793–798, 1990.

diZerega GS: The peritoneum and its response to surgical injury. In diZerega GS, Malinak LR, Diamond MP, and Linsky CB (eds): Treatment of Post Surgical Adhesions: Proceedings of the First International Symposium for the Treatment of Post Surgical Adhesions, held in Phoenix, AZ, September 15 to 17, 1989. New York, Wiley-Liss, 1990, pp 1–11.

Eissa MK, Sawers RS, Docker MF, et al: Characteristics and incidence of dysfunctional ovulation patterns detected by ultrasound. Fertil Steril 47:603–612, 1987.

Hamilton MP, Fleming R, Coutts JRT, et al: Luteal cysts and unexplained infertility: Biochemical and ultrasonic evaluation. Fertil Steril 54:32–37, 1990.

Hulka JF: Adnexal adhesions: A prognostic staging and classification system based on a five-year survey of fertility surgery results at Chapel Hill, North Carolina. Am J Obstet Gynecol 144:141–148, 1982.

Hulka JF: Laparoscopy and culdoscopy. In Garcia C-R, Mastroianni L Jr, Amelar RD, and Dubin L (eds): Current Therapy of Infertility, 1982–1983. Trenton, NJ, Decker, 1982, pp 102–107.

Koninckx PR, Meuleman C, Demeyere S, et al: Suggestive evidence that pelvic endometriosis is a progressive disease, whereas deeply infiltrating endometriosis is associated with pelvic pain. Fertil Steril 55:759–765, 1991.

Marik J and Hulka JF: Luteinized unruptured follicle syndrome: A subtle cause of infertility. Fertil Steril 29:270–274, 1978.

Raj SG and Hulka JF: Second-look laparoscopy in infertility surgery: Therapeutic and prognostic value. Fertil Steril 38:325–329, 1982.

Rawson JMR: Prevalence of endometriosis in asymptomatic women. J Reprod Med 36:513–515, 1991.

Ripps BA and Martin DC: Focal pelvic tenderness, pelvic pain and dysmenorrhea in endometriosis. J Reprod Med 36:470–472, 1991.

Semm K: Technique of second look pelviscopic surgery: Prevention of recurrence of adhesions. Abstract no. 82 in Third World Congress on the Fallopian Tube, July 3 to 6, 1990, Kiel, West Germany.

Trimbos-Kemper TCM, Trimbos JB, and van Hall EV: Adhesion formation after tubal surgery: Results of the eighth-day laparoscopy in 188 patients. Fertil Steril 43:395–399, 1985.

Tulandi T, Falcone T, and Kafka I: Second-look operative laparoscopy 1 year following reproductive surgery. Fertil Steril 52:421–424, 1989.

PAIN

Baker PN and Symonds EM: The resolution of chronic pelvic pain after normal laparoscopy findings. Am J Obstet Gynecol 166:836–843, 1992.

Cunanan RG, Courey NG, and Lippes J: Laparoscopic findings in patients with pelvic pain. Am J Obstet Gynecol 136:589–591, 1983.

Frangenheim H and Kleindienst W: Chronic pelvic disease of unknown origin. In Phillips JM and Keith L (eds): Gynecological laparoscopy: Principles and Techniques. Selected papers and discussion from the First International Congress of the American Association of Gynecological Laparoscopists in New Orleans, Louisiana. New York, Stratton Intercontinental, 1974, pp 43–53.

Jacobson L: Differential diagnosis of acute pelvic inflammatory disease. Am J Obstet Gynecol 7:1006–1011, 1980.

Koninckx PR, Meuleman C, Demeyere S, et al: Suggestive evidence that pelvic endometriosis is a progressive disease, whereas deeply infiltrating endometriosis is associated with pelvic pain. Fertil Steril 55:759–765, 1991.

Kresch AJ, Seifer DB, Sachs LB, and Barrese I: Laparoscopy in 100 women with chronic pelvic pain. Obstet Gynecol 64:672–674, 1984.

Leape LL and Ramenofsky ML: Laparoscopy in infants and children. J Pediatr Surg 12:929–938, 1977.

Leape LL and Ramenofsky ML: Laparoscopy in children. Pediatrics 66:215–220, 1980.

Peters AAW, van Dorst E, Jellis B, et al: A randomized clinical trial to compare two different approaches in women with chronic pelvic pain. Obstet Gynecol 77:740–744, 1991.

Rapkin AJ: Adhesions and pelvic pain: A retrospective study. Obstet Gynecol 68:13–15, 1986.

Ripps BA and Martin DC: Focal pelvic tenderness, pelvic pain and dysmenorrhea in endometriosis. J Reprod Med 36:470–472, 1991.

Sellors J, Mahony J, Goldsmith C, et al: The accuracy of clinical findings and laparoscopy in pelvic inflammatory disease. Am J Obstet Gynecol 164:113–120, 1991.

Steege JF and Stout AL: Resolution of chronic pain after laparoscopic lysis of adhesions. Am J Obstet Gynecol 165:278–281, 1991.

Stout AL, Steege JF, Dodson WC, and Hughes CL: Relationship of laparoscopic findings to self-report of pelvic pain. Am J Obstet Gynecol 164:73–79, 1991.

Stovall TG, Ling FW, and Crawford DA: Hysterectomy for chronic pelvic pain of presumed uterine etiology. Obstet Gynecol 75:676–679, 1990.

Walker E, Katon W, Harrop-Griffiths J, et al: Relationship of chronic pelvic pain to psychiatric diagnoses and childhood sexual abuse. Am J Psychol 145:75–80, 1988.

Special Gynecologic Procedures

After proper entry is ensured, the patient should be placed in the Trendelenburg position, with the uterus anteverted and elevated. The true pelvis can be emptied of bowel contents by pushing on the uterine manipulator, using the uterus as a scoop. Inspection of the tubes and ovaries is facilitated by elevating and stretching the anteverted uterus toward the contralateral pelvic wall. Even with these maneuvers, a second puncture instrument, preferably a grasping forceps, is needed to elevate the tubes to see the fimbriae positively in their entirety (see Atlas, Plate 9); to elevate and flip the ovary to see the undersurface (see Atlas, Plate 8); and to stretch adhesions, when present, to evaluate their consistency and therefore their resectability (see Atlas, Plate 11).

Diagnostic laparoscopies present two opportunities to improve diagnosis but markedly increase complications, and these will be discussed.

DISSECTION OF ADHESIONS

In an abdomen with adhesions, it is quite tempting to try to "take down" these adhesions with operating forceps or scissors to reach the pelvis and see pelvic structures. Alternatively, when adhesions are seen they may be considered to be causally related to the patient's pain or infertility, and the temptation to free them therapeutically at the time of laparoscopy may be great. Although these are all legitimate and fre-

quent indications, certain limits in dissection should be kept in mind to minimize complications.

Dense, vascular adhesions or omentum should be coagulated before division. The bipolar forceps creates a wide and short band of coagulation and is useful if there is room for it between the adherent structures. This effectively coagulates and seals tissue and allows for division after coagulation. If there is the slightest danger of bowel injury at the time of coagulation, the dissection may be abandoned since such adhesions can be better managed by laparotomy.

Thin, avascular adhesions can in many cases be lysed bluntly with grasping forceps pulling tubes or ovaries away from them. Multiple trocars can be used for visualization with a laparoscope, pulling adhesions on a stretch with a grasping forceps through an operating channel and a second puncture, and dividing the stretched avascular adhesions with scissors through a third puncture. This can be surgically quite gratifying and should be embarked on if the exercise has any therapeutic or diagnostic value. Extensive lysis of adhesions is beyond the scope of the standardly trained gynecologist and is dealt with under advanced laparoscopic surgery in Chapter 15.

OVARIAN BIOPSY AND CYST ASPIRATION

Patients with primary amenorrhea, elevated follicle-stimulating hormone (FSH) levels, or chromosomal abnormalities may be good candidates for laparoscopic evaluation. Abnormal or streaked ovaries should be biopsied to evaluate the presence of testicular elements or primary follicles. Although surgical removal is often indicated to avoid malignant changes, a laparoscopic biopsy prior to removal may avoid a serious diagnostic error in these difficult cases.

If diagnostic laparoscopy is performed during the second half of the patient's menstrual cycle, in the midluteal phase, a very vascular corpus hemorrhagicum should be present as normal (see Atlas, Plate 5). Attempts to biopsy this structure to document it as a corpus hemorrhagicum can lead to uncontrollable bleeding. In cycling women below 35 years of age, small, simple cysts that have completely avascular surfaces do not require a biopsy but can be aspirated to enhance visualization of the rest of the structures. Thick-walled cysts that resist puncture and are more than 5 cm in diameter may need laparotomy for eventual pathologic diagnosis and treatment as probable dermoid cysts, endometriomas, or serous adenomas. An ovarian biopsy is possible if laparoscopic cystectomy is not possible. The information gained by submitting a sample of tissue to a pathologist is worth the possible risk involved, since the gross appearance of the cyst and ovary may not correlate with the microscopic diagnosis.

The risk of inadvertently puncturing ovarian carcinomas while performing a laparoscopy and manipulating ovarian cysts must always be kept in mind. Carcinoma of the ovary is rare but possible in women younger than 30 to 40 years of age. Any papillary excrescences on the surface of a small cyst should undergo frozen section before further surgery is decided. The patient's recent endocrine history should be kept in mind: If the patient has been under clomiphene citrate therapy, the possibility that a cyst seen at laparoscopy is anything but an overstimulated follicle is extremely remote. In general, in a young woman with a small cyst (< 5 cm) with a clear wall through which clear fluid can be seen, aspiration can be safely achieved to aid in visualization of the rest of the ovary and pelvis. The finding of an ovarian cyst in a patient with an acute abdomen is one of the few indications for therapeutic aspiration of the cyst, since the cyst is probably the cause of the patient's symptoms and aspiration of this tense structure will result in a prompt relief of pain (see Atlas, Plates 27 and 28). The controversy concerning ovarian masses managed by laparoscopy is presented in Chapter 21.

BIOPSY OF ENDOMETRIOSIS

The diagnostic description by the laparoscopist should suffice to make the clinical diagnosis of endometriosis (see Atlas, Plate 8), and pathologic confirmation may not be worth the additional risk involved. If the endometriosis is adjacent to a blood vessel, or near the ureter, biopsy leading to bleeding that requires coagulation may become disastrous. Because of this desire to minimize hazard while maximizing diagnostic capacity, the role of photography comes into play. The argument that a permanent record is needed to document the diagnosis of endometriosis (or, for example, a benign ovarian cyst) should make it necessary for busy diagnostic laparoscopy services to have video taping or photography routinely available for permanent records of diagnoses. Placing photographs in the patient's chart is an excellent exchange for the risk of biopsying to obtain tissue for permanent record in the pathology laboratories.

REMOVAL OF AN INTRAUTERINE DEVICE

Intra-abdominal intrauterine devices (IUDs) rarely cause symptoms or complications that justify their removal for medical reasons, but patient anxiety, together with the opportunity to achieve permanent contraception by laparoscopic sterilization, causes most of these IUD users to choose laparoscopy.

Inert plastic or medicated IUDs are often free in the peritoneal cavity. Grasping the end of the IUD with a strong forceps in a 10-mm operating laparoscope with a 5-mm channel allows the surgeon to free the IUD bluntly and bring it to the edge of the 10-mm sleeve. An assistant should then hold the sleeve down and its trumpet valve open as the surgeon withdraws the laparoscope, holding the forceps and IUD under direct vision at all times. This technique enables retrieval of most IUDs, since the 10-mm sleeve allows most awkwardly grasped IUDs to pass.

Copper IUDs stimulate an inflammatory response that leads to dense adhesions. The patient should be scheduled for laparoscopy and possible laparotomy, since the IUD may not be dislodged from its bed of adhesions by the forceps, and bleeding resulting from avulsing the IUD from its bed may require suturing.

EXPLORATION OF THE UPPER ABDOMEN

Diagnostic laparoscopy should not be considered complete unless all laparoscopists, regardless of their specialty, explore all of the abdominal structures available. The gynecologist should be as familiar as the surgeon is with the normal appendix, liver, and gallbladder, and the surgeon should be familiar with normal uterus, tubes, and ovaries. For proper inspection of the upper abdomen, the patient should be taken out of the Trendelenburg position briefly, so that the pneumoperitoneum can elevate the diaphragm away from the liver.

Rare hazards of stretching and tearing of the liver because of adhesions between the liver and the diaphragm have been reported in the gastroenterology literature. This condition has caused fatal hemorrhages, leading to the universal recommendation that distention of the upper abdomen be done gently and slowly (especially under general anesthesia) until the absence of these adhesions can be verified.

Liver biopsies can and should be performed with visual direction of the biopsy needle toward nodules suspected to be metastatic disease. As in the case of ovarian pathology or endometriosis, the question of whether a needle biopsy need be performed in the presence of obvious cirrhosis of the liver is moot. By visually directing the area from which biopsies are obtained, hemangiomas and large vessels can be avoided, and the clinical experience with laparoscopically directed liver biopsies of tumor nodules is remarkably free of major hemorrhagic complications. All liver biopsy sites will bleed for 4 to 5 minutes, after which they usually stop with a total blood loss of less than 50 ml intra-abdominally.

Sterilization Techniques

Laparoscopic sterilization has evolved in the United States from the unipolar coagulation that Palmer and Steptoe originally described to the bipolar techniques that Rioux and Kleppinger developed (see Chapter 1). The Silastic band and spring clip are nonelectric alternatives. These alternatives were developed in response to the mysterious bowel burns that occurred in the 1970s with unipolar coagulation. Today, it is thought that these injuries resulted from capacitative complied energy in the operating laparoscope itself, insulated from the skin and with a unipolar electrode inside its operating channel. Unipolar techniques still have their advocates and skilled practitioners in whose hands patients will be well served, but the techniques and precautions are no longer taught.

FIGURE 11–1 Controlling forceps

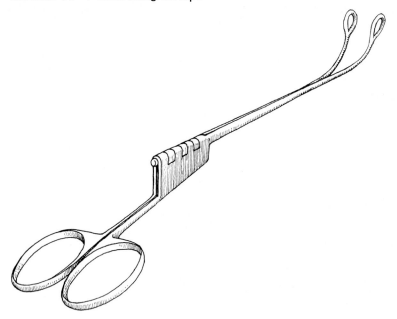

TIMING OF STERILIZATION

Laparoscopic tubal occlusion is the most common method of interval sterilization in the United States today, and approximately 200,000 procedures are performed annually. (An interval is defined as a nonpregnant state, at least 4 to 6 weeks after the completion of the previous pregnancy.) Use of the laparoscope for early postpartum sterilization has been demonstrated to be feasible but technically risky. After vaginal delivery, a postpartum minilaparotomy with Pomeroy tubal occlusion is standard procedure. For a number of considerations (e.g., assurance of the health of the baby, unavailability of anesthesiologists for tubal ligation, indecision by the patient, preference of the physician), a "postpartum" sterilization is usually planned 4 to 6 weeks after delivery by laparoscopy.

After Abortion

Laparoscopic sterilization combined with vacuum aspiration abortion in the first trimester has no increased hazard or decreased efficacy. A special controlling forceps is needed to manipulate the recently evacuated pregnant uterus (Fig. 11–1), since standard intrauterine manipulators do not offer maximal uterine control and may lacerate the soft myometrium. The actual number of combined abortion-sterilization procedures is small, because the stressful situation in which most women are seeking abortion is usually an inappropriate time for the patient to decide upon permanent sterilization.

The evacuated midtrimester uterus is large and may be injured by the trocar. The tubes may be more difficult to elevate and may be close to dilated vessels. For these reasons, laparoscopic sterilization after midtrimester abortion is more risky in terms of safety and efficacy and, although feasible, should only be considered occasionally.

Risk of Luteal Phase Pregnancy

The occlusion of a tube in a woman in her luteal phase may lead to a pregnancy if a fertilized egg is already present. This risk has been managed in different ways. In a review of routine dilatation and curettage (D & C) with laparoscopic sterilization to eliminate such pregnancies, a small but significant number of pregnancies persisted despite the D & C. The D & C was considered to provide a false sense of security to patients and physicians and was not recommended (Grubb and Peterson, 1985). A better intraoperative approach may be destruction of an active corpus luteum by excision, desiccation, or fulguration. Another option is to schedule the operation only during menses or within the first 2 weeks of the cycle. This creates scheduling problems for the physician and the patient and does not completely eliminate the risk. For women whose sexual, contraceptive, and menstrual history suggests that pregnancy is possible, a urine pregnancy test can be obtained on the morning of surgery, and if the result is positive the patient can be offered a simultaneous abortion. If the result is negative, the surgeon can proceed with the operation as scheduled but should advise the patient to return if signs of intrauterine or ectopic pregnancy occur. With this policy, the few intrauterine pregnancies that we have had were managed either by early interruption or, in a few cases, by delivery of this unexpected and gratefully received gift!

FIGURE 11–2 Bipolar coagulation

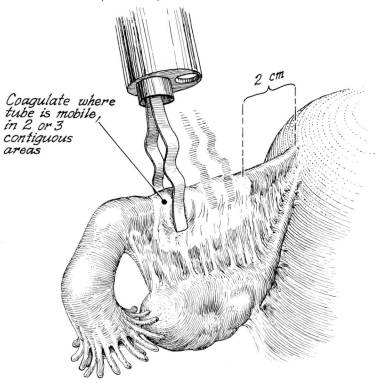

Coagulate where tube is mobile, in 2 or 3 contiguous areas

2 cm

FIGURE 11–3 Output of bipolar Wolf "2075" generator during coagulation

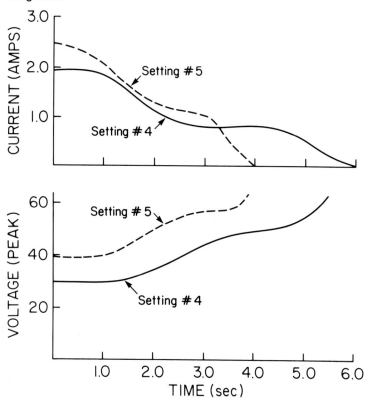

BIPOLAR COAGULATION

In the words of Richard K. Kleppinger:

As the fallopian tube is grasped and situated within the concavity of the forceps, the serrated duck-bill tongs grasp the mesosalpinx. The generator is activated and the grasped portion of the fallopian tube is coagulated. The tube is released. This procedure is repeated at a minimum of three adjacent areas (Fig. 11–2). Rarely is there any adherence of tissue. For that occasion, the forceps is gently twisted clockwise and counterclockwise while decreasing the grasping pressure. The serrations on the tongs prevent slipping or escape of the mesosalpinx, ensuring adequate coagulation for division if desired. The serrations may also be used to grasp only the tube if a severely limited area of coagulation is desired. With such applications the mesosalpinx will show only a hint of coagulation. Because these serrations allow the forceps to be used as an atraumatic grasping tool, a complement of ancillary procedures is possible.

The No. 2075 Wolf Bipolar Generator (Richard Wolf Medical Instruments Corp., Rosemont, IL) was designed specifically for use with the Kleppinger bipolar forceps.

This system has output characteristics across the fallopian tube of 30 to 40 V of nonmodulated current, 24 to 28 W, and 1.9 to 2.4 amperes, which are demonstrated by the accompanying graph (Fig. 11–3). Its solid-state isolated circuitry and limited power output provide for coagulation without tissue adherence to the forceps. An exclusive feature of this generator is an optical control meter, enabling the operator to pre-check the generator and bipolar forceps for proper function. The ammeter also indicates the endpoint of complete tissue coagulation. Additionally, an audible tone change is noticeable at completion of adequate coagulation, which is so critical to the prevention of pregnancy (Kleppinger, 1977, pp 145 to 146).

This succinct and thorough statement describes the most popular method of laparoscopic sterilization in the United States today. The description emphasizes the *system* of forceps and generator designed as a unit for maximum safety (through the use of specifically designed currents in terms of appropriate volts and watts) and efficacy (the optical ammeter indicating proper current flow) (Fig. 11–4).

The *endpoint of coagulation* is *complete cessation of current flow* as monitored by the ammeter.

The tube should be grasped 2 to 4 cm away from the uterus to minimize the risk of uteroperitoneal fistula (see Atlas, Plate 4). The clinical simplicity of identifying, isolating, and occluding the tube with this technique accounts for its popularity. Failures with bipolar coagulation have been documented as attributable to improper matching of forceps and generators. Bowel burns have occurred when bowel was mistaken for tube and coagulated (e.g., a uterine-bowel adhesion after a previous salpingo-oophorectomy), but no deaths from peritonitis because of unrecognized bipolar coagulation of bowel have been reported in the United States.

FIGURE 11–4 Bipolar systems available

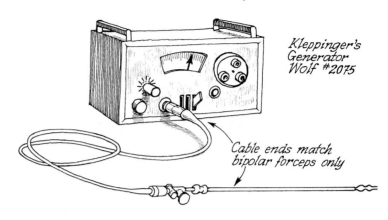

Matched generator and forceps

Kleppinger's Generator Wolf #2075

Cable ends match bipolar forceps only

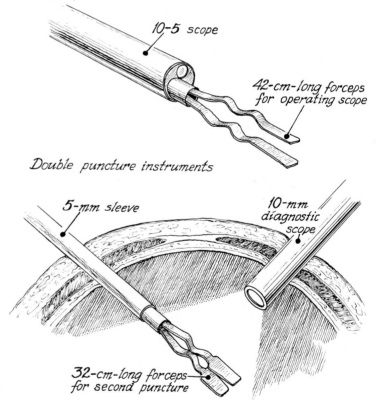

Single puncture instruments

10–5 scope

42-cm-long forceps for operating scope

Double puncture instruments

5-mm sleeve

10-mm diagnostic scope

32-cm-long forceps for second puncture

FIGURE 11–5 Silastic band application

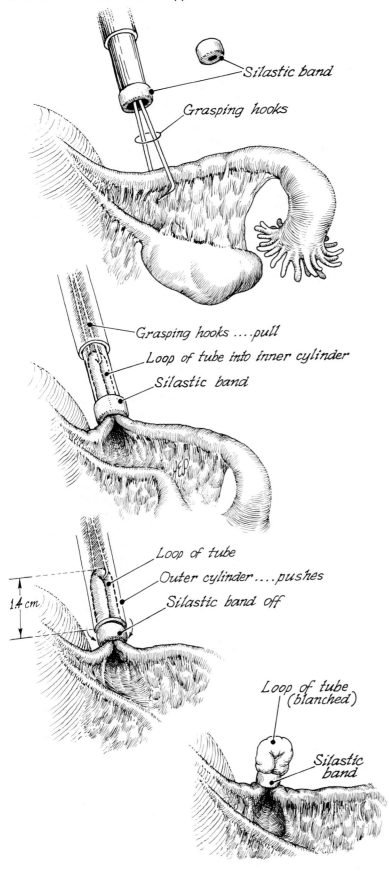

Silastic band

Grasping hooks

Grasping hooks ....pull

Loop of tube into inner cylinder

Silastic band

Loop of tube

Outer cylinder....pushes

Silastic band off

1.4 cm

Loop of tube (blanched)

Silastic band

SILASTIC BAND

According to Yoon and associates (Yoon et al, 1974):

On location of the fallopian tubes, the grasping forceps is employed to pick up one of the tubes, 1 to 2 inches from the cornu of the uterus (Fig. 11–5). The tube is then drawn into the inner cylinder of the ring applicator device. Thereafter either 1 or 2 silicone rubber bands are applied to the grasped segment of the fallopian tube by moving the outer cylinder forward. After the application of the silicone rubber band, the grasping forceps is moved forward out of the inner cylinder to release the occluded segment of tube. In a similar manner, the opposite tube is grasped and the silicone rubber band is applied. . . . After both tubes have been occluded, indigo carmine dye is injected through the Rubin's cannula (which had been previously inserted into the uterine canal for manipulation of the uterus) to confirm tubal lumen occlusion (pp 134 to 135).

Yoon and colleagues make five important points in connection with their Silastic band technique:

1. Patients should practice effective contraceptive measures until the operation has been completed.

2. The surgeon should inspect the pelvic organs completely to determine accurately the location of the fallopian tubes by observing the fimbriae of each tube. One should demonstrate the absence of acute or chronic salpingitis.

3. The fallopian tube should be picked up 3 cm from the uterotubal junction using the laparoscope forceps to lift the entire segment of tube without grasping very much mesosalpinx. A sufficient knuckle of tube should be pulled into the instrument so that after the band has been placed, it clearly contains two complete lumens of tube.

4. As the fallopian tube is drawn into the inner cylinder of the Falope ring laparoscope, the instrument should be moved toward the mesosalpinx to minimize tension on the tube and avoid transection.

5. A significant percentage of these patients require oral analgesic agents for 1 to 2 days after the procedure (Yoon et al, 1977).

The Silastic band technique gained popularity in the 1970s as an alternative to the unipolar coagulation technique that was being promoted throughout the world by the United States Agency for International Development (USAID). See Figure 11–6 for applicators that are now available. Most initial series have experienced a tubal transection or mesosalpingeal bleeding rate of 2.5%, minimizing but not eliminating the need for electrocoagulation for hemostasis. Postoperative pain from the anoxic tissue within the band constrictions can be severe enough to warrant the patient's admission to the hospital for medication and observation. Subsequent pregnancy rates, intrauterine and ectopic, appear to be in ranges comparable with all other laparoscopic methods.

FIGURE 11–6 Silastic band applicators available

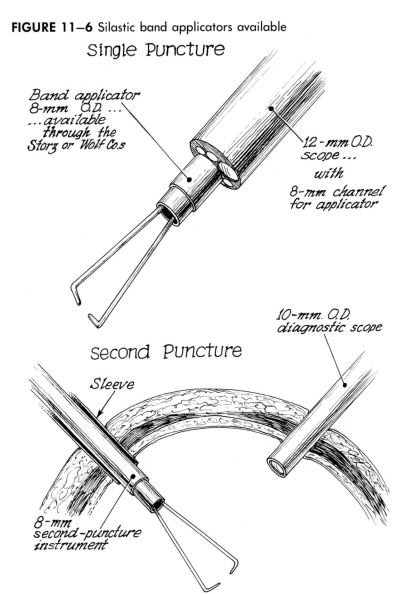

Single Puncture

Band applicator 8-mm O.D. ...available through the Storz or Wolf Co.s

12-mm O.D. scope ... with 8-mm channel for applicator

second Puncture

Sleeve

10-mm O.D. diagnostic scope

8-mm second-puncture instrument

FIGURE 11–7 Spring clip

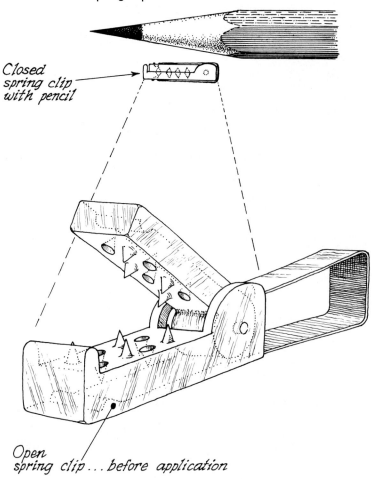

Closed spring clip with pencil

Open spring clip...before application

SPRING CLIP

As the process of laparoscopic sterilization developed, it became clear that certain risks are inherent in the methods of electrocoagulation and Silastic band application. The most frequent complication of both techniques is hemorrhage from the mesosalpinx. In addition, electrocoagulation is associated with rare, but nonetheless severe, bowel-burn complications. The spring clip was developed to eliminate the risk of bowel burn and to reduce the risk of hemorrhage by making it unnecessary to divide the tube or pull it through a Silastic band (Fig. 11–7).

The first clip was applied to humans in 1972. It was tested in a multicenter collaborative study from 1973 to 1975 with more than a 90% 1-year follow-up in 1000 patients. Certain difficulties in the surgical procedure, as well as design defects in the clip itself, were identified, and the final version of the clip was manufactured in 1976.

International multicenter studies have yielded a method-failure pregnancy rate of two to four for each 1000 clip applications. This rate is comparable with the other techniques of laparoscopic sterilization.

Clip application requires particular surgical skill of the surgeon, who must manipulate both tube and clip applicator to ensure correct application of the clip across the isthmus of the tube. A double-puncture technique, described in detail, results in a more secure application in most operators' hands.

Clip application postpartum is a simple matter of elevating the isthmus (right next to the uterus) through a subumbilical incision similar to the one used for a Pomeroy tubal occlusion, stretching the isthmus between two Babcock clamps, and applying the clip with the thumb and third finger controlling the jaws and the index finger pushing the spring. Kleppinger has called this method the "bargain basement applicator" (every surgeon has one), and a comparison of a Pomeroy tubal occlusion to clip application postpartum showed less operative time and considerably less patient recovery time (26 days versus 7 days) using the clip (Lee and Jones, 1991).

Functions of the Clip and Applicator

Figure 11–8 illustrates the functions of the clip and applicator designed by Hulka and Clemens (Richard Wolf Medical Instruments Corp.).

FIGURE 11–8 Functions of the spring clip application

A. Movement without resistance

1. SAFE OPEN

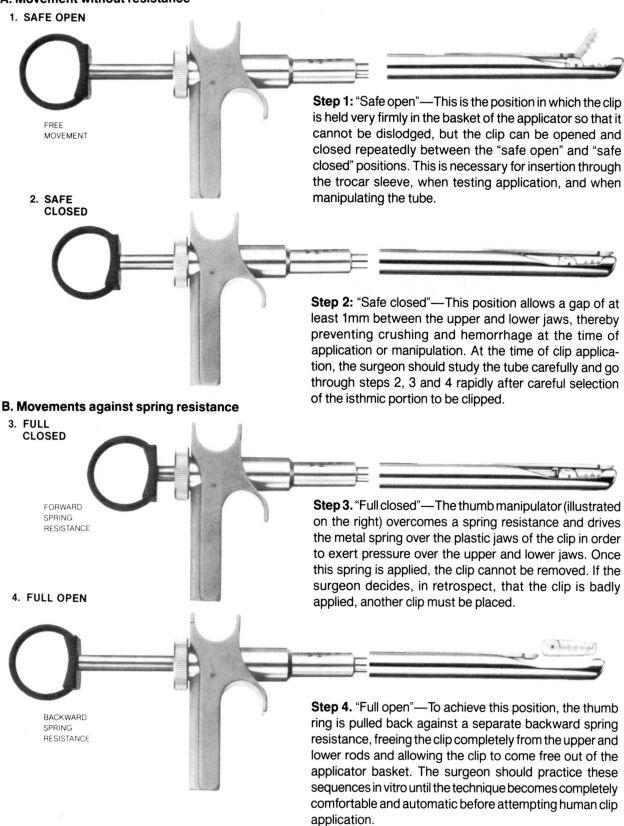

FREE
MOVEMENT

Step 1: "Safe open"—This is the position in which the clip is held very firmly in the basket of the applicator so that it cannot be dislodged, but the clip can be opened and closed repeatedly between the "safe open" and "safe closed" positions. This is necessary for insertion through the trocar sleeve, when testing application, and when manipulating the tube.

2. SAFE CLOSED

Step 2: "Safe closed"—This position allows a gap of at least 1mm between the upper and lower jaws, thereby preventing crushing and hemorrhage at the time of application or manipulation. At the time of clip application, the surgeon should study the tube carefully and go through steps 2, 3 and 4 rapidly after careful selection of the isthmic portion to be clipped.

B. Movements against spring resistance

3. FULL CLOSED

FORWARD
SPRING
RESISTANCE

Step 3. "Full closed"—The thumb manipulator (illustrated on the right) overcomes a spring resistance and drives the metal spring over the plastic jaws of the clip in order to exert pressure over the upper and lower jaws. Once this spring is applied, the clip cannot be removed. If the surgeon decides, in retrospect, that the clip is badly applied, another clip must be placed.

4. FULL OPEN

BACKWARD
SPRING
RESISTANCE

Step 4. "Full open"—To achieve this position, the thumb ring is pulled back against a separate backward spring resistance, freeing the clip completely from the upper and lower rods and allowing the clip to come free out of the applicator basket. The surgeon should practice these sequences in vitro until the technique becomes completely comfortable and automatic before attempting human clip application.

FIGURE 11–9 Controlling the position of the uterus

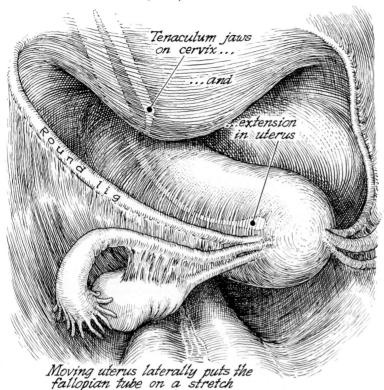

Tenaculum jaws on cervix...

...and

...extension in uterus

Round lig.

Moving uterus laterally puts the fallopian tube on a stretch

Manipulating the Uterus

Figure 11–9 illustrates the technique of manipulating the uterus to put the tube on stretch (for maximal clip application). A controlling instrument, with the features of a uterine sound and tenaculum, is inserted into the uterus and the uterus is anteverted. During surgery, the surgeon should move the uterus laterally with the tenaculum in such a way as to put the fallopian tube on stretch. In contrast to electrocoagulation or band application, this maneuver often requires that the uterus be drawn down into the pelvis, so that the infundibulopelvic ligaments cause the tube to be stretched horizontally deep in the true pelvis rather than protruding into the abdominal cavity at an angle oblique to the applicator. Thus, the most advantageous manipulation with the combined tenaculum-sound is a downward and sideward displacement of the uterus into the true pelvis so that the tube is stretched across the midline.

For physicians who have been performing coagulation by grasping the tube and lifting, it is important to point out that the clip is not applied in this manner. Rather, the tube should be stretched laterally for its maximum availability to the clip applicator. Misapplications, attributed to limited visibility, accounted for pregnancies in early experiences with the clip.

The following illustrations show the second-puncture Wolf clip applicator. For the technique using the 10–7 optic with a single-puncture approach, the optics should be close to the clip during application to permit careful observation of the details of correct clip application.

Identifying the Tubes

When the uterus is anteverted and stretched to the patient's right, her left tube will be visible and partially stretched. The surgeon looks at the entire adnexa to identify three structures positively (Fig. 11–10):

1. Round ligament
2. Tube
3. Utero-ovarian ligament

Under local anesthesia, the isthmic portion of a normal tube may look remarkably flabby like a peritoneal fold. In the postabortion patient, sometimes broad ligament varicosities look like convoluted tube. The surgeon should touch the structure that appears to be the tube to see if it is mobile. The tube is traced to the fimbriae using the clip itself as a grasping forceps. It helps to remember that the structure just over the ovary is usually the tube.

Grasping the Tubes

The fallopian tube is fully grasped deep in the angle between the jaws of the clip, which is in the safe open position (Fig. 11–11). It is important to note that the tube is not elevated, as it is in electrocoagulation and band sterilization. The operation requires practice and coordination of the clip applicator and the uterine manipulator. The tube can be gently slid deep into the jaws of the applicator with a sideways "snuggling" motion until the mesosalpinx abuts the angle of the hinge of the clip.

FIGURE 11–10 Identifying the tube

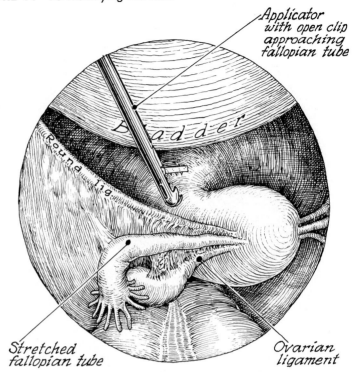

FIGURE 11–11 Grasping the tube

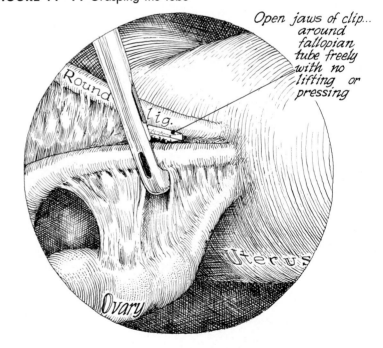

FIGURE 11–12 Stretching the tube with grasping forceps in an operating channel

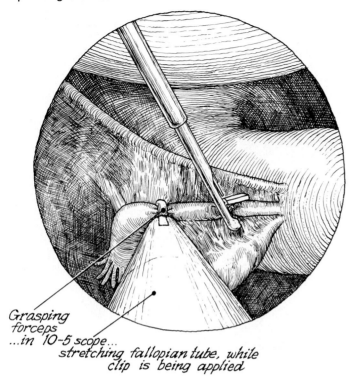

Grasping forceps ...in 10-5 scope... stretching fallopian tube, while clip is being applied

If the uterus cannot be manipulated to provide an easy approach for the clip applicator, a grasping forceps can be introduced through the operating channel of a 10–5 optic. The forceps can elevate the tube and stretch the isthmus. The second-puncture clip applicator can then apply a clip securely, with the assistant holding the uterus and laparoscope steady while the operator manipulates the clip applicator and forceps (Fig. 11–12).

Applying the Clip

The upper ram is pushed forward by the thumb (Fig. 11–13), closing the clip into the safe closed position. If the surgeon has any reservation with regard to the correct application of the clip, the upper ram can be pulled backward at this point into the safe open position and a new application can be tried (see Fig. 11–8). When the clip is applied correctly, as illustrated here, the tube appears to fill the jaws of the clip all the way up to the hinge.

FIGURE 11–13 Applying the clip

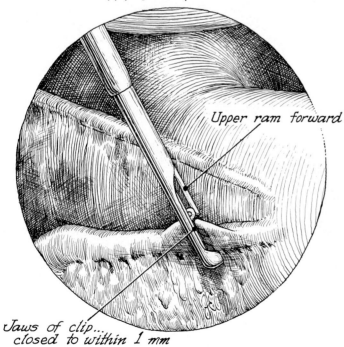

Upper ram forward

Jaws of clip... closed to within 1 mm

Closing the Clip

The lower ram is now moved forward, against spring resistance, closing the C-shaped spring over the upper and lower jaws of the clip (Fig. 11–14). At this point, the clip cannot be removed because it is permanently latched in place onto the tube. Care must be taken to push the lower rod completely forward until the spring snaps in place in the locked position over the jaws. Once the spring is in place over the jaws, both lower and upper rods can be rapidly drawn back into the full open position (see Fig. 11–8), after which the clip will be free to disengage itself from the applicator. A "Japanese bow" of moving the applicator downward and away from the tube will ensure easy disengagement of the clip from the applicator at this point.

Correct Application

The correct application of the clip across the isthmic portion of the tube is illustrated in Figure 11–15. One can see Kleppinger's "envelope" sign of the mesosalpinx on the surface of the tube pulled upward to resemble the flat triangular shape of an envelope flap (see Atlas, Plate 3). Again, the tube and its mesosalpinx occupy the entire clip all the way up to the hinge.

FIGURE 11–14 Closing the clip

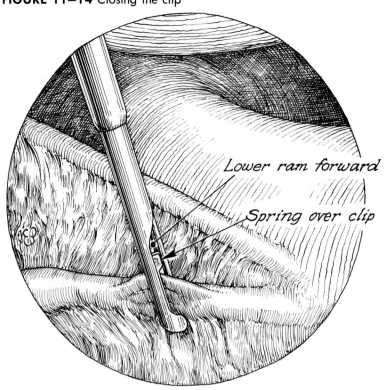

FIGURE 11–15 Correct application of the clip

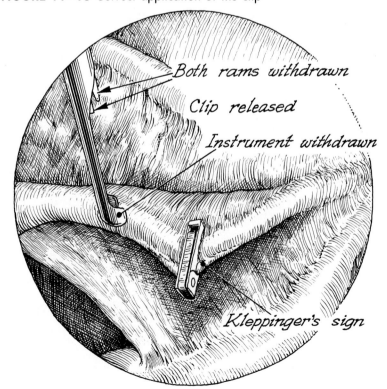

FIGURE 11–16 Correct and incorrect clip applications

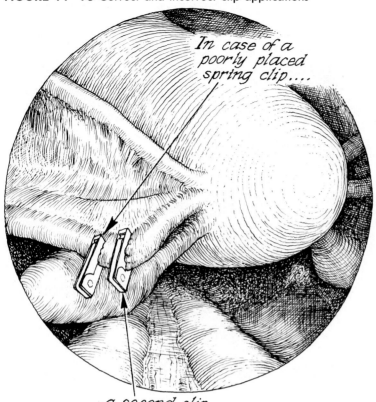

In case of a poorly placed spring clip....

...a second clip is applied to ensure sterilization

An incomplete clip application is shown on the left in Figure 11–16. The inner longitudinal musculature of the tube was not caught in the upper and lower jaw, and the tube remains patent. A second correct application of the clip on the right ensures that the tubal lumen and its very hard longitudinal musculature are enclosed between the jaws and that tubal occlusion will be accomplished.

Practice

One clip per tube, well applied across the isthmus, is effective (see Fig. 11–15). Because the technique described earlier requires practice, we recommend the application of two clips on each tube for the first dozen patients only of a beginning laparoscopist's clip experience. This accelerates the learning process and gives the surgeon greater assurance that the learning experience will not result in pregnancies. Many physicians continue to apply two clips per tube on a routine basis.

Clip Loss

There have been reports of clips (in the open and closed position) having been dropped inside the abdomen. Loss of an open clip can be avoided by always opening and closing the applicator once or twice outside the abdomen after a clip has been loaded. If the clip has been improperly loaded, it will fall out onto the drapes at this time and can be properly reloaded. The applicator has been carefully designed and manufactured with close tolerances to make it almost impossible for a properly loaded clip to be dislodged in the "safe open" position.

If this rare problem nevertheless occurs, retrieval efforts should include grasping the gold-plated spring at the end with a 5-mm grasping forceps in a 10-mm operating laparoscope and withdrawing it through the sleeve as described for removal of an IUD. If the plastic clip is dislodged in this process, it can be retrieved separately by grasping at the hinge end.

OPEN CLIPS. Despite these precautions, clips have become dislodged in the open position and fall into the abdomen, with unsuccessful laparoscopic retrieval attempts. We are not aware of any medical complications or symptoms ever reported from this situation. The clip is light and rapidly surrounded by omentum, where it has occasionally been found when medicolegal concerns or the patient's anxiety led to laparoscopic retrieval.

CLOSED CLIPS. If not retrievable, closed clips can confidently be left within the abdomen because they are rapidly peritonealized and remain asymptomatic, according to animal and human experience.

Available Instrumentation

Although a variety of applicators is now on the market, the clip has been held uniform in dimensions by the two manufacturers (Richard Wolf Medical Instruments Corp. and Rocket of London, Ltd.). Single- and double-puncture applicators of the Wolf Corp. are illustrated as examples of the choices available (Fig. 11–17). The "original" applicator is a single-puncture instrument designed to go through a 10-mm sleeve. It houses a 5-mm optic that can be used separately for diagnostic work with a 5-mm sleeve. The 10–7 optic has a remarkably bright 1-mm optic chain, allowing a 7-mm channel for clip or bipolar applicators. World experience has revealed that fewer anatomic errors are made with a second-puncture technique.

FIGURE 11–17 Clip applicators available

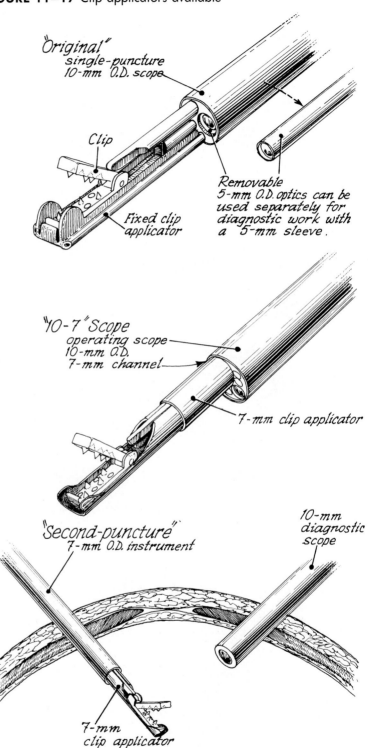

FIGURE 11–18 True cautery techniques

Semm Endotherm :

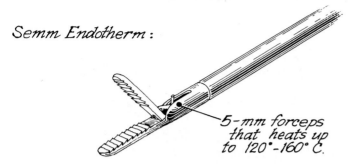

5-mm forceps
that heats up
to 120°–160° C.

Waters Device :

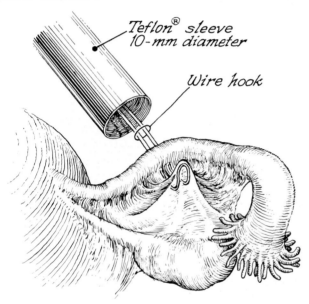

Teflon® sleeve
10-mm diameter

Wire hook

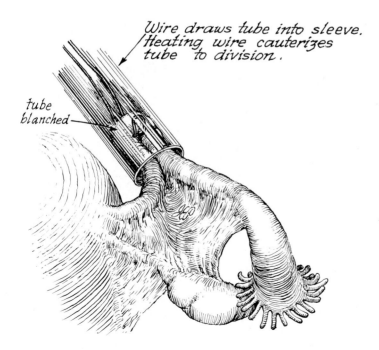

Wire draws tube into sleeve.
Heating wire cauterizes
tube to division.

tube
blanched

OTHER TECHNIQUES

True cautery is used in two techniques. The Semm endotherm consists of a slender 1-cm–long forceps that is directly heated by electric current to 120 to 160°C, causing the tube within the forceps to coagulate over 60 to 90 seconds (Fig. 11–18). Another technique is the Waters device described by Valle and Battifora (1978): A hook brings the fallopian tube into a protective plastic-coated sleeve, where it is cauterized by heating the hook. The safety of this contained cautery device is counterbalanced by the large second puncture necessary to insert the insulating protective sleeve.

A plastic clip designed by Waldemar Bleier in Germany was withdrawn from the American market because of pregnancies apparently caused by the tube's rolling out of its jaws and into space in the latch area.

Another plastic and tantalum clip designed by Marcus Filshie in England is still undergoing evaluation.

COMPARISON OF METHODS

Trends in Laparoscopic Sterilization Techniques

The American Association of Gynecological Laparoscopists (AAGL) has conducted surveys of its membership since 1971. One of the surveys, for the year 1976, revealed how many bipolar, unipolar, band, and clip procedures were done that year. The identical survey has been carried out since then at 3-year intervals, revealing the trends shown in Figure 11–19. The unipolar method has been replaced by the bipolar method as the most common method used, with a small but consistent increase in clip usage.

Subsequent Pregnancies

All sterilization methods have a failure rate between 2 and 10 pregnancies per 1000 operations. The largest comparative study reported to date (based on 24,439 operations) has failed to detect consistent differences among coagulation, band, and clip methods (Bhiwandiwala et al, 1982).

Bipolar failures are mostly ectopic pregnancies. They appear to occur with low frequency, but they do occur throughout the long-term follow-up period at the rate of about one per 1000 per year. A report of 1437 bipolar sterilizations reveals subsequent extrauterine pregnancies spread over a 6-year follow-up period. The cumulative failure rate was 1.18%, and all pregnancies were extrauterine (Makar et al, 1990). We have urged the preservation of a 2-cm proximal isthmic stump to reduce chances of subsequent fistula and ectopic pregnancies. Holt and associates found that the risk of ectopic pregnancy after interval sterilization was 3.7 times as great as among women using oral contraceptives, mostly because of electrocoagulation methods (Holt et al, 1991).

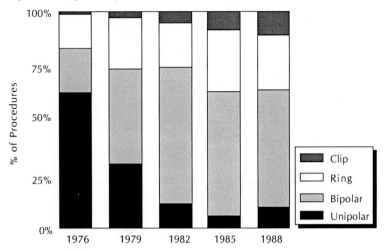

FIGURE 11–19 Trends in laparoscopic sterilization: changing techniques. (From the American Association of Gynecological Laparoscopists survey data.)

TABLE 11–1. RISK OF ECTOPIC PREGNANCY FOLLOWING STERILIZATION METHODS*

Method	Intrauterine No.	Ectopic No.	Rate of Ectopics to Total Pregnancies (%)
Pomeroy	657	145	18
Unipolar, coagulation, division	107	76	41
Unipolar, coagulation only	61	57	48
Bipolar, coagulation, division	46	37	44
Bipolar, coagulation only	151	61	29
Silastic ring	180	33	15
Spring clip	24	1	4
Total	1226	410	33

*From Phillips JM, Hulka JF, Hulka B, and Corson SL: 1979 AAGL membership survey. J Reprod Med 26:529–533, 1981.

Ectopic pregnancies seem to be associated with the more destructive techniques. Extensive coagulation and division have a subsequent rate of ectopic pregnancies of half of all pregnancies. Ectopic pregnancy rates for the mechanical methods are 15% (band) and 4% (clip) of all pregnancies. In Table 11–1 we present a representative comparative study.

Pregnancies after clip application appear to occur mostly within the first year or two of application and are mostly intrauterine. Long-term follow-up studies show that the clip is not associated with ectopic pregnancies or a continuing risk of failure after this initial period. Thus, long-term cumulative pregnancy rates with bipolar sterilization and the clip are similar.

In an unpublished review of his personal experiences with 6763 bipolar and 1588 clip sterilizations over 5 to 10 years, Kleppinger noted 76% ectopic pregnancies after bipolar sterilization and 11% after clip sterilization. The cumulative pregnancy rate was 2.8 per 1000 with a bipolar technique and 5.7 per 1000 with the clip. Kleppinger's clinical impressions from this experience are similar to those presented here.

Coagulation

Unipolar coagulation still has advocates and skilled practitioners, in whose hands patients will be well served. The extensive tissue destruction by this technique renders it inappropriate for women younger than 30 years of age. The poorly understood occurrences of bowel burns and deaths with this technique, in contrast to the absence of such deaths with the more frequently used bipolar coagulation, has reduced this once dominant technique to a small portion of the current practice in the United States.

Bipolar coagulation has the combined advantages of simplicity of instrument design, ease of performance (the tube is simply picked up in the forceps), and safety in terms of reducing the area of electron flow to the tissue held by the forceps. When properly done, approximately 3 cm of tissue is destroyed. The technique is comparable with the Pomeroy or band techniques in terms of tissue destruction and subsequent success of reversal by isthmic-ampullary anastomosis.

The Band

The band technique was widely taught in the United States in the 1970s by hospitals receiving help from the USAID and is therefore well known to many practitioners. There is a risk of mesosalpingeal or tubal tears in approximately 2.5% of cases, requiring occasional electrocoagulation for hemostasis. Postoperatively, this is the most uncomfortable technique, and pelvic cramps continue for 2 days. These cramps are not a complication but are an occasional source of complaint by the patient.

The Spring Clip

The *spring clip* is the most reversible of the techniques, destroying between 0.5 and 0.7 cm of tube when correctly applied in the isthmic portion. Using the clip requires more careful attention to surgical anatomy and technique to ensure that the isthmus is completely occluded. Reversal by isthmic-isthmic anastomosis has led to a worldwide experience of 87% intrauterine pregnancies. In our service, we recommend the clip to women younger than 30 years of age because of this potential for reversal (see the following discussion on reversibility).

We have consistently recommended that physicians choose the technique with which they are most comfortable and that they continue to provide this service to their patients until surgical misadventure or compelling reasons in the literature motivate a change of techniques.

FIGURE 11–20 Reversibility of tubal sterilization

Tubal damage   *Tubal repair*

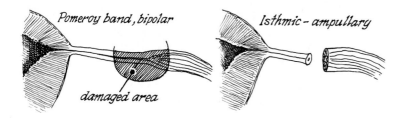

Pomeroy band, bipolar — damaged area

Isthmic – ampullary

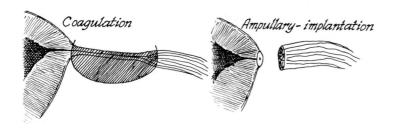

Coagulation

Ampullary – implantation

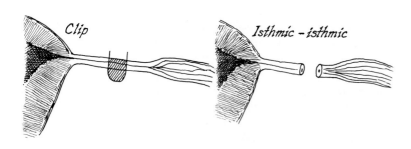

Clip

Isthmic – isthmic

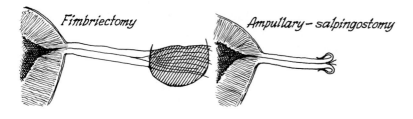

Fimbriectomy

Ampullary – salpingostomy

REGRET AND REVERSIBILITY

The average age of most women requesting sterilization is 30 years, indicating that half of the requests are in women below this age. Winston (1977) and Gomel (1978) observed that women sterilized below 30 years of age run the highest risk of returning later and requesting reversal, usually after divorce and remarriage. A prospective study of women in the United States by the Centers for Disease Control confirmed this finding (Wilcox et al, 1991). The obstetrician or gynecologist thus faces a dilemma: should he or she deny sterilization to the hundreds of younger women who would benefit in order to protect the reproductive ability of the few who may change their minds? Recent experience with reversal operations has provided an outlet for this dilemma since reversibility appears to be correlated with the amount of tissue damage inflicted at the time of sterilization.

As illustrated in Figure 11–20, different sterilization methods require different reversal procedures. The Pomeroy, bipolar, and band techniques are most commonly used in the United States today and usually destroy the most mobile midportion of the tube, including the isthmic-ampullary portion. Anastomosis of the isthmus to the larger ampulla is required for reversal. Unipolar coagulation results in more extensive destruction of the isthmus and ampulla and usually requires an ampullary-cornual anastomosis or implantation if sufficient tissue remains. An isthmic application of the clip, in contrast, requires an isthmic-isthmic anastomosis after excision of the clip and adjacent scar tissue (see Atlas, Plate 7). Fimbriectomy can be reversed with a salpingostomy, but successful reversals are sparse in the literature.

The personal experience of Winston (1980) (Table 11–2) reveals that anastomoses of isthmus to isthmus, requiring microsurgical techniques but involving the least amount of tubal damage, resulted in his highest success rate. This experience was confirmed in a review of the literature on reversibility (Siegler, 1985).

Silber and Cohen (1980) made a similar observation (Table 11–3) that success rates were directly related to the length of tubal tissue remaining after sterilization. A review of our experience with anastomosis (Hulka and Halme, 1988) confirms this important prognostic factor.

TABLE 11–2. **RESULTS OF TUBAL ANASTOMOSIS FOR REVERSAL OF STERILIZATION***

Site	Operations	Pregnancies	Ectopic Pregnancies	Pregnancy Rate (%)
Cornu-isthmus	17	12	0	71
Isthmus-isthmus	16	12	0	75
Cornu-ampulla	26	14	1	54
Isthmus-ampulla	27	17	2	63
Ampulla-ampulla	19	8	0	42
Miscellaneous†	21	10	(1)	48
Total	126	73	3	58

*Adapted from Winston RML: Microsurgery of the fallopian tube: From fantasy to reality. Fertil Steril 34:521–530, 1980. Reproduced with permission of the publisher, The American Fertility Society.

Notes: Operations classified according to site of anastomosis; for asymmetrical sterilizations, operation classified according to the site of anastomosis in the longer tube.

†Refers to different sites in tubes of similar length, double anastomoses, and implantation on one side combined with cornual anastomosis on the other. The number in parentheses indicates one tubal gestation that occurred in an implanted tube; cornual anastomosis on other side was patent.

TABLE 11–3. **RELATIONSHIP OF TOTAL TUBAL LENGTH AND SUBSEQUENT PREGNANCY***

	Tubal Length				
	0–2 cm	2–3 cm	3–4 cm	4–5 cm	>5 cm
Total no. of patients	2	5	7	4	7
Pregnant	0	0	4	4	7
Not pregnant	2	5	3	0	0
Normal intrauterine pregnancy rate	0%	0%	43%	100%	100%

*From Silber SJ and Cohen R: Microsurgical reversal of female sterilization: The role of tubal length. Fertil Steril 33:598–601, 1980. Reproduced with permission of the publisher, The American Fertility Society.

TABLE 11–4. RESULTS AFTER CLIP REVERSAL*

Clinician	Attempts	Ectopic	Intrauterine
		Pregnancies	
Owen	21	1	20
Winston	15	0	15
Wheeless	12	0	10
Noble and Letchworth	12	0	9
Imrie (with splint)	8	0	6
Loeffler and Lieberman	5	1	4
Taft	4	0	2
Gomel	3	0	3
Hulka	3	0	3
Haney	2	0	2
Total	85	2	74

*From Hulka JF, Noble AD, Letchworth AT, et al: Reversibility of clip sterilization. Lancet 2:927, 1982.

TABLE 11–5. SAFETY AND EFFICACY: COMPARISON OF STERILIZATION METHODS*

Measure	Coagulation	Band	Clip
	Method		
Safety			
Days re-admission for complication	10.5	5.5	2.1
Late ectopic rate (%)	29–44	15.0	4.0
Reversibility			
Term pregnancies following reversal (%)	41	72	84
Efficacy			
1-year method failure (rate per 1000)	1.9–2.6	3.3–4.7	1.8–5.9

*From Chi I, Potts M, and Wilkens L: Rare events associated with tubal sterilization: An international experience. Obstet Gynecol Surv 41:7–19, 1986 and Siegler AM, Hulka JF, and Peretz A: Reversibility of female sterilization. Fertil Steril 43:499–510, 1985. Reproduced with the permission of the publisher, The American Fertility Society.

In June 1982 we completed a survey of microsurgeons who had performed reversals after spring clip sterilizations (Table 11–4) and found that after 85 such reversals 74 patients had achieved intrauterine pregnancy, for a reversal rate of 87%. (This total included at least three women who were not trying to get pregnant after the reversal!)

The selection of a sterilization technique appropriate to a particular patient thus can include preserving the option of reversal by choosing a minimally destructive method. In presenting this issue to the patient, it is important to stress to her that all sterilization procedures are permanent; thus if a woman is contemplating more pregnancies later in life all current sterilization techniques, including the clip, are not advisable. However, honest mistakes are made by physicians and patients as life presents its surprises, and the younger patient at greater risk of returning for reversal after divorce and remarriage may be best served with keeping the option of reversibility in mind when choosing a sterilization method. This is the single area in which the spring clip appears to offer a clear advantage over other methods.

SUMMARY

In Table 11–5 we present a summary of the best available comparative data concerning safety and efficacy of the three popular methods: coagulation, band, and clip. Safety is defined and compared in terms of the length of stay of hospitalizations subsequent to the procedure for complications. Another measure is the long-term risk of ectopic pregnancy after sterilization. Efficacy is defined as the known cumulative pregnancy rate. Reversibility is included as an important factor for choosing a procedure in the case of young women.

REFERENCES

Bhiwandiwala PP, Mumford S, and Feldblum PJ: A comparison of different laparoscopic sterilization occlusion techniques in 24,439 procedures. Am J Obstet Gynecol *144*:319–331, 1982.

Gomel V: Profile of women requesting reversal of sterilization. Fertil Steril *30*:39–41, 1978.

Grubb GS and Peterson HB: Luteal phase pregnancy and tubal sterilization. Obstet Gynecol *66*:784–788, 1985.

Holt VL, Chu J, Daling JR, et al: Tubal sterilization and subsequent ectopic pregnancy. JAMA *266*:242–246, 1991.

Hulka JF and Halme J: Sterilization reversal: Results of 101 attempts. Am J Obstet Gynecol *159*:767–774, 1988.

Kleppinger RK: Female outpatient sterilization using bipolar coagulation. Bull Post-Grad Comm Med, Univ Sydney, pp 144–154, Nov. 1977.

Lee SH and Jones JS: Postpartum tubal sterilization: A comparative study of the Hulka clip and modified Pomeroy technique. J Reprod Med *36*:703–706, 1991.

Makar AP, Vanderheyden JS, Schatteman EA, et al: Female sterilization failure after bipolar electrocoagulation: A 6 year retrospective study. Eur J Obstet Gynecol Reprod Biol *37*:237–246, 1990.

Siegler AM, Hulka JF, and Peretz A: Reversibility of female sterilization. Fertil Steril *43*:499–510, 1985.

Silber SJ and Cohen R: Microsurgical reversal of female sterilization: The role of tubal length. Fertil Steril *33*:598–601, 1980.

Valle RF and Battifora HA: A new approach to tubal sterilization by laparoscopy. Fertil Steril *30*:415–422, 1978.

Wilcox LS, Chu SY, Eaker ED, et al: Risk factors for regret after tubal sterilization: 5 years of follow-up in a prospective study. Fertil Steril *55*:27–33, 1991.

Winston RML: Microsurgery of the fallopian tube: From fantasy to reality. Fertil Steril *34*:521–530, 1980.

Winston RML: Why 103 women asked for reversal of sterilisation. BMJ *2*:305–307, 1977.

Yoon IB, King TM, and Parmley TH: A two-year experience with the falope ring sterilization procedure. Am J Obstet Gynecol *127*:109–112, 1977.

Yoon IB, Wheeless CR Jr, and King TM: A preliminary report on a new laparoscopic sterilization approach: The silicone rubber band technique. Am J Obstet Gynecol *120*:132–136, 1974.

FURTHER READINGS

SPRING CLIP

Hulka JF: Spring clip sterilization. The Pelvic Surgeon *1*(5):1–4, 1980.

Hulka JF, Mercer JP, Fishburne JI, et al: Spring clip sterilization: One year follow-up of 1,079 cases. Am J Obstet Gynecol *125*:1039–1043, 1976.

Hulka JF, Omran KF, Lieberman BA, and Gordon AG: Laparoscopic sterilization with the spring clip: Instrumentation development and current clinical experience. Am J Obstet Gynecol *135*:1016–1020, 1979.

COMPARISON OF METHODS

Chi I, Potts M, and Wilkens L: Rare events associated with tubal sterilization: An international experience. Obstet Gynecol Surv *41*:7–19, 1986.

Hulka JF: Relative risks and benefits of electric and nonelectric sterilization techniques. J Reprod Med *21*:111–114, 1978. Also in Phillips JM (ed): Endoscopy in Gynecology. The Proceedings of the Third International Congress on Gynecologic Endoscopy, San Francisco, CA. Downey, CA, American Association of Gynecologic Laparoscopists, 1978, pp 291–295.

Hulka JF, Peterson HB, and Phillips JM: American Association of Gynecological Laparoscopists' Membership Survey of Laparoscopic Sterilization. J Reprod Med *35*:584–586, 1990.

Phillips JM, Hulka JF, Hulka B, and Corson SL: 1979 AAGL membership survey. J Reprod Med *26*:529–533, 1981.

Shain RN, Miller WB, Holden AEC, and Rosenthal M: Impact of tubal sterilization and vasectomy on female marital sexuality: Results of a controlled longitudinal study. Am J Obstet Gynecol *164*:763–771, 1991.

REVERSIBILITY

Hulka JF, Noble AD, Letchworth AT, et al: Reversibility of clip sterilizations. Lancet *2*:927, 1982.

Assessing Patient Risk

Patients who wish to have laparoscopic sterilization or in whom diagnostic laparoscopy would be useful may not be appropriate candidates for the procedure. The following discussion presents various contraindications, as well as a few favorable indications, by which the physician can select appropriate patients with the objective of minimizing complications in these elective procedures.

ABSOLUTE CONTRAINDICATIONS

Multiple Laparotomies

Most experienced laparoscopists agree that an occasional patient with multiple previous abdominal surgery is not suitable for laparoscopy. This includes patients with multiple laparotomies for chronic conditions such as diverticulosis, peritonitis (which may have involved creating and taking down colostomies), or laparotomies at which time the previous surgeon had described multiple abdominal adhesions involving the anterior abdominal wall. In these situations arising from previously surgically created adhesions and scars, a direct laparotomy is the preferred method if the abdomen must be entered.

Class IV Cardiac Disease

Severe cardiac disease remains a contraindication if the patient cannot tolerate the supine or Trendelenburg position. This is seen in class IV cardiac patients and in some class III patients. In general, such severe cardiac illness may of itself be a contraindication to considerations of elective sterilization. If a procedure must be performed, only patients who can stand the Trendelenburg position (pretested) for 15 minutes should undergo surgery by very skilled and experienced surgeons to minimize the period of blood flow derangement and anesthesia. Local anesthesia is preferred to maximize the body's management of respiratory function and to minimize chance for arrhythmias occurring because of medications. One report of five class III and class IV patients undergoing sterilization emphasizes these points (Snabes and Poindexter, 1991).

Peritonitis

ACUTE PERITONITIS WITH BOWEL DISTENTION AND OBSTRUCTION. Bowel distention and obstruction with acute peritonitis is a contraindication for laparoscopy since the patient will need a laparotomy to relieve the obstruction. The insertion of a needle against the distended bowel is almost ensuring bowel injury by the penetrating needle.

PERITONITIS AND DOCUMENTED HEMOPERITONEUM. In the presence of unstable blood pressure, a direct laparotomy is rapidly needed to control an actively bleeding blood vessel such as a laceration, splenic rupture, or ectopic pregnancy. Performance of laparoscopy in such a situation will only delay the need for surgical correction.

PERITONITIS AND DOCUMENTED PELVIC MASS. A large solid mass palpable under anesthesia is also a contraindication, since the pelvic mass is usually causally associated with peritonitis in conditions such as ruptured endometrioma and requires direct surgical therapy to manage the mass and peritonitis.

HIGH-RISK PATIENT

Previous Abdominal Surgery

Even though multiple previous operations may be a contraindication, one or two previous elective procedures may pose no problem. We have been favorably impressed by the surgical skill of our colleagues who have performed cholecystectomies, gastrectomies, cesarean sections, or laparotomies for tubal or ovarian disease and who have left a clean abdominal wall through which a needle and trocar can be safely inserted. In these situations, the patient should be informed that laparoscopy will be attempted and will probably be successful but that possible bowel injury will require laparotomy and repair may be necessary. The bowel injury in these cases is usually not extensive but consists of a relatively small laceration by a needle or trocar of a bowel adherent to the abdominal wall. A small incision can be made directly over the abdominal wall entry (since the injured bowel will be adherent to the wall and easily found); the injury can be identified and closed directly, usually without requiring resection. A patient with previous pelvic surgery may similarly be advised that although laparoscopy may be successful in the sense of successful entry into the abdomen, the pelvic surgery may not be performed because of adhesions generated by her previous surgery or disease. Thus, patients seeking tubal sterilization after previous cesarean sections or history of inflammatory disease should be counseled that a laparotomy may be necessary to complete their wishes if the pelvic structures are unavailable because of pelvic adhesions.

Anticoagulation Therapy

Patients under anticoagulation therapy for cardiac or thrombotic disease may not be appropriate candidates. Since laparoscopy is a surgical procedure, complete reversal of anticoagulation therapy is necessary before this invasive procedure is performed. If the reversal constitutes a threat to the patient's life (e.g., patients with artificial mitral valves on anticoagulation therapy to prevent arterial emboli), direct laparotomy with direct visual management of bleeding points may be preferred. One death in our experience occurred in the case of a patient who was anticoagulated because of artificial aortic and mitral valves. At the time of laparoscopic sterilization incompletely reversed anticoagulation therapy led to the slow development of hemoperitoneum and death days later from coronary occlusion by an embolus after the coagulation was reversed.

Peritonitis

The diagnostic use of laparoscopy can be extremely useful in patients with an unclear cause for peritonitis. Although the best of clinical skills must always be used in the differential diagnosis of the acute condition of an abdomen, there are situations in which one cannot clinically distinguish among the following abdominal conditions:

- Normal pelvis
- Unruptured ovarian cyst
- Ruptured endometrioma
- Ruptured corpus luteal cyst
- Torsion of the adnexum
- Endometriosis
- Ectopic pregnancy
- Active suppurative salpingitis
- Pelvic abscess
- Diverticulitis
- Regional enteritis
- Appendicitis
- Perforated viscus

Since management of these conditions is so obviously different and several conditions need no laparotomy, diagnostic laparoscopy is useful in peritonitis of unclear etiology. Pelvic examination under anesthesia is always recommended because the patient may have a large pelvic mass, including an otherwise unsuspected intrauterine pregnancy, that might be inadvertently perforated by the needle or trocar.

Abdominal Hernias

Abdominal hernias are not as strong a contraindication as was once thought. If careful attention is paid to maintaining appropriate intra-abdominal pressures (see Chapter 4), inguinal or umbilical hernias will not be disrupted. A diaphragmatic true hernia (sacculation of the diaphragmatic wall) is not a contraindication, because low pressures will not force the stomach or bowel into the chest cavity past the chronic hernial sac. The absence of a hernial sac, or a defect in the diaphragm, is a contraindication but is rarely seen in adults. At the time of laparoscopy, direct and indirect inguinal hernias can be diagnosed and documented, as well as the presence or absence of incisional or diaphragmatic hernias. With prior knowledge, the elective sterilization or diagnostic procedure can be planned together with an elective hernia repair.

Obesity

Obesity is an occasional reason for operative failure but is not a contraindication to attempt laparoscopy. The success of laparoscopy in the obese patient is a direct function of the physician's skill and experience as well as occasional good luck. Laparoscopic sterilization may be the method of choice in the extremely obese, when considering the morbidity associated with the alternatives of vaginal approach, laparotomy, or hysterectomy. Furthermore, if one attempt at laparoscopy fails in the obese patient, she can be scheduled for surgery another day provided that the laparoscopist is forewarned to attempt a second laparoscopy and possible laparotomy to accomplish the intra-abdominal surgery.

Thinness and Nulliparity

Surprisingly, the nulliparous patient in exceptional good health who follows a program of exercise and weight reduction may be at higher risk than normal. We have experienced difficulty in abdominal entry in women as well as men who have had a vigorous athletic program of jogging, dancing, or horseback riding. The abdominal wall muscles and fascia in these patients are strong and resistant to elevation with towel clips or other methods and may present difficulties in entry in a way that avoids the underlying vessels. Placing a finger on the umbilicus of these patients may indicate the pulsations of the aorta less than 1 in. below the finger. General anesthesia may be required if the patient cannot relax sufficiently to allow elevation of the abdomen for performance of laparoscopy under local anesthesia. In a review of aortic and other large vessel lacerations, the incidence of these complications is surprisingly high among this category of patients, when the physician was not sufficiently circumspect about the anatomic hazards presented by the thin, athletic patient.

Diabetes, Thyroid, and Other Metabolic Diseases

Elective sterilization may be truly indicated in the chronically ill patient, but the selection of anesthesia should be local if possible. In these situations, skilled laparoscopists experienced in local anesthesia can perform the sterilization procedure in less than 10 minutes in a manner that constitutes no stress to the patient's metabolic system and that allows for resumption of medications immediately after surgery.

Concomitant Uterine Disease

Laparoscopy may not be indicated in patients who have coexistent pelvic pathology. For example, patients with chronic pelvic pain or menometrorrhagia may be better served by a careful review of their history and consideration of a hysterectomy rather than sterilization, particularly if the patient may be inclined to consider the laparoscopic procedure as having made her pain or bleeding worse subsequently. Similarly, patients with a history of abnormal Papanicolaou smears in the past, combined with other pelvic pathology such as cervicitis or pelvic pain, may be well served by hysterectomy to relieve their anxieties about cancer as well as pregnancy. Patients with stress incontinence may similarly be best served by vaginal hysterectomy and plastic repair than by sterilization alone. Newly appearing fibroids, although small and asymptomatic, may lead to hysterectomy later. Hysterectomy should now be discussed. These conditions are not contraindications to laparoscopy, and after counseling, the patient may elect sterilization by laparoscopy in the presence of these diseases, in which case a clear record with regard to her choice at the time after presentation of the alternatives should be entered in her chart.

LOW-RISK PATIENT

Characteristics

Patients who have none of the aforementioned considerations can be considered low-risk patients. Specifically, they:

- Have no systemic disease
- Are anesthetic class I status
- Have had no previous abdominal surgery
- Have no history suggestive of pelvic inflammatory disease
- Are not obese (abdominal wall less than 2 in. thick)
- Are multiparous, preferably having delivered awake vaginally
- Are comfortable and relaxed during bimanual pelvic examination

These characteristics describe the majority of American women seeking elective sterilization. For such selected patients, several clinics in the United States have started providing laparoscopic sterilization under local anesthesia in a facility other than an operating room. Caution must be strongly advised, however, before considering such a service. The surgeon should be skilled and experienced and should have performed at least 100 laparoscopies, half of which were under local anesthesia conditions in an operating room. This volume of experience will begin to provide those clinical judgments as to patient selection, as well as surgical judgment as to when to proceed in the face of unsuspected findings and when to abandon the procedure as inappropriate under the circumstances. The facility should be fully equipped for all laparoscopic procedures, including coagulation power sources and forceps, even though a mechanical method of sterilization is being offered. If a major vessel is entered, the patient should be able to be wheeled to an ambulance for transport to a hospital within 10 minutes; the surgeon should have admitting privileges in such a hospital and should be on good terms with the vascular surgery service.

These conditions are recommended after reviewing the circumstances surrounding complications and death as they have occurred in the United States and England. When such conditions are met, a facility can provide a low-cost sterilization service to most American women without compromising safety, since low-risk patients under these circumstances do not need the full range of anesthesia and equipment that a more costly traditional operating room provides.

Suitability for Local Anesthesia

Complications can arise if a patient judged to be suitable for local anesthesia turns out to be unsuitable. Patients who have undergone deliveries under local anesthesia are ideal candidates for local anesthesia for laparoscopy since they are experienced and presumably comfortable with surgical manipulation of their bodies. On the other hand, nulliparous patients, who are not comfortable during the pelvic examination, will certainly not be comfortable during a laparoscopic procedure. One very useful way of screening for the degree of relaxation that the patient can provide is to try elevating the abdomen at the time of the preoperative pelvic examination. The patient should be told that this is the most uncomfortable aspect of the procedure that she will experience. If the patient cannot relax her abdomen in the examining room before surgery, she will not be able to relax during surgery, and general anesthesia should be recommended.

INFORMING THE PATIENT

Because lack of information about risks is a principal complaint in legal action when complications occur, the method of ensuring informed consent prior to surgery is discussed in detail. As mentioned earlier, patients known to be at high risk should be informed beforehand of their special risk and should be advised that a laparotomy may be necessary.

Most patients undergoing laparoscopy in the United States are healthy young women undergoing elective sterilization or relatively unpressured diagnostic laparoscopy for chronic pelvic pain or infertility. Since sterilization is completely elective and one of a number of options in fertility management, the patient needs to be fully informed of all alternatives and risks prior to the procedure. As complications were occurring in the 1970s, patients expressed their dissatisfaction with results through their lawyers and brought to the sharp attention of the medical community the need for proper informed consent prior to the procedure. Laparoscopy today is the second most frequent cause for suing obstetricians and gynecologists (the most frequent being unfavorable outcome of delivery).

Many aids to ensure patients' informed consent were rapidly generated, such as audiovisual packets (available through Planned Parenthood of America); pamphlets prepared by the Department of Health and Human Services (DHHS) (available and required in some states for patients whose sterilization will be paid for with federal funds); and pamphlets written for the healthy private patient (available through the American College of Obstetricians and Gynecologists). A "jury friendly" 20-minute video describing sterilization procedures in a simple manner has been used as an informed consent. This video, available from the Department of Obstetrics and Gynecology at the University of North Carolina at Chapel Hill, has been in use for

many years. These materials should form the basis for informing the patient of the risks and alternatives of the procedure but should not be the sole attempt to inform her. Extensive counseling by the physician and nurse prior to the elective sterilization procedure is strongly recommended to ensure that the patient is comfortable and happy with her decision before the operation and is aware of the risks involved, especially the possibility of subsequent pregnancy.

COUNSELING IN CHOOSING STERILIZATION

The question of which patient is appropriate for elective sterilization has been a difficult one to address. Although DHHS has institutionalized their prerequisites to patients over 21 years of age who have waited at least 72 hours between signature and performance and are mentally competent, these rules apply in most states only to patients whose sterilization will be paid for with federal funds. Private patients are usually not under these constraints. Recommendations for the performance of sterilization on these patients include that the patient be *unpressured, informed,* and *mature.*

Unpressured implies that the patient should not be under any known emotional stress when she makes the decision. Some reasons for postponing this decision include considering a combination of abortion and sterilization. Abortion is a known crisis situation in which permanent prevention of future pregnancies by sterilization may be regretted after the stress of the unwanted pregnancy is over. However, women who have completed their family plans a long time ago and who find themselves unexpectedly and unacceptably pregnant in their mid-30s or later can be offered combined abortion and sterilization with little fear of error. Pressure is also present if sterilization is first offered in circumstances of labor and delivery. Postpartum sterilization is best discussed months before delivery as part of prenatal counseling. Emergency cesarean section may be a very good indication for sterilization, but if there is any hesitancy on the part of the patient, this permanent decision should be postponed. Patients in the process of separation or divorce are similarly under emotional pressure and may not be appropriate candidates for sterilization, since the most common pattern in the United States following divorce is remarriage with possibly the desire to have children with the new spouse.

It is very important that the patient be informed. As has been mentioned earlier, the alternatives to sterilization (including vasectomy) as well as the main risks of sterilization (complications and risk of subsequent pregnancies) should be fully presented to the patient by the physician as well as in pamphlet form.

Being mature implies that the patient has made a seasoned choice appropriate to her reproductive plan. There are mature 19-year-old mothers in whom the sterilization decision is utterly appropriate; similarly, there are relatively immature 28-year-old women whose decision is inappropriate.

The question of involuntary sterilization of mentally incompetent patients is relatively clear in today's society. North Carolina has model legislation concerning the process. Severely mentally defective children whose parents fear seduction and pregnancy can be sterilized if the county judge is presented with objective evidence that the patient is irretrievably mentally incompetent. The clerk of court acts as the patient's defense counsel in this proceeding. In this situation the judge issues an order to the physician to perform an involuntary sterilization. Parents cannot impose involuntary sterilization on their children directly.

POSTOPERATIVE CARE

For outpatient laparoscopy, a number of routine preoperative and postoperative instructions have been carefully written, tested, and rewritten by the nursing staff at The University of North Carolina Hospitals and are available through the Department of Obstetrics and Gynecology at this university. These instructions address the most common concerns and ensure that the patient is informed how to deal with postoperative problems.

Patients should be given written postoperative instructions since they may be too groggy from surgical excitement and medication to remember verbal instructions. In addition, the hospital or physician's office should telephone the patient postoperatively to ensure that normal recovery is occurring. A return clinic visit and examination are necessary only if the patient is experiencing some complication requiring examination. We routinely schedule a return visit for 1 week later, but we instruct the patient to cancel this appointment if she is well–and most patients do.

REFERENCE

Snabes MC and Poindexter AN III: Laparoscopic tubal sterilization under local anesthesia in women with cyanotic heart disease. Obstet Gynecol 78:437–440, 1991.

ADVANCED LAPAROSCOPIC SURGERY

Diagnostic laparoscopy is the most common gynecologic procedure performed today. It may confirm normal anatomy or indicate the need for further surgical or medical therapy. Its greatest impact has been to replace exploratory laparotomy for accurate diagnosis of pelvic pain or infertility.

Operative laparoscopy implies the performance of a therapeutic procedure that is usually accomplished by laparotomy. Major advantages of a laparoscopic approach over laparotomy include a short period of hospitalization, rapid recuperation, superior cosmetics, easier intraoperative access to the vagina and rectum, confirmation of complete hemostasis and evacuation of all blood clots at the close of the procedure by direct visualization in a liquid medium following the replacement of CO_2 pneumoperitoneum with lactated Ringer's solution, and results at least equivalent to those obtainable by laparotomy.

Most gynecologic surgery can be performed using laparoscopic visualization. The method of treatment is the same regardless of whether laparoscopic or laparotomy visualization is used. Laparoscopy is only another method of access and is not a method of treatment. While the surgeon's hands are much further from the area being treated than during laparotomy, his or her eye (or eyes with video) is right on top of it, much like when using the operating microscope for pelvic reconstructive surgery, except that the laparoscope is easier to manipulate than an operating microscope.

The surgeon must know pelvic anatomy, pathology, and available instrumentation. Every laparoscopic procedure should be an anatomy lesson, especially the easy cases, with identification of the ureters, the common iliac vessels and their branches, the liver and gallbladder, the bowel, and the appendix. The location of pelvic retroperitoneal structures should be second nature for surgeons performing advanced gynecologic endoscopy.

The ability to perform operative laparoscopy is not laser dependent, although for most Americans, these techniques evolved with the laser. In Europe, operative laparoscopy paralleled the development of surgical instruments and suture capable of being applied endoscopically. Laparoscopic electrosurgery has been used safely for many years by skilled surgeons throughout the world.

Laparoscopic surgical procedures can last from 1 to 6 hours, and schedules for operating rooms must be prepared accordingly. In some hospitals, prolonged operating room time may become the major problem limiting wider acceptance of laparoscopic surgery. Yet, complex plastic surgical procedures like muscle transposition can last for 24 hours. Should prospective patients be denied a laparoscopic procedure because it would take too long, or should there be special centers geared toward long cases with "teams"? The anesthetic risk associated with a 20- to 30-degree Trendelenburg position and high-flow CO_2 pneumoperitoneum has yet to be determined. Potential anesthesia risk, operating room time, reimbursement, and liability limit the extent to which gynecologic procedures are managed endoscopically. When these problems are resolved, advanced surgical training will produce the proficiency necessary to implement extensive operative laparoscopy. If these problems are not solved by the gynecologist, the general surgeon will become the operative laparoscopist of the future, because informed patients will seek surgeons who can perform laparoscopic surgery on an ambulatory basis.

In this section we present the special considerations and techniques pertinent to all advanced laparoscopic surgery. Although scientific documentation of the advantages of laparoscopy over laparotomy is incomplete for many procedures (Grimes, 1992), the procedures included have gained general acceptance as appropriately performed by laparoscopy.

Appendix A contains a complete list of the instruments and equipment required to perform laparoscopic surgery.

REFERENCE

Grimes DA: Frontiers of operative laparoscopy: A review and critique of the evidence. Am J Obstet Gynecol *166*:1062–1071, 1992.

13

Special Requirements

Operative laparoscopy requires another level of skill, facilities, and equipment far beyond the standard diagnostic and sterilization procedures of the 1970s and 1980s. Diagnostic procedures are useful to study the wide range of normal anatomy found in the pelvis, and the video camera is an effective teaching tool for both techniques and findings with standard laparoscopy.

A suction-irrigator (aquadissector), special forceps, scissors, high-flow insufflator, 30-degree tiltable operating table, and an electrosurgical generator are indispensable tools for advanced surgical procedures. The video camera and monitor facilitate assistance, documentation, and comfort. Just as no surgeon would contemplate a laparotomy using only two clamps and one pair of scissors, the laparoscopist needs a full selection of instruments and ancillary equipment to carry out these procedures safely and effectively. In this chapter we present these considerations in detail.

TRAINING OF THE SURGEON

Differences in surgical skill have always existed among gynecologic surgeons. The same is true for laparoscopic surgery; the interpretation of three-dimensional spatial relationships on a two-dimensional screen may be beyond the capabilities of many surgeons who have not played Nintendo video games with their children. Gynecologists doing advanced laparoscopic surgery need a particularly detailed knowledge of the anatomy of the pelvic wall and its con-

tents. Such knowledge is usually acquired by extensive prior experience in laparotomies for endometriosis and microsurgical lysis of adhesions. Most gynecologists in practice today have reserved such laparotomies as the next step after diagnostic laparoscopy; the gynecologists of tomorrow may not have that opportunity if operative laparoscopy is done at the same time that endometriosis or adhesions are found.

At present, there is no formal set of prerequisites or criteria for licensing or recognizing a physician as capable of advanced gynecologic laparoscopy. For private practitioners who are eager to expand their skills, many workshops exist to demonstrate the basic hand-eye coordination required for video-assisted laparoscopy, dissection, suture ligatures, laser use, and so forth. Although mechanical and animal models serve these purposes well and some courses provide ample "hands-on" opportunity to learn these skills, experience with patients remains the best way to gain the detailed judgment and skills necessary for good surgery. Such clinical training is currently available through personal preceptorships arranged by gynecologists and some operative laparoscopists, varying in length from days to months of operative experience.

Although laparoscopy is presently used more by reproductive surgeons than by oncologists, and the Society of Reproductive Surgeons could be the group to develop and transmit the skills and standards of advanced operative laparoscopy, the experience of the general surgeon with chole-

FIGURE 13–1 Surgeon's old, painful posture

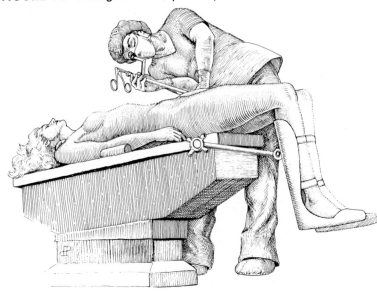

cystectomy indicates that the general gynecologist will be the laparoscopic surgeon of the future.

FACILITIES

Cameras, Light Sources, and Recorders

An operating room dedicated to video endoscopic surgery can have an efficient moveable overhead platform (similar to the monitors in radiology suites) for the video monitor, camera, and light source with multiple heads for different light cables. The room can be wired to direct the video signal to a video cassette recorder (VCR) or color printer away from the operating table for recording purposes. The camera, light source, and monitor are currently designed to function as an integral unit for maximum visual resolution. Having this expensive and delicate electronic equipment mounted permanently in a moveable holder overhead saves it from considerable wear and tear, because it otherwise must be wheeled from storage to surgery. If the hospital has no room dedicated to video endoscopy, large carts holding all visual equipment need to be located close to the operating table so that the light cables and camera cables can reach the operative field.

Video Arrangements

Video enables the surgeon to stand comfortably watching the monitor, compared with bending awkwardly and painfully for hours looking directly through the optics (Fig. 13–1). Video monitors, laser generators, and assistants add to the standard laparoscopic arrangement described in Chapter 5. The operating staff should be quite familiar with laser and light sources, video cameras and recorders, special suction-aspiration equipment, and so forth, preferably as a standing endoscopy team. The special demands for space around the patient for the surgeon, the video monitors, and surgical assistants have led to a variety of practical arrangements.

VIDEO OPPOSITE THE SURGEON (Fig. 13–2). This arrangement is the one that we prefer, because only one monitor is necessary. The monitor is on the patient's (1) right; the surgeon (2) is on her left; and the assistant (3) is located between the patient's legs where the monitor can be viewed. The anesthesiologist (4) can also view the monitor. Both the surgeon and the assistant have access to instrument tables beside or behind them, and a scrub nurse is not necessary if the assistant is specially trained. When a deep Trendelenburg position is used, the assistant will need elevating stands for comfort. One or more circulating nurses (5,6) tend the video recorder, irrigation supply, laser, and so forth. Laser and suction-irrigation come most conveniently from behind the surgeon: laser from above the operative field and cephalad, suction-irrigation from below the field with the tubing attached to the patient's left leg drapes to minimize tangles.

This arrangement requires some hand-eye adjustment for the surgeon, since the monitor is rotated 90 degrees from the plane of surgery. However, it avoids neck and back strain from twisting to see a monitor placed between the patient's legs, especially if the surgeon operates with instruments in the left hand and a laparoscope in the right hand in the same plane. Hand-eye coordination (almost mirror-image) is extremely difficult for the assistant, however, who often assumes a passive role of maintaining retraction or grasper positions achieved by the surgeon. Mirror-image operating skills are attainable after extensive training and greatly increase the efficiency of the surgical team.

FIGURE 13–2 Operating room setup

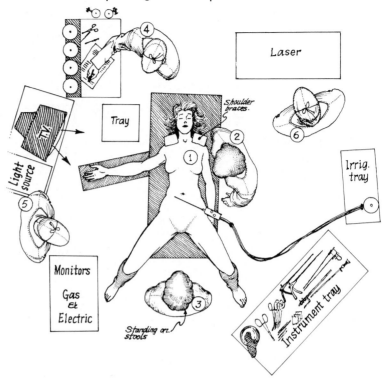

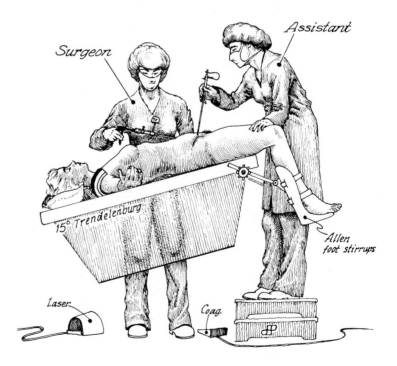

FIGURE 13–3 Double video monitors

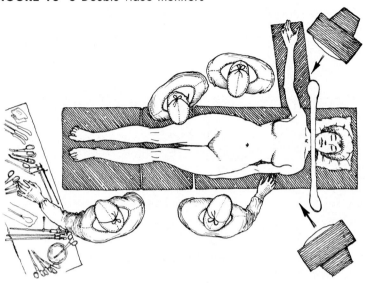

FIGURE 13–4 Video at the foot of the table

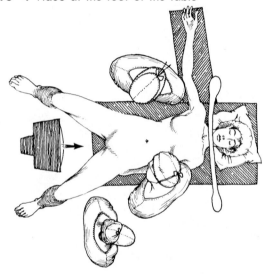

FIGURE 13–5 Surgeon at the foot of the table

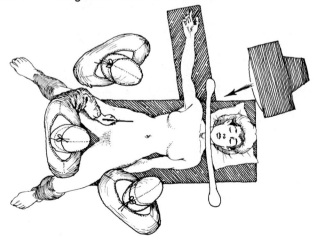

DOUBLE VIDEO MONITORS (Fig. 13–3). This arrangement is preferred by most surgeons for cholecystectomy. Two monitors are placed on either side of the patient above chest level, allowing the surgeon (usually at the patient's left) and first assistant (opposite) to have comfortable views cephalad and across the patient. A second assistant can hold the camera or retract.

VIDEO AT THE FOOT OF THE TABLE (Fig. 13–4). Some pelvic surgeons prefer the video monitor to be at the foot of the table, allowing the assistant (opposite the surgeon) an equally good view and eliminating the difficult hand-eye coordination problems for surgeon and assistant that are inherent with one monitor opposite the surgeon. The surgeon and assistant cannot share instrument tables, and a scrub nurse is necessary with this arrangement.

SURGEON BETWEEN THE PATIENT'S LEGS (Fig. 13–5). Some European surgeons performing cholecystectomies find that with the reverse Trendelenburg position, the table can be lowered enough for them to sit between the patient's legs and operate looking cephalad at the monitor with both hands comfortably positioned over the abdomen. The first and second assistants are on the patient's left and right.

PREOPERATIVE PREPARATION

Laparoscopy is done prior to ovulation if possible. Leuprolide acetate for depot suspension (Lupron Depot) 3.75 mg intramuscularly (IM) is often administered after ovulation in the cycle preceding surgery to avoid operating on ovaries containing a corpus luteum cyst. Another approach is to administer norethindrone acetate, 10 mg/day, starting on the first day of menses until surgery. Endovaginal ultrasound is performed to evaluate the ovaries in cases involving a pelvic mass, retrocervical nodules, or fibroids. Intravenous pyelograms (IVP) are rarely obtained preoperatively but are ordered frequently postoperatively if abdominal pain persists following surgery on or near the ureter. Lower abdominal, pubic, and perineal hair is not shaved. Patients are encouraged to hydrate and eat lightly for 24 hours before admission to the hospital.

Bowel Preparation

Laparoscopic surgery is usually done on a same-day or 24-hour basis, except when serious medical conditions exist or postoperative difficulties are anticipated. Patients are asked to take magnesium citrate and a Fleet enema on the evening before surgery. When extensive bowel dissection is anticipated, such as with cul-de-sac dissections, a mechanical bowel preparation is useful. Polyethylene glycol–based isosmotic solution (GOLYTELY or Colyte) is dissolved in water to a volume of 4 liters. Oral administration induces diarrhea, which rapidly cleanses the bowel (usually within 4 hours). This solution is usually taken by the patient on the afternoon before surgery so sleep is not disturbed. Metoclopramide hydrochloride (Reglan), 10 mg by mouth (PO) taken 30 minutes earlier, helps to promote gastric emptying time and thus reduce abdominal bloating and distention.

When extensive small bowel adhesions are expected, 90 ml or 6 tablets of charcoal is administered on the night before surgery. If accidental small bowel enterotomy occurs, identification and repair are simplified by the intraluminal charcoal.

FIGURE 13–6 Patient positioned on the table

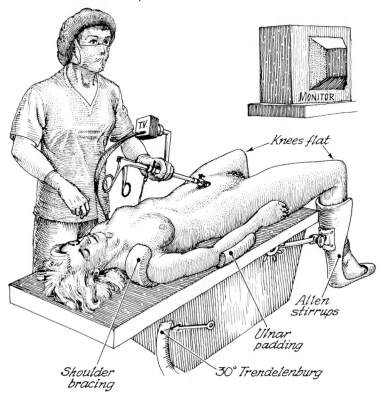

Knees flat

Allen stirrups

Ulnar padding

30° Trendelenburg

Shoulder bracing

MONITOR

TV.

Bladder

Just prior to surgery, patients are encouraged to void, and a Foley catheter is inserted only if the bladder is distended during surgery and in procedures lasting for more than 2 hours. It is easier to identify a distended bladder, and in difficult cases, the bladder is filled with 100 ml of indigo carmine solution to make accidental entry apparent. The catheter is not removed until the patient is awake and aware of its presence, usually 1 to 2 hours after surgery; this precaution avoids early overdistention with resultant urinary retention and overflow incontinence.

Positioning on the Operating Table

Extensive pelvic surgery may require a steep Trendelenburg position for prolonged periods, as well as rapid reversals of these angles for irrigation and aspiration. The table chosen should be capable of attaining a 30-degree Trendelenburg position and should preferably be electric for rapid reversals during surgery. Affiliated Tables Champagne Model 600, ObGyn version, has manual control but is capable of attaining a 30-degree position. Because of these positions and the surgeon's inevitable leaning on the patient's limbs, special precautions are necessary (Fig. 13–6). The surgeon should not lean against the patient's extended arm. Rather, prior to the induction of general anesthesia, bilateral ulnar pads (Zimfoam: laminectomy arm cradle set, Zimmer) are applied and both arms are tucked at the patient's side, with the patient's right arm on a padded arm board. Shoulder braces are placed over the acromioclavicular joint to prevent brachial plexus injury. The legs are positioned and checked for comfort while the patient is awake. Knee stirrups with careful lateral padding (to protect the peroneal nerve and avoid foot-drop) or Allan stirrups to support the heel with no pressure points around the free knee are used. Allan stirrups allow the thighs to be placed in an extended (not elevated) position, facilitating manipulation of instruments when operating in the upper abdomen through lower quadrant incisions.

The buttocks are placed to protrude slightly from the table edge in the lithotomy position.

ANESTHESIA

All videoendoscopic procedures are performed under general anesthesia. No preoperative medication is given, but intravenous (IV) sedation is considered if indicated. Anesthesia is induced and maintained as has been described in Chapter 7. For prolonged cases, in addition to the usual monitors, an end-tidal CO_2 monitor is placed, and an oral gastric tube is inserted to empty the stomach contents. Anesthesia evaluation is always done prior to preparing the patient.

General anesthesia is maintained with 100% oxygen, an inhalational anesthetic (N_2O or isoflurane [Forane]), a continuous infusion of short-acting narcotic (alfentanil infused at a rate of 1 µg/kg/min), and a muscle relaxant (vecuronium bromide infused at a rate of 1 µg/kg/min). After reversal of the neuromuscular blockade, the patient usually wakes in 5 to 10 minutes. The administration of an antiemetic preinduction and the placement of an oral gastric tube may help to decrease postoperative nausea. With the rapid recovery from anesthesia and decreased amount of postlaparoscopic nausea in procedures lasting longer than 3 hours, the time taken from the end of the procedure to the patient's discharge from the hospital is usually 2 to 4 hours.

INSTRUMENTS

Insufflators and Irrigators

High-flow CO_2 insufflation up to 15 l/min is used to compensate for the rapid loss of CO_2 during suctioning. Models are available that filter the CO_2 gas, allowing it to recirculate after removal of smoke produced by electrosurgery or laser. The ability to maintain a constant intra-abdominal pressure between 10 and 15 mm Hg during long laparoscopic procedures is essential. Higher pressure settings may be used during initial insertion of the trocar, and the setting is lowered thereafter to diminish the development of subcutaneous emphysema.

Optics

Three laparoscopes are essential: a 10-mm 0-degree straight-viewing laparoscope, a 10-mm laser laparoscope with 5-mm laser channel and 5-mm operating channel adaptor to convert to an operative laparoscope, and a 5-mm straight-viewing laparoscope for introduction through 5-mm trocar sleeves. If possible, the laserscope should be aligned before surgery and should be kept on a separate table for immediate use, and a second operative laparoscope should be available for operative work. Oblique-angled scopes are useful for upper abdominal procedures. A HydroLaparoscope (Circon-ACMI) is now available with a built-in lens-washing and irrigation system to clean the distal lens during surgery and to rinse the operative site.

FIGURE 13–7 Self-retaining sleeve (Reich)

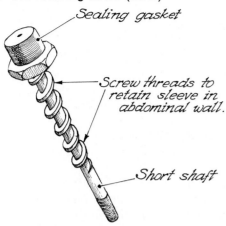

Sealing gasket

Screw threads to retain sleeve in abdominal wall.

Short shaft

Trocar Sleeves

Trocar sleeves are available in many sizes and shapes. For most instruments, 5.5-mm cannulas are adequate. Newer electrosurgical electrodes that eliminate capacitance and insulation failures (Electroshield from Electroscope) require 7- to 8-mm sleeves. Laparoscopic stapling is performed through 12- to 13-mm ports; fascial closure is often necessary to prevent incisional hernias from occurring in incisions larger than 5 mm.

We use trocar sleeves of a special design: short, self-retaining secondary to a screw wound around its external surface, and without a trap (Reich self-retaining sleeve, Richard Wolf Medical Instruments Corp.) (Fig. 13–7). These trocar sleeves facilitate efficient instrument exchanges and eliminate time spent reinserting sleeves removed during these exchanges. Once placed, their portal of exit stays fixed at the level of the anterior abdominal wall parietal peritoneum, permitting more room for instrument manipulation. A disposable, all-plastic version is available (Hunt-Reich trocar, Apple Medical).

Traditional lower quadrant trocar sleeves are too long for free access to pelvic structures with available instruments—the trocar sleeve falls into the operative field and must be lifted to open scissors or biopsy forceps when operating on structures directly beneath it. Slippage out of the peritoneal cavity is a concern during intraoperative instrument removal resulting in additional time spent re-establishing the second-puncture site. The traps or valves interfere with efficient instrument exchange and prohibit the introduction and removal of suture material and evacuation of tissue.

Aquadissector Pump and Accessories

The *aquadissector pump* is best positioned behind the surgeon with its handle either draped over the patient's left leg or on a sterile table within easy reach of the surgeon (see Fig. 13–2). Depending on the experience of the surgeon's assistant, it may be easier for the surgeon to make personal instrument exchanges from a sterile table behind him or her.

The usual irrigant is lactated Ringer's solution in 1-liter square plastic pour bottles (Travenol Labs). A screw cap facilitates bottle exchange; trocar puncture tube caps should be avoided. For suction, the Medi-Vac CRD Suction System (Baxter) with four 3000-ml canisters mounted on a carousel and hooked to wall suction at 200-mm Hg negative pressure is preferred. The canisters have a built-in filter that effectively traps aerosolized microorganisms and particulate matter. In addition, a shut-off valve prevents overflow. A laser plume filter (Baxter) is placed between the Medi-Vac CRD Suction System and wall suction.

Proficient use of aquadissection often requires the availability of many bottles of lactated Ringer's solution and specially trained surgical personnel to change them. Fortunately, most hospitals in the United States require a separate laser nurse to be available in the operating room throughout a procedure in which the laser may be used. In addition to turning the laser on and off, this nurse's ability to change 1-liter bottles rapidly makes aquadissection possible. An average of 10 liters of lactated Ringer's is used per case; more than 30 liters have been used occasionally. In the future, the development of compatible irrigant bottles with larger capacities will make this task easier.

Aquadissectors

Aquadissectors (suction-irrigators with the ability to dissect using pressurized fluid) should have a single channel to maximize suctioning and irrigating capacity. Separate suction and irrigation channels, either side by side or one inside the other, result in diminished suction capacity and reduced hydraulic effect. Clots stuck at the bifurcation of the single channel are dislodged by flushing through the tip of a 50-ml syringe.

The aquadissector should be designed so that the surgeon can operate with minimal upper arm and shoulder strain—with the upper arm at the surgeon's side. Complicated finger movements to activate the device rapidly lead to fatigue; thus large buttons are preferable to small valves. Arm comfort is essential because the aquadissector should convey "feel" through indirect manual contact with tissue.

An aquadissector with a solid (not perforated) distal tip is necessary to perform atraumatic suction-traction-retraction, irrigate directly, and develop surgical planes (aquadissection). Small holes at the tip impede these actions and serve no purpose. In addition, the shaft of the aquadissector should be bead blasted to produce a dull finish to minimize reflection when operating the CO_2 laser.

FIGURE 13–8 Aquadissector (Semm)

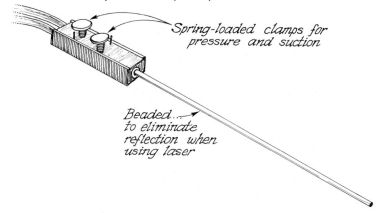

Spring-loaded clamps for pressure and suction

Beaded... to eliminate reflection when using laser

FIGURE 13–9 Wolf irrigator-aspirator

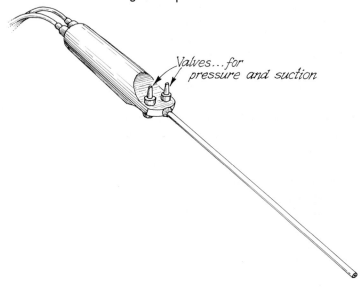

Valves...for pressure and suction

FIGURE 13–10 Eder aquadissector

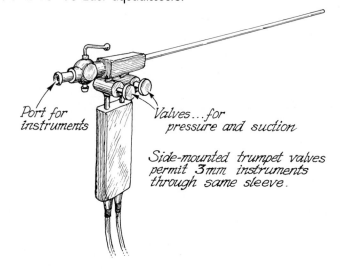

Port for instruments

Valves...for pressure and suction

Side-mounted trumpet valves permit 3mm instruments through same sleeve.

The Aqua-Purator (WISAP) was the first of the aquadissection devices (Fig. 13–8). It delivers fluid under 200-mm Hg pressure at a rate of 250 ml/10 sec. One liter can be instilled in 35 seconds. The handle of the Aqua-Purator uses large staples to occlude the suction and irrigation tubing, each of which funnels into a single-channeled tube. Problems frequently arise from malocclusion of the tubing, resulting in persistent leaking of irrigant or suctioning of pneumoperitoneum. It is not uncommon to require more than one handle to complete a difficult laparoscopic surgical procedure, and multiple handles should be available to ensure that one is in proper working order. The Wolf (Richard Wolf Medical Instruments Corp.) irrigator-aspirator is a less clumsy design, but the small valves are difficult to depress and tend to malfunction over time (Fig. 13–9).

Other aquadissection devices are available. The Irrivac (Baxter-Travenol), Pump-Vac systems (Gynescope), and Gyne-Flo Irrigator/Aspirator Cannula (Bard) are disposable devices, and in some the pressure can be controlled and varied by pushing on the automatically filling vacuum bulb or syringe in the system. The bag containing the irrigant is held at table level, usually attached to the patient's leg brace. These systems are particularly useful when attached to the cleaning channel of the Vancaillie microbipolar forceps (Storz) to obtain hemostasis from small arteriolar and venous bleeding sites near the end of the procedure.

WISAP has introduced a nonelectric CO_2-powered Aqua-Purator. Fluid is delivered at between 50 and 750 mm Hg of pressure. At 300 mm Hg of pressure, 1 liter can be instilled in 20 seconds.

Probes with an irrigation channel inside a suction channel studded with openings produce more efficient smoke evacuation for CO_2 laser surgery but hinder suction-traction and aquadissection. Many companies manufacture this type of device.

Several versions of combined suction-aspiration devices exist, consisting of 5-mm channels that allow a 3-mm needle electrode or scissors to pass through them for combined cutting, coagulation, irrigation, and aspiration (Fig. 13–10).

Pulsatile water jet irrigators (Gyne-Flo pump, Bard) generate high-pressure liquid pulsations by compressed nitrogen at a recommended pressure of 80 psi. This produces very efficient aquadissection. In addition, a dual spike adapter allows a multiple irrigation bag setup. Pulsatile aquadissection may also be possible with ultrasonic dissectors (CUSA: Valley Lab; Olympus). These devices vibrate at 23 kHz frequency with adjustable amplitude up to 350 μm and can selectively fragment soft, firm, and even tough, fibrous tissue. They have suction, irrigation, and electrosurgical cutting and coagulation abilities.

Forceps

Self-retaining, atraumatic forceps are the retractors of operative laparoscopy, maintaining exposure and position for surgery (Fig. 13–11A). At least two such instruments should be available. Blunt lead-shot–tipped forceps (see Fig. 13–11B) (WISAP) are used to retract small bowel. Strong atraumatic ovarian forceps, solid tipped (see Fig. 13–11C) or ring tipped, are applied to the uteroovarian ligament to stabilize or retract the ovary. Smooth-tipped, smooth-bodied atraumatic grasping forceps (see Fig. 13–11D) are used for ureteral dissection.

Single-tooth cupped biopsy forceps (see Fig. 13–11E) have been used extensively in laparoscopic surgery for more than 20 years and still grasp and hold tissue better than other forceps. This forceps is used to grasp the ovarian cyst wall firmly for dissection and avulsion. Two of them work well to separate the normal ovary from cyst walls. These forceps with teeth (see Fig. 13–11C) are used for grasping and pulling specimens through trocar sleeves during their removal.

Laparoscopic 5-mm corkscrews are the best instruments to place large solid masses on traction during myomectomy or hysterectomy. The 11-mm corkscrew inserted vaginally aids in all morcellation procedures.

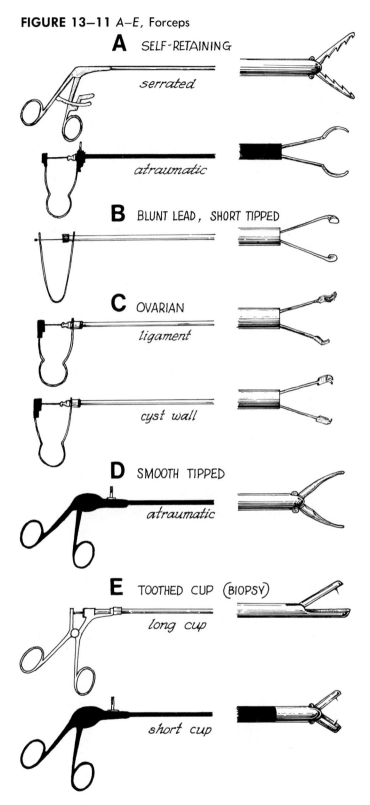

FIGURE 13–11 A–E, Forceps

A SELF-RETAINING
serrated
atraumatic

B BLUNT LEAD, SHORT TIPPED

C OVARIAN
ligament
cyst wall

D SMOOTH TIPPED
atraumatic

E TOOTHED CUP (BIOPSY)
long cup
short cup

FIGURE 13–12 Scissors

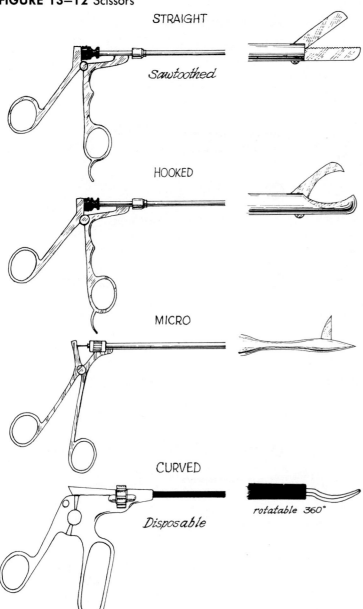

STRAIGHT

Sawtoothed

HOOKED

MICRO

CURVED

Disposable

rotatable 360°

Scissors

Sharp dissection is the primary technique used for adhesiolysis to diminish the potential for adhesion formation; electrosurgery and laser are usually reserved for hemostasis. Hooked, straight, and microscissors (3 mm and 5 mm) are used to lyse thin and thick bowel adhesions sharply (Fig. 13–12). Since scissors notoriously become dull after processing between operations, a large number and variety should be available to ensure that some will cut. Blunt-tipped, sawtooth scissors and disposable scissors hold their cutting edge. Hooked scissors are used when the surgeon can get completely around the structure being divided, but these scissors rarely maintain their sharpness. Microscissors, when sharp, are excellent for distal tubal work (e.g., fimbrioplasty and salpingostomy).

Electrosurgical Instruments

Electrosurgery is the mainstay of laparotomy surgery today. Because techniques for laparoscopic surgery are patterned on laparotomy, it seems logical that the instruments should match. The old FDA recommendation suggesting a low-power limit of under a 100-W and 600-V peak is outdated, because it prohibits fulguration with electrodes or the argon beam coagulator.

A 3-mm knife or 1-mm needle electrode is an excellent instrument for lysing adhesions and draining cysts (Fig. 13–13). The effective power density of the electrode can be modified by applying either the sharp tip or the wider body to the tissue being treated to gain the desired effect. The electrode is connected to an electrosurgical generator (Aspen Lab or Valley Lab Force 2 or 4). For lysing adhesions or draining cysts, nonmodulated "cutting" current (40 to 80 W) is used. Cutting current (and rarely coagulation current) through a knife, hook, or button electrode is used for coagulating specific blood vessels or hemorrhagic ovarian cysts. The vessel should be compressed to occlude it before coagulation. A quick application of cutting current following coagulation often avoids pulling off the char that results. Cutting current is used to produce varying degrees of coagulation during the cutting process with multiple different shaped electrodes—knife, hook, straight and curved spatula, spoon, and button (see Fig. 13–13). Coagulation current is used primarily to fulgurate in the noncontact application with high-voltage coagulation current.

Valley Lab has introduced a laparoscopic hand switch that provides electrosurgical, suction, and irrigation capabilities in one hand-piece and is compatible with six different electrode configurations. Other electrodes are available from Electroscope and Kirwin Surgical. Electroscope has introduced the Electroshield, a reusable sheath that surrounds existing laparoscopic electrodes to detect any insulation faults or capacitive coupling. This sheath should eliminate the potential for electrical burns beyond the view of the laparoscope.

FIGURE 13–13 Electrosurgical instruments.

NEEDLE ELECTRODE

KNIFE ELECTRODE

HOOK

CURVED SPATULA

BUTTON

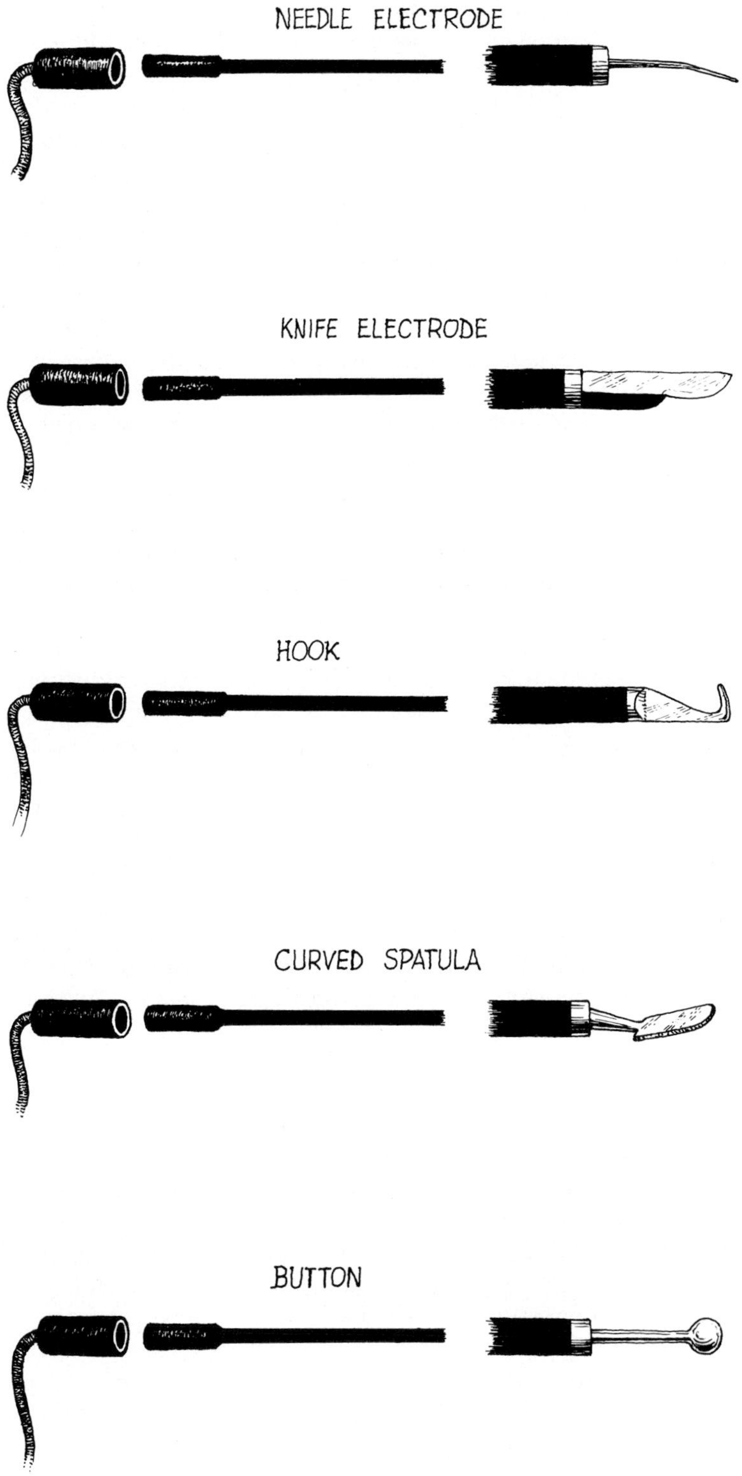

The Kleppinger bipolar forceps (see Fig. 11–4) with matched power source is an indispensable tool in all operative laparoscopies. The visual current flowmeter (Electroscope, Wolf) ensures that desiccation of tissue held by the forceps is complete. Although initially designed only to desiccate fallopian tubes, it has proved to be reliable for compressing and desiccating blood vessels that are too large to manage by surface coagulation or laser alone. Wolf Corp. has introduced a narrower version of this versatile forceps. Bipolar instruments with opposing forceps that do not touch may burn through vessels during desiccation, allowing the vessel to slip into its pedicle and making retrieval difficult.

The argon beam coagulator can be used to provide more powerful fulguration; spray coagulation current at 80 W will arc approximately 1 cm through the argon gas with resultant superficial charring and hemostasis. Uses include intraovarian bleeding after cystectomy and uterine hemostasis after myomectomy.

Laser

Use of the CO_2 laser through a laser laparoscope converts the umbilical incision into a portal for performing surgery, reducing the need for an additional incision. This delivery system results in a panoramic field of vision and allows the surgeon to reach otherwise inaccessible locations in the deep pelvis perpendicular to this field. The invisible CO_2 laser beam, composed of photons of electromagnetic radiation of 10.6-μm wavelength, is delivered to the laparoscope through mirrors fixed in an articulating arm. This beam then travels down the 5- to 8-mm–diameter operating channel of an operating laparoscope, with a focal point approximately 2 cm from the end of the laparoscope, remaining in focus for several centimeters beyond this point. This beam is adjusted into a 1-mm helium-neon spot with a micromanipulator joystick from which the tissue effect will be slightly greater than 1 mm (1.5 mm).

The passage of CO_2 gas through the laparoscope lumen, presently a necessity to purge this channel of debris, results in a decrease in power delivered to tissue and power density at tissue because of the 10.6-μm wavelength of the laser beam and the purge gas. Power is reduced by 30 to 50% with a 7.2-mm laparoscopic operating channel and by 60% with a 5-mm operating channel (see Table 3–1). Although it is desirable to operate at high-power density for a short time to minimize damage to surrounding tissue, the passage of CO_2 gas through the laparoscope lumen results in an increase in spot size and thus a reduction in power density (the concentration of laser energy on the tissue) at higher power settings. Considering these limitations with a Sharplan 1100 laser through a 5-mm operating channel, a setting of 20 to 35 W in superpulse mode is used for most procedures (<1000 W/cm^2 at the tissue) and between 80 and 100 W continuous mode to obtain a diffuse hemostatic effect for myomectomy and culdotomy. The Coherent Company has advanced CO_2 laser technology by modifying the 10.6-μm wavelength to 11.1 μm resulting in little interference in power transmission from the purge gas. With this modification, settings of 10 to 20 W ultrapulse are used for precise cutting and 50 to 80 W for extirpative procedures. Also little power is lost in the coherent coupler from the 6-mm raw beam. An ice-pack between the laserscope coupler and the surgeon's hand may be necessary to prevent skin burns when using lasers with larger raw beams and beam-coupler mismatches.

Fiber lasers (e.g., KTP, argon, and Nd:YAG) are not used because they hold no advantage over the cutting and coagulation possible with electrosurgery, CO_2 laser, and scissor combinations. The light energy from these lasers is converted to heat in tissue through light absorption by the proteinaceous structure of the tissue. This creates a much larger volume of tissue involved in the laser thermal effect, with coagulation initially and vaporization occurring only after protein is heated to greater than 100°C. In contrast, energy from the CO_2 laser is totally absorbed by water and rapidly converted to thermal energy with a much smaller volume of tissue involved in the laser thermal effect as cutting proceeds.

Suture Instruments

Laparoscopic needle holders are introduced through abdominal puncture sites to manipulate suture, needle, and involved tissue. Conventional laparoscopic needle holders have grooves at right angles to the longitudinal axis of the device and can grasp only straight needles securely (Fig. 13–14A). These straight needles are introduced by grasping the suture 2 cm from the needle and pulling the needle flattened out against the needle holder through a 5-mm cannula. The suture, 4–0 polydioxanone (PDS) on a tapered ST4 needle (Ethicon Z-420), 5–0 Vicryl (D-7676), or Vicryl, silk, or Gore-Tex on a manually straightened needle, is tied outside the peritoneal cavity using a Clarke knot pusher and pushed to the desired tissue. Average operating time for placing and tying a suture is less than 5 minutes.

An endoscopic curved needle driver (see Fig. 13–14B) (Cook OB/GYN, WISAP) is designed to hold a curved needle at 90 degrees to the shaft with little lateral motion. Oblique versions, right and left, hold the needle at a 45-degree angle to the shaft and are especially valuable for suture placement because of the fixed positions of the abdominal puncture sites. Special steps to insert curved needles through 5-mm puncture sites are described in Chapter 16. This device grasps the curved needle (CT-1, CT-2, or SH) and completes the suture needle placement with Gore-Tex or Vicryl (2–0: J-339, J-333, J-317; 3–0: J-316).

A pelviscopic loop ligature (Endoloop, Ethicon) consists of a 0-gauge chromic catgut with a preformed slipknot at its end (Fig. 13–15). The loop is placed around tissue to be ligated; the proximal tip of the introducer is broken off; and the suture is pulled through the introducer to tighten the loop.

FIGURE 13–14 A and B, Needle holders

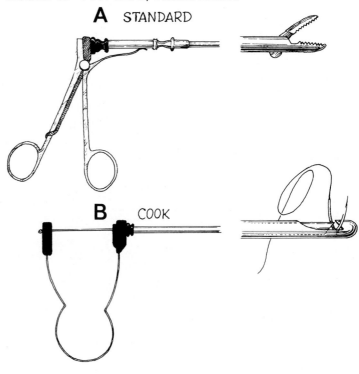

A STANDARD

B COOK

FIGURE 13–15 Endoloop

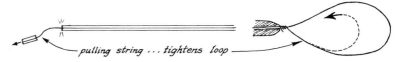

pulling string ... tightens loop

FIGURE 13–16 Clips.

A Hemostasis clip: single or multiple.

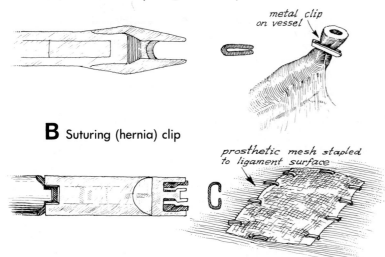

metal clip
on vessel

B Suturing (hernia) clip

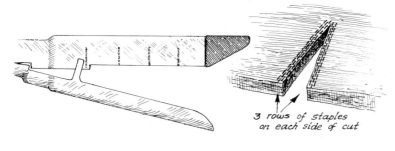

prosthetic mesh stapled
to ligament surface

FIGURE 13–17 Staples.

A Straight (ENDO GIA 30) for tissue division.

3 rows of staples
on each side of cut

B Circular (Premium CEEA) for rectosigmoid anastomosis

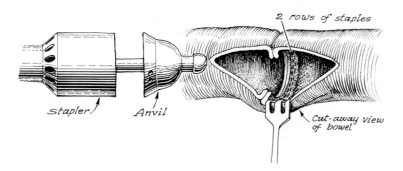

2 rows of staples

Stapler

Anvil

Cut-away view
of bowel

Clips and Staples

Disposable clip and stapling instrumentation for laparoscopic surgery is valuable for large-vessel hemostasis in procedures such as oophorectomy, hysterectomy, and cholecystectomy.

Individual clip applicators are available and may be appropriate when a few clips are used in a procedure (Fig. 13–16A). An automatic clip applier stacks 20 medium- or large-sized clips (9 mm long when closed) made of titanium, which is an inert, nonreactive metal. These disposable staplers are designed for introduction through a 10-mm trocar sleeve. Skeletonization of vessels is necessary before application of this staple. When applied to vessels with overlying peritoneum, the staple may slip off during further manipulation of the tissue.

A stapler designed for hernia repair (see Fig. 13–16B) will fix mesh to underlying fascia with a metal staple, thus acting as a metal suture. The final configuration of the staple is similar to the common paper staple.

A multiple stapler applicator (ENDO GIA Stapler) places six rows of staples, 30 mm in length, and divides the stapled tissue (Fig. 13–17A). This instrument functions similarly to the gastrointestinal anastomosis stapler that thoracic and general surgeons have used for the last 25 years. It is used for more rapid division of the adnexa during laparoscopically assisted hysterectomy.

A multiple staple applicator in a circular design (Premium CEEA) is intended for rapid end-to-end anastomosis of the rectosigmoid (see Fig. 13–17B). Introduced through the rectum, this large device fires off a circle of staples into aligned proximal and distal stumps of a rectosigmoid resection. The procedure can be done during laparoscopic resections of cul-de-sac endometriosis if there is a bowel constriction because of scarring.

Rectal, Vaginal, and Uterine Probes (Manipulators)

To define the rectum and posterior vagina in endometriosis and adhesion cases with some degree of cul-de-sac obliteration, a No. 3 or 4 Sims blunt curette or Hulka uterine elevator (Fig. 13–18A) is placed in the endometrial cavity to antevert the uterus markedly and stretch out the cul-de-sac. To define or open the posterior vagina (culdotomy), a sponge on a ring forceps (see Fig. 13–18B) is inserted into the posterior vaginal fornix and a No. 81 French rectal probe (see Fig. 13–18C) is placed in the rectum. A Valtchev uterine mobilizer with 100-mm long, 10-mm thick obturator is the best available single instrument to antevert the uterus and delineate the posterior vagina throughout complicated cases.

FIGURE 13–18 A–C, Probes for cul-de-sac dissection

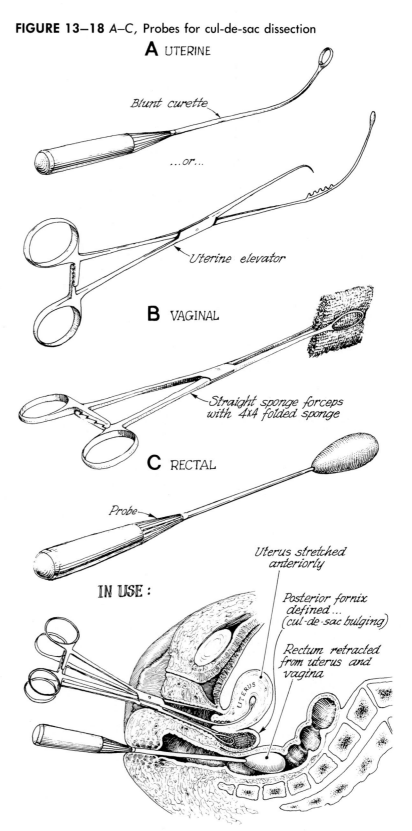

A UTERINE

Blunt curette

...or...

Uterine elevator

B VAGINAL

Straight sponge forceps with 4x4 folded sponge

C RECTAL

Probe

IN USE:

Uterus stretched anteriorly

Posterior fornix defined... (cul-de-sac bulging)

Rectum retracted from uterus and vagina

UTERUS

Lower Abdominal Incisions and Specimen Removal Techniques

Operative laparoscopy with video monitoring allows the surgeon and assistants to use multiple instruments under visual control. For most pelvic procedures, we prefer to limit the operative incisions to three: 10-mm umbilical and 5-mm right and left lower quadrant. Others add a fourth incision in the midline above the symphysis to allow four-handed surgery similar to laparotomy. More or larger incisions can lead to incisional hernias. In removing larger specimens, incisions need to be extended or created, and closed with sutures. In this chapter we review the choices and techniques of these incisions.

FIGURE 14–1 Lower quadrant incisions: optimal view

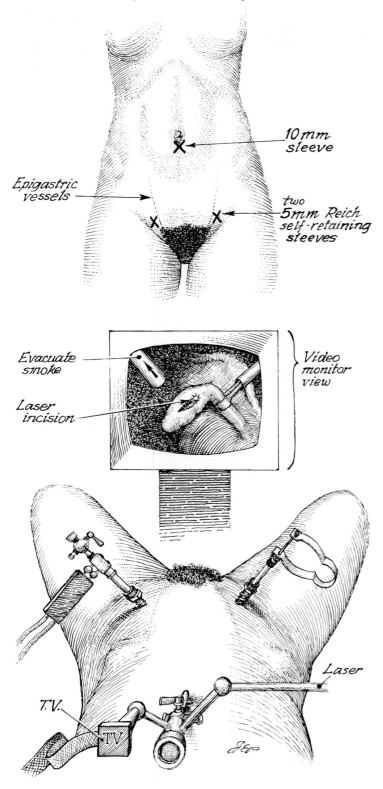

LOWER QUADRANT INCISIONS

Laparoscopic puncture sites should be kept to a minimum because deep fascia never fully regains its previous strength after division. Three puncture sites in the anterior abdominal wall are sufficient for 90% of laparoscopic procedures. Large puncture sites or incisions bordering on minilaparotomy should be replaced by an umbilical extension or by a laparoscopic culdotomy approach (see later).

Two uniform lower quadrant incisions are made regardless of the pathology involved. Consistency with incisions results in a spatially reproducible procedure with less time consumed making intraoperative decisions.

Lower quadrant incisions are made with a No. 11 blade near the top of the pubic hairline, adjacent to the deep inferior epigastric vessels (Fig. 14–1). These vessels, an artery flanked by two veins (venae comitantes), are located by direct inner laparoscopic inspection of the anterior abdominal wall. They are found lateral to the umbilical ligaments (obliterated umbilical artery) and generally cannot be consistently found by traditional transillumination. Placement of the trocar sleeves lateral to the deep epigastric vessels is preferred.

A 5-mm lower quadrant puncture is always made on the patient's left and is the major portal for operative manipulation. Mechanical malfunctions from the aquadissector are avoided by draping it over the patient's left leg and by connecting the tubing to wall suction and to a pressurized source of lactated Ringer's solution behind the surgeon. The tubing of the aquadissector, which is normally manipulated with the surgeon's left hand, is more likely to become kinked when stretched across the abdomen to a right-sided abdominal puncture site. Other instruments used through the left 5-mm puncture site include bipolar forceps, biopsy forceps, grasping forceps, scissors, and laparoscopic needle holders. Laparoscopic procedures are performed by the left hand; the right hand is the surgeon's "eye": it guides and focuses the optics and aims the laser beam. The recent availability of personnel trained to follow surgical procedures while holding the laparoscope makes it now possible for the surgeon to operate with two hands and should reduce the learning curve previously required to gain one-handed expertise.

A 5-mm trocar sleeve is inserted on the right side, and through it, atraumatic grasping forceps are used to retract tissues as needed.

NINTH INTERCOSTAL SPACE

Special entry techniques are necessary in patients who have undergone multiple laparotomies or who may have extensive adhesions either suspected clinically or known from another physician's operative record. If CO_2 insufflation is not obtainable through the umbilicus, a Veress needle puncture is done in the left ninth intercostal space, anterior axillary line (Reich, 1992). The trocar is then inserted at the left costal margin in the midclavicular line, giving a panoramic view of the entire peritoneal cavity. Likewise when extensive adhesions are encountered initially surrounding the umbilical puncture, the surgeon should immediately seek a higher site. Thereafter, the adhesions can be freed down to and just beneath the umbilicus, at which time it becomes possible to establish the umbilical portal for further work.

CLOSURE

The umbilical incision is closed with a 4–0 Vicryl suture opposing deep fascia and skin. The knot is buried beneath the fascia. Suture material is avoided in the lower quadrant skin incisions because their prolonged dissolution results in scarring. The lower quadrant 5-mm incisions are loosely approximated with Javid vascular clamps (V. Mueller) and covered with collodion (AMEND) to allow drainage of excess lactated Ringer's solution if increased intraabdominal pressure is present. Patients are instructed to expect leakage from the incision for 24 hours and to wait 1 week for the collodion to slough off. These wounds heal by secondary intention because they are clean, free from pressure, surrounded by mobile tissue, and have good blood supply. Minimal scarring results. Any other incisions that are larger than 5 mm require

fascial closure, since herniation with bowel obstruction can occur if these fascial defects are left unrepaired. Large incisions through the rectus muscle may require peritoneal closure to prevent herniation into the rectus sheath.

ALTERNATE INCISIONS FOR OVARY, MYOMA, AND GALLBLADDER EXTRACTION

Surgeons should be aware that incisional hernias can occur from lower quadrant incisions longer than 7 mm, since primary repair of deep fascia at these incisions is not always possible. Because of our bias against large lower quadrant incisions, techniques for umbilical incision enlargement and laparoscopic culdotomy were developed to remove ovaries from the peritoneal cavity. Postmenopausal cystic ovaries should be removed intact through the culde-sac, as should perimenopausal cystic ovaries that do not drain "chocolate"-like material on mobilization from their respective pelvic sidewall or uterosacral ligament. Large endometriomas in women not desiring future childbearing are usually sufficiently cystic and pliable so that, once separated from the pelvic sidewall, they can be removed through the umbilical incision.

Biopsies 8-mm or less in diameter are removed through laterally placed 5-mm lower quadrant incisions. After grasping a specimen larger than the 5-mm channel, the sleeve is slipped upward on the biopsy forceps shaft out of the peritoneal cavity; the biopsy forceps with the specimen is then pulled out in one motion through the soft tissue of the anterior abdominal wall. Biopsy forceps are then reinserted through their exit tract, and the sleeve is pushed back into the peritoneal cavity over the forceps. Initial placement of the sleeves lateral to the deep epigastric vessels facilitates this procedure, because it avoids going back and forth through the rectus muscle. The trocar penetrates the external oblique, internal oblique, and transversalis fascia only, leaving an easily identifiable tract.

For small ovaries, ruptured cysts without any solid components, or the appendix, an operating laparoscope is used. Biopsy forceps in the operating channel grasp the tissue, which is then partially delivered into

FIGURE 14–2 Umbilical incision extension

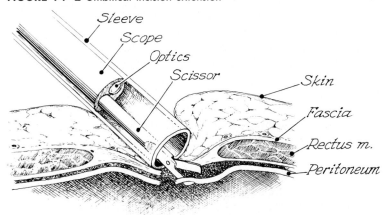

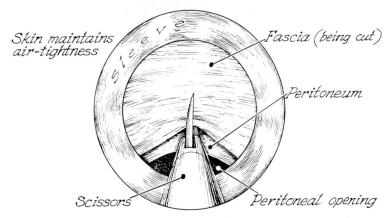

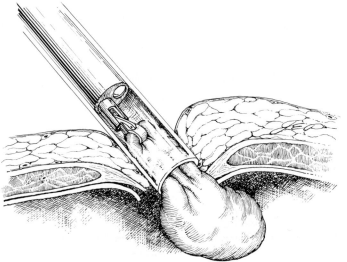

Specimen grasped, pulled into sleeve...

Sleeve, scope, and specimen removed...

*Skin and fascia further enlarged,
    as necessary.*

the tip of the 10-mm umbilical sleeve. Holding the biopsy forceps steady, the sleeve and laparoscope are popped out of the umbilicus in one motion, after which the protruding tissue is grasped with hemostats or Kocher clamps and is gently teased out of the peritoneal cavity. Alternatively a 5-mm laparoscope can be used for visualization through the 5-mm lower sleeve, and the tissue to be removed can be grasped with an 11-mm grasping forceps inserted through the umbilicus and extracted.

UMBILICAL EXTENSION

For gallbladders, ovaries (benign pathology), and small fibroids, the umbilical incision can be enlarged, especially if the initial skin incision was vertical intraumbilical overlying the area where skin, deep fascia, and parietal peritoneum of the anterior abdominal wall meet as described earlier. The operating laparoscope is used with scissors in the operating channel (Fig. 14–2). The tip of the laparoscope is placed 1 cm above the tip of the sleeve, which is then carefully removed from the peritoneal cavity. The peritoneum is visualized first and incised downward in the midline with the scissors in the operating channel of the operating laparoscope. Next, deep fascia is identified and incised to add another centimeter or more to the incision. Finally, the skin incision inside the umbilicus can be extended upward to incorporate the superior wall of the umbilical fossa. Most gallbladders and decompressed ovaries can be removed through this incision. The fascia and skin are closed with a single 4–0 Vicryl suture, opposing deep fascia and skin with the knot buried beneath the fascia.

An alternative is the selection of an open laparoscopy method (see Chapter 8) when removal of a large specimen is anticipated. The fascia and skin can be extended and repaired under direct vision using the standard laparotomy technique (Silva et al, 1991).

LAPAROSCOPIC CULDOTOMY

Ovarian cysts of unknown pathology separated intact from the pelvic sidewall are best removed through the cul-de-sac. A posterior *culdotomy* incision using a CO_2 laser or electrosurgery through the cul-de-sac of Douglas into the vagina (Fig. 14–3) is preferable to a *colpotomy* incision with scissors through the vagina and overlying peritoneum, because complete hemostasis is obtained while making the incision. The anatomic relationship between the rectum and the posterior vagina must be confirmed to avoid cutting the rectum while making the laparoscopic culdotomy incision. A curette or controlling forceps is placed in the uterus for elevation; a wet sponge at the end of a ring forceps is placed just behind the cervix to identify the posterior vaginal fornix; and a rectal probe (Reznik Instruments) ensures that the rectum is out of the way and aids in the dissection required if the rectum covers the posterior vagina. Alternatively, a Valtchev uterine mobilizer (Conkin Surgical Instruments) can be inserted to antevert the uterus and delineate the posterior vagina. With this device, the cervix sits on a wide acorn that is readily visible between the uterosacral ligaments when the cul-de-sac is inspected laparoscopically.

Before the rectal probe is removed, it may be necessary to reflect the rectum off the posterior vaginal fornix. This is performed using either cutting current through a spatula electrode or the laparoscopic CO_2 laser at 35-W superpulse or 20-W ultrapulse. The peritoneum at the junction of the rectum and vagina is incised. Using the aquadissector, the plane between the rectum and the vagina is developed and the rectum is pushed downward.

Following these maneuvers, and when it is clear that the rectum has been separated off the posterior wall of the vagina or vaginal apex if the uterus has been removed, the upper vagina or posterior fornix is distended by the wet sponge on ring forceps (see Fig. 14–3). The transverse laparoscopic culdotomy incision is made with the spatula electrode at 80 W of cutting current or the CO_2 laser with power set at 50 to 100 W continuous or ultrapulse. This incision is usually bloodless, and the sponge in the posterior vagina rapidly comes into view.

FIGURE 14–3 Laparoscopic culdotomy

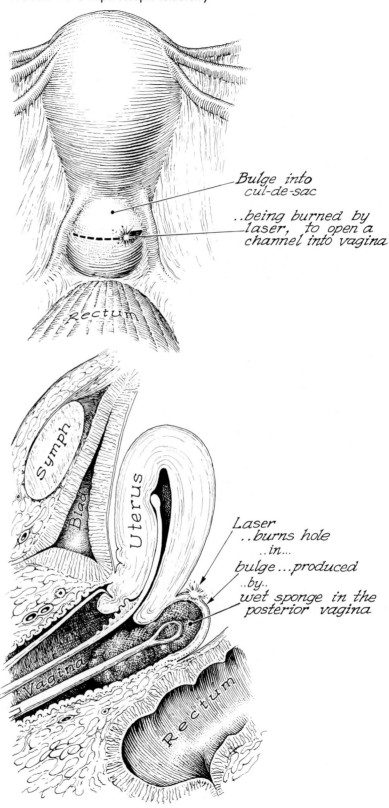

Bulge into cul-de-sac

..being burned by laser, to open a channel into vagina

Rectum

Symph

Bla...

Uterus

Vagina

Rectum

Laser ..burns hole ..in... bulge...produced ..by.. wet sponge in the posterior vagina

FIGURE 14–4 Large ovarian cyst removed through a cul-de-sac

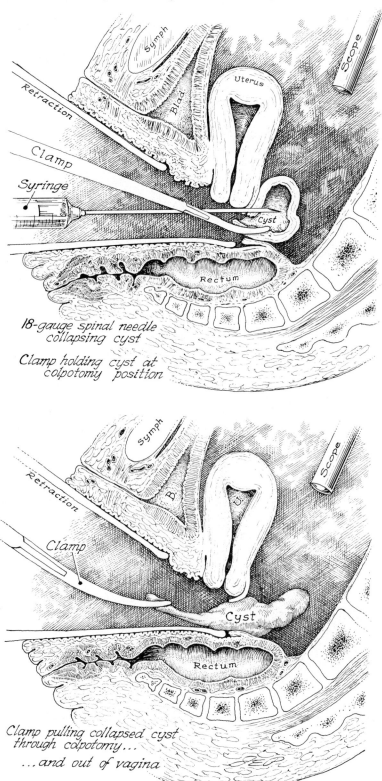

18-gauge spinal needle collapsing cyst

Clamp holding cyst at colpotomy position

Clamp pulling collapsed cyst through colpotomy...

...and out of vagina

Some difficulty may be encountered maintaining adequate pneumoperitoneum once the vagina is entered, but a damp sponge in contact with the incision is usually adequate for this purpose. A culpotome designed to allow electrosurgical entrance of the cul-de-sac from below while monitoring from above is being developed. A long, disposable 10- or 11-mm diameter trocar without the sleeve can also be inserted vaginally under laparoscopic control. Ring forceps are then used to enlarge the incision with blunt dissection by opening the forceps. Further enlargement is done vaginally with Mayo scissors. The incision and enlargement take 1 minute or less (Childers et al, 1993). Laparoscopic biopsy or ring forceps can then be inserted through the vagina, using the damp sponge to prevent peritoneal gas loss, and used to grasp the ovary and pull it out through the culdotomy incision. Alternately, a 5-mm lower quadrant grasping forceps can be used to push the mass through the culdotomy incision. On occasion, the operator's fingers can be inserted into the peritoneal cavity and used to grasp the ovary.

The potential danger of grasping bowel with a sharp grasper through the vagina is always present if the surgeon loses sight of the lesion to be extracted. Following culdotomy, a sponge, pack, or 30-ml Foley balloon should be kept in close contact with the vaginal incision to avoid the loss of pneumoperitoneum and to facilitate the extraction of large masses.

For removal of large ovarian cystic masses (Fig. 14–4), a 14- to 18-gauge needle on a needle extension adapter (Crown Brothers) directed through the vagina is used for decompression or, if a dermoid is present, the mass can be incised so that the contents of the thick cyst drain into the vagina until the mass is small enough to be pulled through the incision (Levine, 1990).

Our most recent technique is to insert an impermeable sac (LapSac: Cook OB/GYN) intraperitoneally through the culdotomy incision. This 5- by 8-in. nylon bag has a polyurethane inner coating and a nylon drawstring. It is impermeable to water and dye. The ovary with intact cyst is placed in the bag, which is closed by pulling its drawstring. The sac is delivered by the drawstring through the posterior vagina; the bag is opened, and the intact specimen is visually identified, decompressed, and removed.

For fibroids, a tenaculum or 11-mm corkscrew (WISAP) is inserted through the vagina by maneuvering it around the sponge to minimize loss of pneumoperitoneum. The fibroid is grasped under direct laparoscopic vision. In some cases the fibroid can be pushed into the deep cul-de-sac and held there while a second surgeon identifies it from below and applies the tenaculum. An 11-mm corkscrew device is screwed into the myoma vaginally through the culdotomy incision; the myoma is put on traction at the incision and is further morcellated vaginally with scissors or a scalpel if necessary until removal is completed. The culdotomy incision is closed with interrupted or running 0 Vicryl sutures applied vaginally or with a figure-of-eight 0 Vicryl suture laparoscopically. Vaginal suturing is aided by use of a lateral vaginal retractor used to spread the lateral vagina adjacent to the culdotomy incision (Euro-Med, Inc. or Simpson/Basye). This device is self-retaining and has a thumb-ratchet release that keeps it open and in place. Vaginal suturing can be difficult as the vaginal incision frequently becomes edematous during the procedure, making exposure inadequate. In these cases, the surgeon may elect to close the culdotomy incision from above using one to three curved needle sutures (Vicryl on a CT-2 or CT-1) tied extracorporeally with the Clarke knot pusher.

Whereas culdotomy surgery offers an opportunity for invasion by organisms that are already present in the genital tract, the use of an electrosurgical or laser incision, aspiration of all blood clots, and copious irrigation with over 2 liters of irrigant left in the peritoneal cavity at the close of the procedure eliminates the environment necessary for proliferation of these organisms. Pelvic cellulitis and postoperative sepsis with laparoscopic culdotomy using these techniques have not been reported.

FUTURE CONSIDERATIONS

While morcellation of fibroids is too time consuming with presently available instruments, future developments should solve this problem for the gynecologist. Cook Urological has developed a motorized circular saw with suction for laparoscopic nephrectomy. After the kidney is placed in the LapSac, it is morcellated into small soft pieces that are sucked into the device until the LapSac is small enough to be pulled out of the umbilicus. This instrument can be used for myoma morcellation during laparoscopic hysterectomy. A 2-cm version for culdotomy morcellation will soon be available.

Semm and WISAP have developed a manual circular saw to core out 2-cm cylinders of fibromyomatous tissue while the fibroid is still in or attached to the uterus. This device is inserted through a 2-cm cannula and depends on a corkscrew inside it to fixate the fibroid prior to twisting the circular saw into it. Loss of resistance during the twisting indicates the base of the fibroid after which the cylindrical specimen is pulled free by traction, the specimen is removed, and the instrument is reinserted. After the bulk of the lesion is removed in this fashion, a claw forceps is substituted for the corkscrew in the device for traction and the compressible, fenestrated, remaining tissue is removed from the uterus through the 2-cm cannula.

REFERENCES

Childers JM, Huang D, and Surwit EA: Laparoscopic trocar-assisted colpotomy. Obstet Gynecol *81*:153–155, 1993.

Levine RL: Pelviscopic surgery in women over 40. J Reprod Med *35*:597–600, 1990.

Reich H: Laparoscopic bowel injury. Surg Laparosc Endosc *2*:74, 1992.

Silva PD, Kuffel ME, and Beguin EA: Open laparoscopy simplifies instrumentation required for laparoscopic oophorectomy and salpingo-oophorectomy. Obstet Gynecol *77*:482–485, 1991.

FURTHER READINGS

Reich H: Laparoscopic oophorectomy and salpingo-oophorectomy in the treatment of benign tuboovarian disease. Int J Fertil *32*:233–236, 1987.

Reich H: Laparoscopic oophorectomy without ligature or morcellation. Contemp Obstet/Gynecol *9*:34–46, 1989.

Reich H: New techniques in advanced laparoscopic surgery. Baillieres Clin Obstet Gynecol *3*:655–681, 1989.

Reich H, Clarke HC, and Sekel L: A simple method for ligating with straight and curved needles in operative laparoscopy. Obstet Gynecol *79*:143–147, 1992.

Lysis of Adhesions

LAPAROSCOPIC ADHESIOLYSIS

Laparoscopy is replacing laparotomy as the method of choice for lysing most pelvic adhesions. It appears in animal studies (Luciano et al, 1989) and clinical studies (Lundorff et al, 1991) that laparoscopy leads to fewer de novo adhesions as seen at second look compared with laparotomy. This finding may be because of the absence of retraction and packing that can damage peritoneum, gentler handling of tissue, no drying in room air, and no foreign bodies such as glove talc and lint. Also, the excellent visualization and close-up magnification of adhesions possible with laparoscopy compensate for the more difficult exposure and dissection techniques required.

No widely accepted terminology exists for adhesions. Operative reports, current literature, and textbooks all rely on a poorly defined set of descriptive terms. In general, *adhesions* are characterized as dense or filmy, broad or thin, opaque or translucent, and vascular or avascular. Extirpated adhesions are rarely adequate for pathologic examination. In most cases, it is not possible, even with close visual inspection, to relate the physical appearance of an adhesion to its underlying cause, unless the patient's medical or surgical history is relatively simple and well documented. Thus, adhesions from pelvic inflammatory disease and prior surgery may look the same.

Indications for lysis of adhesions are under continuous evaluation and evolution. At diagnostic laparoscopy, all surgeons should be prepared to do some dissection and lysis simply to get to the pathology to make a diagnosis of tubal occlusion or extensive endometriosis. Therapeutic lysis is indicated under some conditions of infertility and pelvic pain.

For Infertility

An analysis of our results and those in the literature have led us to classify patients (see Chapter 9) with adhesions into three groups.

STAGE I. Those who definitely will benefit from laparoscopic lysis in terms of take-home babies (THB). This stage involves adhesions that cover less than half of the ovary and are mostly filmy. The distribution and nature of adhesions elsewhere has little prognostic value for fertility. Tubes should be patent with normal fimbriae. More than half of these patients will have successful pregnancies and their adhesions should be lysed at laparoscopy.

STAGE II. Those who may benefit. This stage includes anything between stages I and III.

STAGE III. Those who will not and should go directly to in vitro fertilization (IVF). This stage involves adhesions of any nature that cover the entire surface of the ovary. Adhesion re-formation on the ovary, even with current preventive efforts, results in successful pregnancy rates of less than 12%, which is less than the rate that can be achieved with IVF. These patients should therefore be spared the expense of extensive lysis and should be directed to an IVF program.

For Pain

Since adhesions form immediately after surgery, postoperative adhesions causing pain usually do so within 1 or 2 months after surgery. Pelvic pain, especially chronic pain over 6 months' duration and arising months or years after surgery, is thus seldom causally related to postsurgical adhesions, and more elusive psychologic trauma and scars need to be sought and dealt with. Adhesions from endometriosis or infection may be progressive over time and causally related to chronic pain, but these adhesions may also be incidental findings in a patient with deeper psychologic origins of chronic pain. Studies of pelvic findings in patients undergoing laparoscopy for chronic pain, compared with patients with infertility and no complaints of pain, have generally shown no statistical difference between the nature or distribution of adhesions or other pathology found (Peters et al, 1991; Rapkin, 1986; Stout et al, 1991; Walker et al, 1988). A suggestion has even been made that laparoscopy has no therapeutic value alone compared with a total pain management program (Peters et al, 1991). Most pelvic pain is relieved after laparoscopy for 3 to 6 months, but pain of central nervous origin is re-established within 1 year in 60% of patients (Steege and Stout, 1991). These considerations should be taken into account by the operative laparoscopist before a second or third attempt is made at relieving chronic pain surgically.

The duration and severity of pain correlate poorly with the extent and location of adhesions. Before the introduction of laparoscopic techniques to lyse adhesions and minimize their recurrence, many surgeons were reluctant to attempt therapy, unless the adhesions caused bowel obstruction.

CHOICE OF TECHNIQUES

Lysis of adhesions by laparoscopy follows the same principles of dissection that lysis by laparotomy requires. Surgeons attempting laparoscopic lysis should be thoroughly experienced, preferably through microsurgery, with the techniques of blunt and sharp dissection, unipolar electrosurgical division, and bipolar electrodesiccation for hemostasis. The following is a brief description of some of these principles and the reasons for choosing different techniques for different problems.

Adhesions are the end result of an old healing process in which normal tissue attempted to provide a blood supply to damaged tissue (see Chapter 6). Recent adhesions may therefore be vascular, but old adhesions may either be dense or surprisingly thin. The nature of these adhesions can best be studied by putting the two adherent structures on a stretch in order to put the fibers of the adhesion under tension. For uterine and some adnexal structures, this can be accomplished laparoscopically with the use of one grasping forceps and the uterine manipulator or with two second-puncture grasping forceps. After studying the adhesion in detail by a close-up and magnified view (better than at laparotomy), the following choices can be made.

Blunt Dissection

Using a forceps, the tip of an aquairrigator, or a blunt-tipped scissors, firm pressure can be put on the adhesion directly, firmly stabilizing one structure (e.g., ovary) and maintaining tension on the other structure to encourage separation. The forceps pulling the adhesion away may supply all the tension necessary to divide the adhesion if it is thin. This is the first approach to adhesion division, since blunt dissection allows thin adhesions to separate along the correct anatomic cleavage planes separating the two structures. A surprising number of abdominal wall adhesions can be lysed this way, since blood supply from the abdominal wall is usually excellent and the adhesions are relatively avascular. How much tension, when to turn to another technique, and so forth are matters of accumulated surgical experience. Adhesions from acute inflammatory processes such as salpingitis with tubo-ovarian abscess or appendiceal abscess can be completely lysed with gentle blunt dissection using a probe or aquadissection, since vascularization and collagen deposition do not begin for at least 7 days. Sharp dissection or laser treatment for hemostasis is rarely necessary.

Sharp Dissection

As adhesive structures are separated, one always sees a few fibrous bands denser than the others that resist blunt dissection. These bands need to be studied carefully by close magnification and temporarily relaxing tension to see if these structures are vascular. Most are not and can be divided most rapidly and safely with sharp scissors. Blunt-tipped scissors with serrated edges are preferred (see Fig. 13–12), since their rounded tips minimize the risk of opening up a hole in the surface being dissected (e.g., peritoneum, bowel). A very small bite of the resistant fiber is taken under full direct vision, and when the scissors are closed the scissor tip is pushed immediately forward to put the remaining adhesion under tension and extend the dissection bluntly. The scissors are held as flat as possible along the surface being dissected to minimize the creation of a false plane between the adhered surfaces.

Omental adhesions to the anterior abdominal wall are divided mechanically using scissors through the operating channel of an operating laparoscope. Electrosurgery and laser should be avoided when the adhesions block identification of the structures behind them because loops of small bowel can frequently be present, fused to the anterior parietal peritoneum. If the surgeon holds the operating laparoscope with the viewing channel in the transverse plane, this results in the scissors exiting it at a 3 o'clock position (Fig. 15–1). Better dissection can often be obtained by swinging the viewing channel to the 6 o'clock position, because the operating scissors then exit at a 12 o'clock position flush with the interface between the omental adhesion and the parietal peritoneum. For dense adhesions near small bowel loops, the aquadissector can be inserted into the laparoscope's operating channel and used to distend the adhesion interface prior to its division. After all of the adhesions are divided, persistent omental and anterior abdominal wall bleeding sites are identified and coagulated with microbipolar forceps.

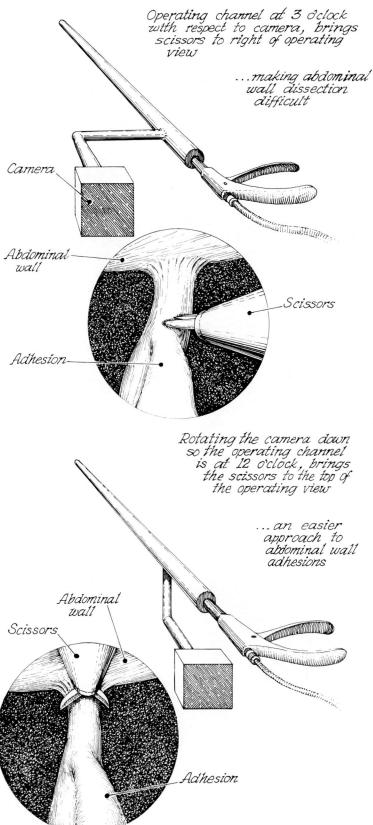

FIGURE 15–1 Scissors at 3 and 12 o'clock positions

FIGURE 15–2 Aquadissection

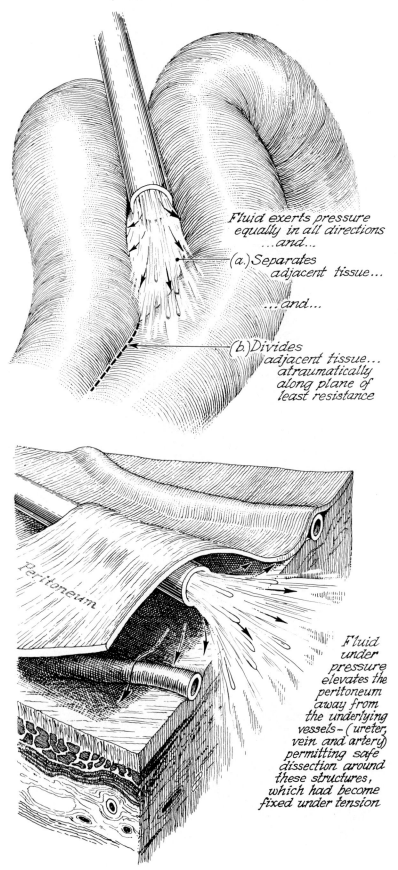

Fluid exerts pressure
equally in all directions
...and...

(a.) Separates
adjacent tissue...

...and...

(b.) Divides
adjacent tissue...
atraumatically
along plane of
least resistance

Peritoneum

Fluid
under
pressure
elevates the
peritoneum
away from
the underlying
vessels–(ureter,
vein and artery)
permitting safe
dissection around
these structures,
which had become
fixed under tension

Aquadissection

A suction-irrigator-dissector (aquadissector) is the first instrument in and the last out for most laparoscopic procedures. Between the beginning and the end of the operation, this device can be used to irrigate; evacuate smoke, clot, and debris; suction-retract; and perform blunt dissection with its tip using the hydraulic pressure of fluid delivered through it.

In the late 1970s, aquadissection was developed as a laparoscopic technique to separate newly formed adhesions at second-look laparoscopy following laparotomy reconstructive surgery, to divide acute adhesions during pelvic abscess surgery, and to free ovaries stuck to the pelvic sidewall and uterosacral ligament (Reich and McGlynn, 1987).

Aquadissection is broadly defined as the use of pressurized fluid to aid in the performance of surgical procedures. The aquadissector can be considered a substitute for the laparoscopic surgeon's fingers, with aquadissection the method of performing blunt or finger dissection.

The technique uses the hydraulic energy of pressurized fluid (Fig. 15–2). This energy differs from the mechanical energy applied with a blunt probe, which is a unidirectional force, the direct prolongation of the surgeon's hands. The force with hydraulic energy is multidirectional within the volume of expansion of the noncompressible fluid. Instillation of fluid under pressure displaces tissue, often resulting in the fluid's creating cleavage planes in the least resistant spaces. In addition, the instillation of fluid under pressure into closed spaces or behind enclosed areas of adhesions produces edematous, distended tissue on tension with resultant loss of elasticity. Thereafter, it is possible to disrupt the tissue safely using blunt dissection, scissors dissection, laser, or electrosurgery.

Aquadissection is performed by placing the tip of the aquadissector against the adhesive interface between bowel-adnexa, adnexa-pelvic sidewall, or gallbladder-liver and using the pressurized fluid gushing from it to develop a cleavage plane that can be extended either bluntly or with more fluid pressure. Often, adhesions can be "weakened" with laser treatment and then taken down with aquadissection using either the hydraulic effect or suction-traction. Aquadissection is used to develop and distend the retroperitoneal spaces to aid in their dissection during the excision of endometriosis on the peritoneal undersurface and for retroperitoneal surgery. Aquadissection into closed adhesive spaces or the retroperitoneum can be considered another way to put the tissue to be dissected on tension.

Suction-traction refers to the use of the suction capability of the aquadissector to retract adhesions and viscera; it can be done only with a solid distal tip device. Suction-traction can be used early in the operation to elevate the bowel to gain better visualization of its attachments and to elevate the gallbladder for a better look at its undersurface. Small bowel and appendix can also be easily lifted to identify intervening adhesions better prior to their division.

Electrodissection

Microsurgeons who are familiar with the use of a fine electrode under magnification may want to try this technique laparoscopically. A fine unipolar needle can dissect dense or vascular adhesions very well, with excellent hemostasis. However, the fine control of microsurgery is not available through the more clumsy laparoscopic technique, and electrodissection is usually reserved for dense adhesions between two relatively safe structures (e.g., uterus, abdominal wall, ovary, or omentum). The risks of unipolar dissection arise from the unpredictable direction in which the electrons flow through tissue to reach the ground plate. If unipolar dissection is used near ureter or bowel, such as on omental adhesions within 1 to 2 cm of bowel, electron flow may pass through the bowel to cause postoperative perforation. At this point, sharp or laser dissection is preferred.

Bipolar Coagulation before Division

Dense, vascular pedicles of adhesions can be well managed by compressing and desiccating them with a bipolar forceps before sharp division with scissors. This procedure is usually feasible with some adhesive systems between the omentum and the abdominal wall or the ovary. The risk with this procedure is that the contents of the omentum may not be fully identified, and a loop of bowel may be involved. If dense, vascular adhesions are on a bowel surface and need dissection, a laparotomy may be indicated at this point to control the bleeding with suture ligatures.

Laser Dissection

The technique of laser dissection is presented last to emphasize that a good deal of laparoscopic dissection can be accomplished with the techniques described earlier and also to emphasize that laser treatment offers no biologic advantage over electrosurgery. Luciano and associates (1987) showed in rabbits that when equal power densities (W/cm^2) are applied to tissue using electricity or laser, the patterns of thermal injury and postoperative adhesion formation are identical. This confirmed the report of Filmar and colleagues (1986) that electromicrosurgery and the CO_2 laser were equally effective in adhesiolysis in the rat model and also supported an important clinical observation made by Tulandi (1986). In a prospective, randomized study comparing the CO_2 laser with electromicrosurgery in patients undergoing salpingo-ovariolysis, there was no difference in subsequent pregnancy rates.

However, there are situations in which the CO_2 laser is preferred for technical advantages.

DIFFICULT EXPOSURE. All available secondary trocars and uterine manipulators may be necessary to expose some of the more difficult adhesions between the ovary and the pelvic sidewall. At this point, a laser laparoscope with the beam coaxial with the line of vision becomes the easiest tool for lysis, since the surgeon uses the laparoscope itself as a scalpel to aim the beam precisely at the adhesion to be dissected. The aquadissector can be well used as both a backstop and a smoke evacuator in these difficult areas.

OOZING ADHESIONS. Dense adhesions between the tube, uterus, and ovary may require the moderate hemostasis that the laser provides in the focused mode. In these situations, great care must be taken with constant checking of the anatomy, since the laser can easily create a false plane into, rather than between, structures. A backstop for the laser is seldom needed in these dense tissues.

BOWEL AND URETER. When adhesions are dense and close to areas where the ureter may be, such as dense ovarian or tubal adhesions in the ovarian fossa, laser treatment is a relatively safe way to separate these structures to minimize bleeding and adjacent tissue destruction. If omental or bowel adhesions need dissection with hemostasis, again the laser will do so with minimal risk of bowel damage, compared with the use of electric current in these situations. For these reasons, some laparoscopists prefer laser treatment for all omental adhesions in which hemostasis may be required.

PREVENTION OF ADHESION RECURRENCE

Our current belief is that minimal tissue compromise at surgery is the key to minimal adhesion reformation. Sharp, clean dissection with scissors or vaporization with a laser leaves few anoxic cells to provoke adhesion formation. Allowing oozing tissue to constrict and clot spontaneously for at least 5 minutes minimizes the need for coagulation hemostasis and its trauma to adjacent normal tissue. Leaving a large volume of lactated Ringer's solution in the abdomen allows dilution of the angiogenic factors arising from operated surfaces, as well as causing some physical separation of normal and compromised structures. The use of 1000 to 2000 ml of lactated Ringer's solution left intraperitoneally postoperatively is widely employed, appears to be retained for the first 3 critical days postoperatively (Rose et al, 1991), but has never been prospectively studied in humans. An animal study comparing Gore-Tex, Interceed, and lactated Ringer's solution showed that lactated Ringer's solution was superior to the others in preventing adhesion formation (Pagidas and Tulandi, 1992). Second-look laparoscopy is effective in further reducing adhesions in most patients but not in improving subsequent fertility rates (Trimbos-Kemper et al, 1985; Tulandi et al, 1989).

Other chemical adjuvants have had mixed reports. Use of both Hyskon (Pharmacia, Inc.) and Interceed (Johnson & Johnson Patient Care, Inc.) has resulted in negative experiences after initial good results (Drollette and Badawy, 1992). Steroids and antihistamines have a similar history and are no longer popular. Ibuprofen is used postoperatively as a safe regimen with little documentation of efficacy in humans.

Prevention of ovarian adhesion re-formation continues to be a challenge for both the surgeon and the pharmacologist.

REFERENCES

LYSIS OF ADHESIONS

Drollette CM and Badawy SZA: Pathophysiology of pelvic adhesions: Modern trends in preventing infertility. J Reprod Med 37:107–121, 1992.

Filmar S, Gomel V, and McComb P: The effectiveness of CO_2 laser and electromicrosurgery in adhesiolysis: A comparative study. Fertil Steril 45:407–411, 1986.

Luciano AA, Maier DB, Koch EI, et al: A comparative study of postoperative adhesions following laser surgery by laparoscopy versus laparotomy in the rabbit model. Obstet Gynecol 74:220–224, 1989.

Luciano AA, Whitman G, Maier DB, et al: A comparison of thermal injury, healing patterns, and postoperative adhesion formation following CO_2 laser and electromicrosurgery. Fertil Steril 48:1025–1029, 1987.

Lundorff P, Hahlin M, Källfelt B, et al: Adhesion formation after laparoscopic surgery in tubal pregnancy: A randomized trial versus laparotomy. Fertil Steril 55:911–915, 1991.

Pagidas K and Tulandi T: Effects of Ringer's lactate, Interceed (TC7) and Gore-Tex Surgical Membrane on postsurgical adhesion formation. Fertil Steril 57:199–201, 1992.

Reich H: Laparoscopic treatment of extensive pelvic adhesions including hydrosalpinx. J Reprod Med 32:736–742, 1987.

Reich H and McGlynn F: Laparoscopic treatment of tuboovarian and pelvic abscess. J Reprod Med 32:747–752, 1987.

Rose BI, MacNeill C, Larrain R, and Kopreski MM: Abdominal instillation of high-molecular-weight dextran or lactated Ringer's solution after laparoscopic surgery: A randomized comparison of the effect on weight change. J Reprod Med 74:537–539, 1991.

Trimbos-Kemper TC, Trimbos JB, and van Hall EV: Adhesion formation after tubal surgery: Results of the eighth-day laparoscopy in 188 patients. Fertil Steril 43:395–400, 1985.

Tulandi T: Salpingo-ovariolysis: A comparison between laser surgery and electrosurgery. Fertil Steril 45:489–491, 1986.

Tulandi T, Falcone T, and Kafka I: Second-look operative laparoscopy 1 year following reproductive surgery. Fertil Steril 52:421–424, 1989.

PAIN

Peters AAW, van Dorst E, Jellis B, et al: A randomized clinical trial to compare two different approaches in women with chronic pelvic pain. Obstet Gynecol 77:740–744, 1991.

Rapkin AJ: Adhesions and pelvic pain: A retrospective study. Obstet Gynecol 68:13–15, 1986.

Steege JF and Stout AL: Resolution of chronic pelvic pain after laparoscopic lysis of adhesions. Am J Obstet Gynecol 165:278–281, 1991.

Stout AL, Steege JF, Dodson WC, and Hughes CL: Relationship of laparoscopic findings to self-report of pelvic pain. Am J Obstet Gynecol 164:73–79, 1991.

Walker E, Katon W, Harrop-Griffiths J, et al: Relationship of chronic pelvic pain to psychiatric diagnoses and childhood sexual abuse. Am J Psychiatry 145:75–80, 1988.

FURTHER READING

Goodman M, Johns A, Levine R, et al: Report of study group: advanced operative laparoscopy (pelviscopy). J Gynecol Surg 5:353–360, 1989.

Hemostasis, Sutures, Clips, and Staples

The realization that secure hemostasis can be achieved at laparoscopy with skilled use of bipolar desiccation, specially designed vascular clips and staples, or suture ligatures has expanded the field of laparoscopic surgery. Manufacturers are producing new and innovative sutures, staples, and other instruments to allow surgeons to accomplish as much excision and repair by laparoscopy as by laparotomy. In this chapter we present the current "state of the art" principles and techniques of hemostasis and suturing, with the understanding that new and improved instrumentation will be available by the time that this edition is printed.

FIGURE 16–1 Clinical currents

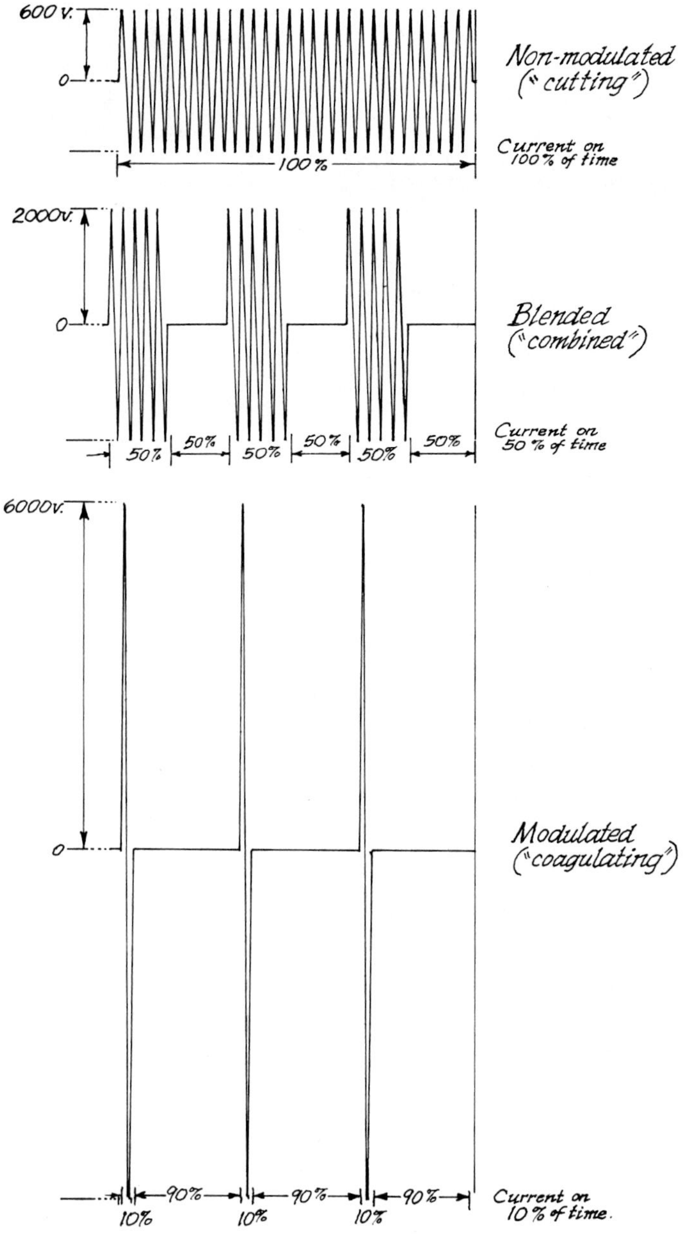

Non-modulated ("cutting")
Current on 100% of time

Blended ("combined")
Current on 50% of time

Modulated ("coagulating")
Current on 10% of time.

ELECTROSURGICAL HEMOSTASIS

Laparoscopy requires a thorough knowledge of electrosurgical techniques for hemostasis. Monopolar electrodes, bipolar electrodes, and thermocoagulation or heater probes use electric current to generate heat that produces hemostasis by coagulating proteins in blood vessels. A common feature of these approaches is the ability to touch and compress the bleeding vessel prior to coagulation.

Electrosurgery means that electric current flows through living tissue. Both monopolar (or unipolar) and bipolar electrosurgery are used for hemostasis. When referring to electrosurgery, the commonly used term *cautery* should be abandoned because it refers to the passive transfer of heat to tissue, usually from the hot tip of a surgical instrument; no electric current flows through the patient's body. The two clinical currents used are an unmodulated "cutting" current and a modulated "coagulation" current with much higher voltage but intermittent in nature (Fig. 16–1).

Monopolar Coagulation

Monopolar electrocoagulation equipment is simple and easy to apply. In many cases, this technique controls bleeding. Concerns about monopolar approaches follow.

EXTENT OF INJURY. The injury resulting from monopolar coagulation is predictable when nonmodulated, low-voltage cutting current is used. Coagulation current may result in deep organ injuries and injuries to adjacent organs (Kivnick and Kanter, 1992).

STICKING. The monopolar electrode often sticks to the coagulated tissue. Removal of the probe may restart the bleeding by pulling off the eschar. As the probe is applied again, char builds up on the probe and on the bleeding site. This char increases electrical impedance and makes the hemostatic process more difficult. Irrigation with sterile water, sorbitol, or glycine at the tip of the electrode may reduce sticking.

SPARKING. Concerns about arcing of unipolar current to sites distant from the operative field are unwarranted. It takes 30% more power to spark or arc in CO_2 than in room air. However, electrosurgical burns may occur in areas outside the surgeon's laparoscopic view from electrode insulation defects and capacitative coupling (see Fig. 3–11).

Nonmodulated cutting current through a knife or spatula electrode is used to cut or coagulate depending on the electrode's configuration in contact with the tissue. The knife-electrode tip is used to cut. The electrode's flat blade is used to tamponade arteriolar bleeding vessels; cutting current is applied to coagulate them. Cutting with some degree of coagulation is done with cutting current using the broad portion of the electrode by increasing power (W). Blended current is avoided because its higher voltages result in deeper tissue damage. Applying 200 W of cutting current through scissors or a spoon electrode in contact with tissue results in cutting with coagulation, used to divide the round ligament, broad ligament, and mesosalpinx, and to seal arterioles and smaller arteries.

Fulguration

Unipolar modulated *coagulation current* is used in close proximity to, but not contacting, tissue, to fulgurate. Diffuse venous and arteriolar bleeding may often be controlled with fulguration, which involves the noncontact application of coagulation current to the tissue via a 1- to 2-mm spark or arc (Fig. 16–2A). Coagulation current uses high voltages that are more than 10 times that of cutting current (see Fig. 16–1). This voltage is used to produce spark-gap fulguration; tissue contact should be judiciously avoided. Uses include intraovarian bleeding after cystectomy, uterine hemostasis after myomectomy, and pelvic hemostasis after hysterectomy and endometriosis surgery.

Argon Beam Coagulation

The argon beam coagulator can be used to provide fulguration from a greater distance; spray coagulation current at 80 W will arc approximately 1 cm through the argon gas flowing at 2 l/min with resultant charring and hemostasis (see Fig. 16–2B). Beacon Labs made the first argon beam coagulator using argon gas at 2 l/min and high voltage coagulation current to increase the distance

FIGURE 16–2 A–C, Fulguration

A Broad electrode, modulated current

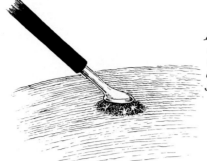

Broad electrode emits a high voltage flow of electrons to char, coagulate and shrink superficial tissue.

B Argon beam, modulated current

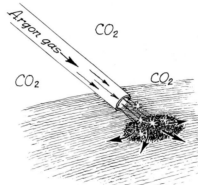

Flowing stream of inert argon gas "conducts" current through more resistant CO_2 gas to "aim" the modulated current on spot to be fulgurated

C CO_2 Laser.

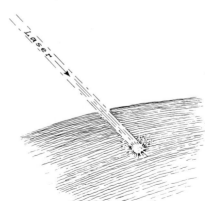

Defocused (2-4 mm diam. spot size) laser will fulgurate surface if set at 50 watts.

FIGURE 16–3 A and B, Large vessel hemostasis

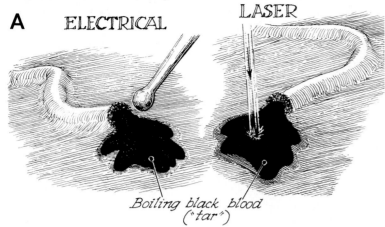

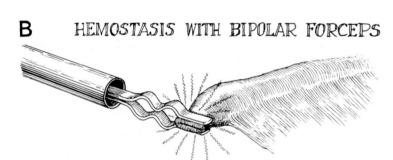

of the fulgurating spark or arc while penetrating the tissue very superficially.

The major advantage of the argon beam coagulator over electrode fulguration in the open abdomen is its ability to clear the operative site of surface blood and fluids, making the bleeding vessel or rent in that vessel visible by the high flow of argon gas as it moves towards the tissue but before it is close enough to activate current.

Bipolar Coagulation for Large Vessel Hemostasis

A large, bleeding vessel cannot be sealed by heating alone, either by electrocoagulation current or by a defocused laser. These approaches result only in obscuring the source of bleeding with "boiling black blood" (Fig. 16–3A). The vessel must first be compressed.

Bipolar desiccation (coagulation) seals arterial blood vessels up to 5 mm immediately (see Fig. 16–3B) so that they can withstand the pulsating arterial pressure until permanent sealing can be accomplished through the healing process (Sigel and Dunn, 1965). Bipolar desiccation for large vessel hemostasis of uterine and ovarian vessels during laparoscopic surgery was first reported in 1986 (Reich, 1987; Reich and McGlynn, 1990). The bipolar forceps use high-frequency, low-voltage non-modulated "cutting" current (20 to 50 W) to coagulate large vessels including the cystic, ovarian, and uterine arteries. Coagulating current is not used because it may quickly desiccate the outer layers of the tissue, producing superficial resistance that may prevent deeper penetration. For large vessel hemostasis using bipolar forceps, electrical current flow must be monitored with a meter to ensure total coagulation of the tissue between the tips of the bipolar forceps. Complete endpoint desiccation results in full-thickness coagulation (Soderstrom and Levy, 1987), fusion of collagen and elastic fibers (Sigel and Dunn, 1965), and vessel weld strength (Harrison and Morris, 1991). The ammeter provides a scientific measurement of complete desiccation, thus allowing the surgeon to make an objective decision with regard to how much current is enough and when it is safest to divide. A designated operating room nurse reports the progress of the ammeter needle to the surgeon during desiccation.

Excision of structures is most easily and safely accomplished by a series of small grasps and cuts of the pedicle with thorough desiccation (Fig. 16–4). This technique closely parallels good open surgical technique: use of the Kelly or Kocher grasping forceps (bipolar forceps) is followed by suturing (desiccation) until the pedicle is divided. Grasps that are too large lead to a wide lateral spread of current beyond the forceps tips and possibly to damage to sensitive adjacent structures. Division of the desiccated pedicle should be close to the side of the specimen so that the compressed and sealed vessels in the area of desiccation remain to provide hemostasis.

We have experience with the Kleppinger bipolar forceps for large vessel hemostasis and specially insulated microbipolar forceps that allow current to pass only through their tips in order to obtain precise small vessel hemostasis. Vancaillie microbipolar forceps contain a channel for irrigation and a fixed distance between the electrodes. With this instrument, irrigation of bleeding sites identifies vessels prior to their desiccation and helps to prevent the sticking of the electrode to the eschar created. Irrigation can be used during underwater examination to push away blood products and clots from the bleeding vessel, thus making its identification prior to coagulation more precise. Large electrodes (e.g., Kleppinger) work poorly underwater because their large surface area encourages current flow through the electrolyte solution, bypassing the tissue between the electrodes. The BICAP irrigation probe (Circon ACMI) has longitudinal stripe electrodes along the probe tip arranged in a circumferential pattern, so that a bipolar field contacts the target tissue upon application of any angle of the circumference of the probe to the tissue. This will soon include the option for a channel recessed proximally to allow washing during coaptation prior to coagulation.

FIGURE 16–4 Excision of organs

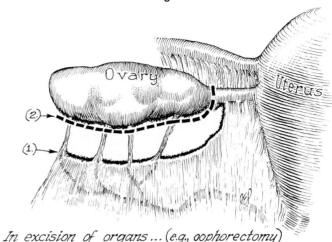

In excision of organs ... (e.g., oophorectomy)

(1.) *Compress and desiccate ("clamp and ligate") the vessel pedicles.*

(2.) *Cut close to the specimen, leaving desiccated pedicle for hemostasis.*

LASER HEMOSTASIS

The CO_2 laser coagulates small blood vessels during cutting or vaporization. Tissue may also be coagulated directly by applying a low power density over a long period of time, elevating the temperature at the tissue surface to between 60 and 100°C. The maximum coagulation depth with CO_2 laser is between 0.5 and 1 mm. The pneumoperitoneum at laparoscopic surgery serves as a minor tamponade to slow or stop oozing from small vessels up to 0.5 mm in diameter. Delayed bleeding may result. These open vessels are recognized as highly reflective red dots, which are often surrounded by a small clot, and a defocused beam can be used to coagulate them. They are also detected at the end of the procedure with low-pressure, underwater examination and coagulated with microforceps. Blood pooling around an actively bleeding vessel may prevent its coagulation.

An effect similar to a blended current is accomplished with the CO_2 laser through the operating channel of an operating laparoscope when used at power settings above 50 W. A large spot size with diameter from 2 to 4 mm is obtained that is extremely coagulative and provides very good hemostatic cutting (see Fig. 16–2C) (Reich et al, 1991). A laparoscopic posterior *culdotomy* incision through the cul-de-sac of Douglas into the vagina is a good example of the hemostatic advantages of using electrosurgery or laser to divide tissue. Complete hemostasis is obtained when making the culdotomy incision. Vaginal bleeding greater than 100 ml is typical before all cuff bleeding is stopped after scissors colpotomy through the vagina and overlying peritoneum.

The argon, KTP-532, and neodymium yttrium aluminum garnet (Nd:YAG) fiber lasers are excellent coagulators. Tissue cutting or vaporization is produced with arteriolar and venous coagulation, especially when using sapphire tips on the Nd:YAG fibers. However, they have no advantage over electrosurgical electrodes for either cutting or coagulation. Their extreme expense may be justified if the user is uncomfortable with electrosurgery. Fibers cannot be maneuvered into places accessible with the CO_2 laser shot through the operating channel of an operating laparoscope perpendicular to the surgeon's field of vision. Less plume occurs with these fiber lasers because the heat is dispersed into the tissue, causing much greater coagulation and tissue necrosis.

UNDERWATER SURGERY AT THE END OF EACH PROCEDURE

Near the end of each operation, hemostasis can be checked in stages using the 10-mm straight laparoscope. Bleeding from vessels and viscera tamponaded during the procedure by the increased intraperitoneal pressure of the CO_2 pneumoperitoneum is detected by discontinuing insufflation and displacing the pneumoperitoneum with 2 to 6 liters of warm (98°F) Ringer's lactate solution. The pelvis is then inspected underwater to detect any further bleeding, which is controlled using microbipolar forceps to coagulate through the electrolyte solution. One microelectrode is placed on the bleeding site, and the current bridges the 1-mm gap between the electrodes through the conductive electrolyte solution with resultant coagulation.

First, complete hemostasis is *established* with the patient in the Trendelenburg position. Next, complete hemostasis is *secured* with the patient supine and in a reverse Trendelenburg position using underwater microbipolar coagulation. Finally, complete hemostasis is *documented* with all instruments removed, including the uterine manipulator (Reich, 1989).

To visualize the pelvis with the patient supine, the laparoscope and the actively irrigating aquadissector tip are manipulated together into the deep cul-de-sac beneath floating bowel and omentum to maintain a clear underwater view in a bloody field. This bloody fluid is diluted, circulated, and aspirated by alternately irrigating and suctioning until the effluent is clear of blood products in the pelvis and upper abdomen, usually after 3 to 10 liters. During this copious irrigation procedure, clear fluid is deposited in the pelvis and circulates into the upper abdomen, displacing upper abdominal bloody fluid that is suctioned after flowing back into the pelvis. An "underwater" examination is then performed to observe the completely separated tubes and ovaries and to confirm complete hemostasis. Individual blood clots are isolated, usually in the pararectosigmoid gutters, and aspirated. A final copious lavage with Ringer's lactate solution is undertaken, and at least 2 liters of lactated Ringer's solution are left in the peritoneal cavity to displace CO_2 and to prevent fibrin adherences from forming by separating raw operated-upon surfaces during the initial stages of reperitonealization. Displacement of the CO_2 with Ringer's lactate diminishes the frequency and severity of shoulder pain from CO_2 insufflation. No other antiadhesive agents are employed. No drains, antibiotic solutions, or heparin are used. The lactated Ringer's solution is absorbed in 2 to 3 days (Rose et al, 1991).

SUTURING

The ability to suture during laparoscopy greatly expands the indications for laparoscopic surgery as well as the confidence of the surgeon performing more difficult procedures. Pioneered by Semm (1978) and Clarke (1972), indications include:

- Ovarian repair after excision of cysts
- Eversion of tubal ostia following salpingostomy
- Closure of salpingotomy following removal of tubal pregnancy
- Excision of omentum
- Reperitonealization of left pelvic sidewall defect with rectosigmoid
- Closure of peritoneal and smooth muscle defects after rectal mobilization during cul-de-sac reconstruction in cases of severe endometriosis
- Ligation of vessels

Two lower abdominal puncture sites are necessary, and through them laparoscopic needle holders are introduced to manipulate suture, needle, and involved tissue. Initial placement of the trocar sleeves lateral to the deep epigastric vessels facilitates this procedure, because it avoids going back and forth through the rectus muscle. The trocar penetrates the external oblique, internal oblique, and transversalis fascia only, leaving an easily identifiable tract.

Suturing is facilitated by using a trocar sleeve without a trap when making the knot outside the peritoneal cavity (extracorporeal). Any available suture material or needle can be used laparoscopically. When curved needle expertise has not been acquired, straight needles are used: 4–0 polydioxanone (Ethicon PDS) on a tapered ST4 needle (Ethicon Z-420); 5–0 Vicryl (Ethicon D7676); or Vicryl, silk, or Gore-Tex on a manually straightened needle. Average operating time for placing and tying a suture is less than 5 minutes.

FIGURE 16–5 A–D, Clarke knot pusher

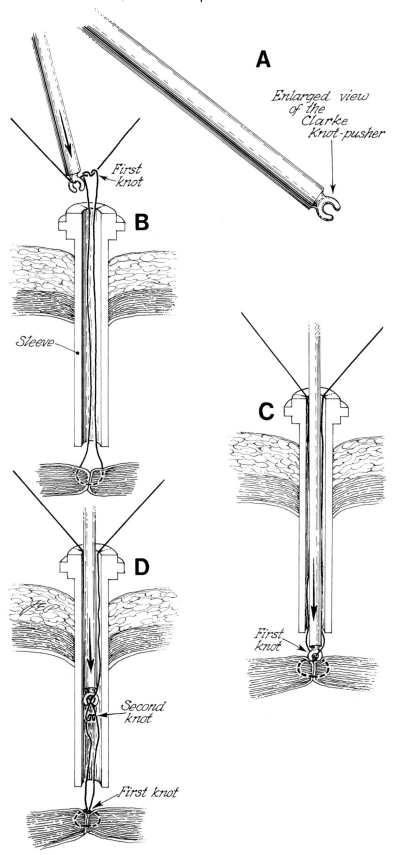

An excellent technique for laparoscopic suturing was developed in 1970 by Clarke using a knot pusher to tie, just as one would hand-tie a suture at open laparotomy: This device is an extension of the surgeon's fingers. Figure 16–5A demonstrates the working tip of the Clarke knot pusher. A simple loop (half-hitch) is tied outside the peritoneal cavity, and the knot pusher is applied to one strand (see Fig. 16–5B). Holding both strands and the knot over the surgeon's index finger facilitates this application. Thereafter, the knot is pushed through the trapless short trocar sleeve, while both ends of the suture are held on tension outside of the peritoneal cavity until the knot has reached the tissue to be ligated (see Fig. 16–5C). The Clarke knot pusher is then removed and applied to a second half-hitch, which is again pushed down to the desired area while tension is exerted from above (see Fig. 16–5D). In most cases a third loop is also pushed downward, and the suture is divided with laparoscopic scissors.

Straight suture needles used laparoscopically are applied using a needle holder designed with grooves to hold the needle at right angles. The straight needle makes insertion through a short trapless trocar sleeve easy. However, curved needles facilitate placement, especially for ligating large vessels and closing deep myometrial defects, bowel, and vagina. To insert a suture with a curved needle into the peritoneal cavity, the 5-mm trocar sleeve is removed from the left lower quadrant incision (Fig. 16–6A). The terminal end of the suture is grasped with the needle holder inserted in the trocar sleeve and pulled through the sleeve (see Fig. 16–6B). Thereafter, the needle holder is reinserted into the sleeve and used to grasp the suture 2 to 4 cm from the needle (see Fig. 16–6C).

FIGURE 16–6 A–J, To tie suture knots externally

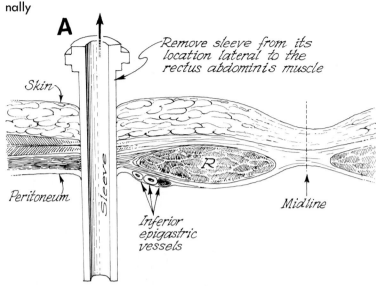

A

Remove sleeve from its location lateral to the rectus abdominis muscle

Skin

Sleeve

Peritoneum

R

Inferior epigastric vessels

Midline

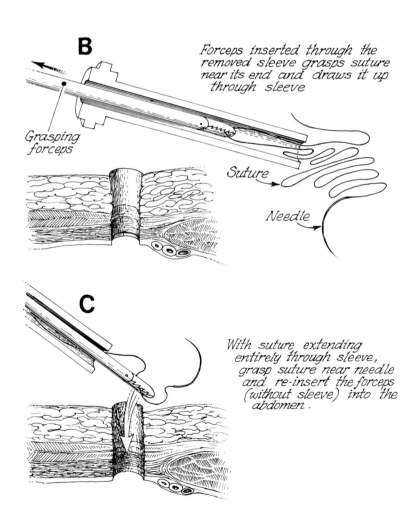

B

Forceps inserted through the removed sleeve grasps suture near its end and draws it up through sleeve

Grasping forceps

Suture

Needle

C

With suture extending entirely through sleeve, grasp suture near needle and re-insert the forceps (without sleeve) into the abdomen.

FIGURE 16–6 Continued

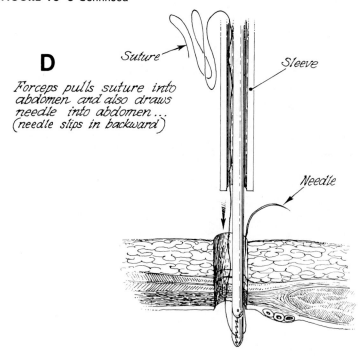

D

Forceps pulls suture into abdomen and also draws needle into abdomen... (needle slips in backward)

Suture

Sleeve

Needle

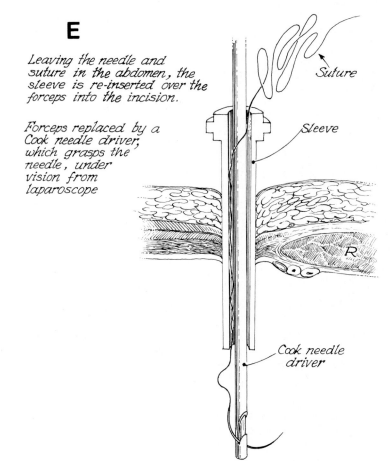

E

Leaving the needle and suture in the abdomen, the sleeve is re-inserted over the forceps into the incision.

Forceps replaced by a Cook needle driver, which grasps the needle, under vision from laparoscope

Suture

Sleeve

R

Cook needle driver

The needle holder is inserted into the peritoneal cavity, and the curved needle follows through the original incision (see Fig. 16–6D). The trocar sleeve surrounding the needle holder is reinserted into the peritoneal cavity over the needle holder (see Fig. 16–6E).

After removal of the conventional needle holder from the sleeve, a Cook endoscopic curved needle driver designed to hold a curved needle with little lateral motion grasps the curved needle and completes the suture needle placement (see Fig. 16–6F). The needle with 2 cm of suture is cut free from the suture and stored for later removal, usually in the parietal peritoneum of the anterior abdominal wall (see Fig. 16–6G). The cut end of the suture is pulled from the peritoneal cavity, where it lies adjacent to the previously inserted terminal end (see Fig. 16–6H).

FIGURE 16–6 Continued

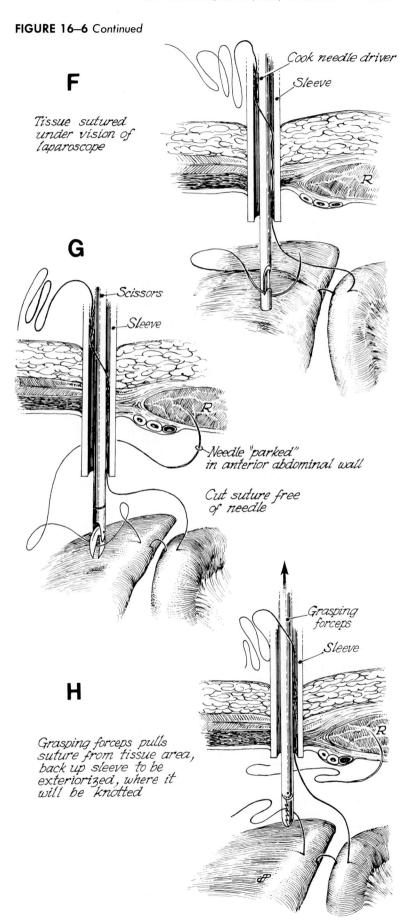

F

Tissue sutured under vision of laparoscope

Cook needle driver

Sleeve

G

Scissors

Sleeve

Needle "parked" in anterior abdominal wall

Cut suture free of needle

H

Grasping forceps

Sleeve

Grasping forceps pulls suture from tissue area, back up sleeve to be exteriorized, where it will be knotted

FIGURE 16–6 *Continued*

I

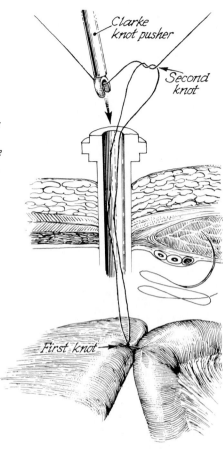

Sutures are tied extracorporeally, and the knot is slid down the length of the suture until it is snugged tightly against the tissue

The second knot is also tied as above, and that knot is slid down until it too is tightly against the first knot

J

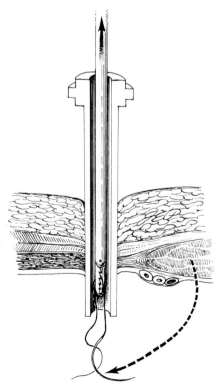

Needle is retrieved from its "parking place" by grasping cut suture, removing trocar sleeve from the incision, and pulling suture with its attached needle up through soft tissue and skin

Forceps and sleeve are then reinserted through the same incision, and the procedure continues

An extracorporeal tie can then be accomplished and pushed to the operative site with a Clarke knot pusher (see Fig. 16–6*I*). After the knot has been secured, the needle is retrieved from the peritoneal cavity by grasping the suture attached to it (see Fig. 16–6*J*), again unscrewing the trocar sleeve to above skin level and pulling the needle out with the conventional needle holder in one motion. The trocar sleeve is reinserted into the same opening with or without another suture, and the operation continues (Reich et al, 1992).

A pelviscopic loop ligature (Endoloop) is available (see Fig. 13–15). It consists of a 0-gauge chromic catgut preformed loop with slipknot, which is designed to fit over vascular pedicles and then be tightened. The device is used through a 5-mm second-puncture trocar sheath to ligate arterial bleeders, vascular pedicles (especially in the area of the mesosalpinx), the utero-ovarian ligament, the infundibulopelvic ligament, omentum, and the appendiceal stump. The most secure knot is obtained by tightening the knot with one pull for 10 seconds. Knot slippage occurs more frequently with each additional pull, as successive pulls seem to weaken the strand of the suture at the base of the knot (Hay et al, 1990). During the last 15 years, this author (H. R.) has used the Endoloop for appendectomies and omentectomies (but never for oophorectomy) because bipolar desiccation is more secure, thus eliminating any chance of slippage. Postoperative pelvic pain is less in desiccated pedicles; a pedicle secured with an Endoloop leaves living cells distal to the loop to necrose and form adhesions.

CLIPS AND STAPLES

Disposable clip and stapling instrumentation for laparoscopic surgery is valuable for large vessel hemostasis in procedures such as oophorectomy, hysterectomy, and cholecystectomy. An automatic clip applier (ENDO CLIP Applier) stacks 20 medium- to large-sized clips (9 mm long when closed) made of titanium, an inert, nonreactive metal. The disposable stapler is designed for introduction through a 10-mm trocar sleeve (Fig. 16–7A). Skeletonization of vessels is necessary prior to application of this staple. When applied to vessels with overlying peritoneum, the staple may slip off during further manipulation of the tissue.

A stapler designed for hernia repair will fix meshes to underlying fascia with a metal staple (see Fig. 16–7B), thus acting as a metal suture. The final configuration of the staple is similar to the common paper staple.

A right-angle clip applier (Origin Medsystems) is now available. This applicator incorporates a small distal hook as an anvil for clip closure after the hook pulls the duct or vessel away from adjacent tissue.

A multiple staple applicator (MULTIFIRE ENDO GIA 30 Stapler) places six rows of titanium staples, 30 mm in length, and divides the stapled tissue (Fig. 16–8A). It consists of a disposable handle and shaft, the end of which contains a replaceable single-use stapling cartridge. The standard staple compresses on firing to 1.5 mm, while the vascular cartridge compresses to 1 mm. The disposable handle is designed to fire up to 4 staple cartridges through a 12-mm cannula (SURGIPORT) before being discarded. It is important to realize that the MULTIFIRE ENDO GIA 30 Stapler is a straight device without staples in its distal 1-cm end and is much wider than a Kelly clamp. This instrument functions similarly

FIGURE 16–7 Clips.

A Hemostatic clip: single or multiple.

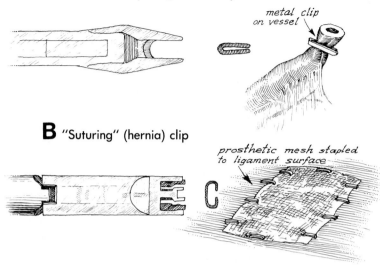

B "Suturing" (hernia) clip

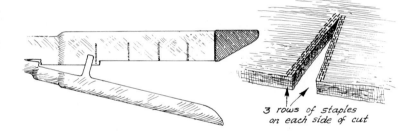

FIGURE 16–8 Staples.

A Straight (ENDO GIA 30).

B Circular (Premium CEEA)

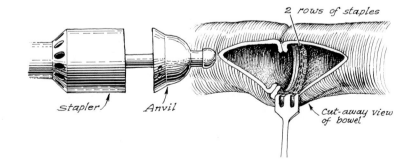

to the gastrointestinal anastomosis stapler that thoracic and general surgeons have used for the last 25 years. It is used for rapid bloodless division of the adnexa or utero-ovarian ligament during laparoscopically assisted hysterectomy.

A multiple staple applicator (EEA) in a circular design is intended for rapid end-to-end anastomosis of the rectosigmoid colon. Introduced through the rectum, this large device fires off a circle of staples into aligned proximal and distal stumps of a rectosigmoid resection. This procedure (see Fig. 16–8B) can be done during laparoscopic resection of cul-de-sac endometriosis if bowel stricture exists.

OTHER TECHNIQUES

Use of vasoconstrictive agents should not be routine for myomectomy surgery. Dilute vasopressin solution (Pitressin; Parke Davis) may cause delayed bleeding from the needle puncture sites when injected into the myometrium, requiring later electrosurgical coagulation. If used, great care is necessary to avoid vessel laceration, penetration, or intravascular injection, which can cause arterial hypertension. Extravascular injection itself can induce an increase in the arterial blood pressure or bradycardia. Vasopressin use has been banned in France after fatalities occurred presumably from cardiac arrhythmias during cervical procedures and *laparotomy* myomectomy.

Surgicel (oxidized regenerated cellulose) application is a very useful, time-saving technique for myoma bed bleeding during myomectomy. A piece is packed into the defect, which is then repaired with a 0-Vicryl suture on CT-1 curved needles to compress the full thickness of exposed myometrium.

Avitene Microfibrillar Collagen Hemostat (MCH) is now available for endoscopic use (Endo-Avitene). Its delivery system negotiates a 10-mm trocar sheath and can be applied directly to the bleeding site with a blunt plunger tip, allowing pressure during placement. Avitene works by mechanical means and by attracting platelets that adhere to its collagen fibrils. Excess Avitene is irrigated and suctioned away.

Bulldog clamps inserted through the 10-mm umbilical cannula may be applied to the infundibulopelvic ligaments to decrease the risk of bleeding and fluid overload during hysteroscopic and laparoscopic myomectomy. Surgical sponges can also be used.

SUMMARY

Hemostasis, an integral component of any surgical procedure, can be secured laparoscopically by employing any number of currently available techniques. New instrumentation is constantly being developed. Underwater examination at the close of each procedure documents comprehensive and complete hemostasis. This increases the confidence of the surgeon and optimizes patient outcome.

REFERENCES

Clarke HC: Laparoscopy: New instruments for suturing and ligation. Fertil Steril 23:274–277, 1972.

Harrison JD and Morris DL: Does bipolar electrocoagulation time affect vessel weld strength? Gut 32:188–190, 1991.

Hay DL, Levine RL, von Fraunhofer JA, and Masterson BJ: Chromic gut pelviscopic loop ligature: Effect of the number of pulls on the tensile strength. J Reprod Med 35:260–262, 1990.

Kivnick S and Kanter MH: Bowel injury from rollerball ablation of the endometrium. Obstet Gynecol 79:833–835, 1992.

Reich H: Laparoscopic oophorectomy and salpingo-oophorectomy in the treatment of benign tubo-ovarian disease. Int J Fertil 32:233–236, 1987.

Reich H: New techniques in advanced laparoscopic surgery. Baillieres Clin Obstet Gynaecol 3:655–681, 1989.

Reich H, Clarke HC, and Sekel L: A simple method for ligating with straight and curved needles in operative laparoscopy. Obstet Gynecol 79:143–147, 1992.

Reich H and McGlynn F: Laparoscopic oophorectomy and salpingo-oophorectomy in the treatment of benign tuboovarian disease. J Reprod Med 31:609, 1986.

Reich H and McGlynn F: Short self-retaining trocar sleeves for laparoscopic surgery. Am J Obstet Gynecol 162:453–454, 1990.

Reich H, MacGregor TS III, and Vancaillie TG: CO_2 laser used through the operating channel of laser laparoscopes: In vitro study of power and power density losses. Obstet Gynecol 77:40–47, 1991.

Rose BI, MacNeill C, Larrain R, and Kopreski MM: Abdominal instillation of high-molecular-weight Dextran or lactated Ringer's solution after laparoscopic surgery: A randomized comparison of the effect on weight change. J Reprod Med 36:537–539, 1991.

Semm K: Tissue puncher and loop-ligature: New aids for surgical-therapeutic pelviscopy (laparoscopy)-endoscopic intraabdominal surgery. Endoscopy 10:119–124, 1978.

Sigel B and Dunn MR: The mechanism of blood vessel closure by high frequency electrocoagulation. Surg Gynecol Obstet 121:823–831, 1965.

Soderstrom RM and Levy BS: Bipolar systems—do they perform? Obstet Gynecol 69:425–426, 1987.

Endometriosis

Treatment of endometriosis is the single most frequent indication for operative laparoscopy in the United States (Peterson et al, 1990). It is therefore important for the laparoscopist to be thoroughly familiar with the current standards of diagnosis and management of this complex disease. Schenken's book (1989) and a review of the role of laparoscopy (Cook and Rock, 1991) give an excellent detailed discussion of the difficult problems concerning diagnosis and choices of therapy in this disease. In this chapter we concentrate on the current techniques of laparoscopic management.

FIGURE 17–1 Peritoneal implant excision

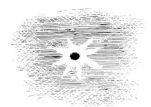

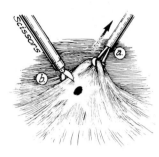

Implants have white, stellate, peritoneal scars encircling the lesion.

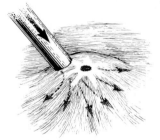

a. Tent peritoneum at a free edge

b. Make a small "nick" incision into peritoneum

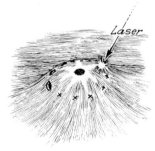

c. Dissection and undermining by fluid under pressure

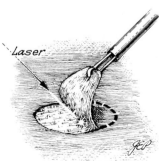

d. Wide excision with laser around scar

e. Lift specimen to free deep fibrotic adherences with laser as excision proceeds.

PERITONEAL IMPLANTS

To treat superficial fibrotic or hemorrhagic peritoneal endometriosis, the endometriosis implant and its adjacent peritoneum are excised, using a CO_2 laser beam at 20- to 40-W superpulse, a knife or a needle electrode at a 20- to 40-W unipolar cutting current, or scissors. An incision is made in normal peritoneum surrounding the lesion (Fig. 17–1A and B); its edge is lifted upward; and the lesion is undermined using the hydraulic effect of pressurized irrigant from an aquadissector (see Fig. 17–1C). This procedure pushes underlying pelvic structures or the rectum away and makes undercutting of the lesion with laser, electrosurgery, or scissors easy and safe. Laser or electrosurgery can then be used to remove fibrotic adhesions (see Fig. 17–1D and E).

Following excision, the ureter, anterior rectal wall, and upper posterior vagina are checked, and superficial endometriosis in these areas is excised or vaporized. The uterus, tube, and ovary do not have loose peritoneum, and implants on these surfaces should be ablated directly (Fig. 17–2).

Small pinpoint lesions can be vaporized using the CO_2 laser or unipolar cutting-current electrosurgery with resultant drainage of hemosiderin-filled fluid in cases in which deposits have progressed to just beneath the peritoneum. The base of the lesion is then vaporized until normal tissue is seen.

FIGURE 17–2 Excision versus ablation

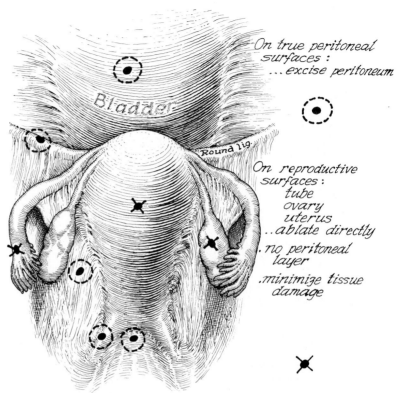

FIGURE 17–3 *A–H,* Dissection of endometrioma

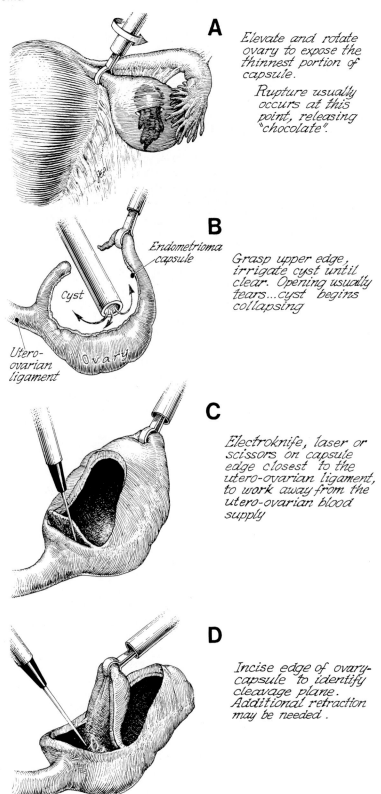

A

Elevate and rotate ovary to expose the thinnest portion of capsule.

Rupture usually occurs at this point, releasing "chocolate".

B

Endometrioma capsule

Cyst

Utero-ovarian ligament

Ovary

Grasp upper edge, irrigate cyst until clear. Opening usually tears...cyst begins collapsing

C

Electroknife, laser or scissors on capsule edge closest to the utero-ovarian ligament, to work away from the utero-ovarian blood supply

D

Incise edge of ovary-capsule to identify cleavage plane. Additional retraction may be needed.

ENDOMETRIOMAS

Leuprolide acetate for depot suspension (Lupron Depot), 3.75 mg intramuscularly (IM), is often administered after ovulation in the cycle preceding surgery to avoid operating on ovaries that contain a corpus luteum. An aquadissector is used to lift up the ovaries if they are attached by adhesions to their respective uterosacral ligament or pelvic sidewall. This maneuver often results in drainage of an endometrioma from the undersurface of the ovary (Fig. 17–3A). If no endometrioma is readily identified, and the patient has "unexplained infertility" or pre- or postmenstrual spotting, a 3-mm knife electrode connected to nonmodulated unipolar cutting current (40 W) is used to incise and drain areas on the ovary with superficial endometriosis and cysts that are suspicious for endometrioma. The clinical distinction between an endometrioma (pathology to be excised) and a corpus luteum cyst (normal, vascular tissue best left alone) is difficult to make, and conservative discretion is advised to avoid the trauma and risk of removing what may be normal tissue.

If a true endometrioma is discovered by either of these two methods, the cyst cavity is rinsed with lactated Ringer's solution (see Fig. 17–3B) and then excised using a 5-mm biopsy forceps, grasping forceps, or scissors. To help delineate the initial plane between normal ovarian cortex and endometrioma cyst wall, cutting current through the knife electrode tip applied at the cyst wall-cortex junction (see Fig. 17–3C and D) results in the development of a dissection plane. This step is particularly useful near the utero-ovarian ligament because rough avulsion can lead to excessive bleeding.

To identify this plane, the laparoscope should be brought close in to the area of dissection to "zoom in" or magnify the area of dissection until the cyst wall is clearly identified (see Fig. 17–3E).

Grasping forceps are then used to stabilize ovarian cortex while the endometrioma cyst wall is avulsed (see Fig. 17–3F and G and Atlas, Plate 21). Excision can be performed with minimal bleeding from the cyst wall bed, and the ovarian wall edges usually reapproximate quite well (see Fig. 17–3H). Bleeding can be controlled with bipolar desiccation or fulguration inside the cyst cavity. If the cyst wall is felt to be incompletely excised, the cyst cavity can be desiccated or fulgurized to destroy any remaining endometrioma. Otherwise, the endometrioma may recur. The ovarian cortex is suture approximated only if the defect is large and asymmetrical. Although suturing is occasionally thought to be necessary for reapproximation, second-look evaluations of cysts left open have revealed remarkable re-establishment of the ovarian surface free of adhesions. This finding is consistent with animal studies.

FIGURE 17–3 Continued

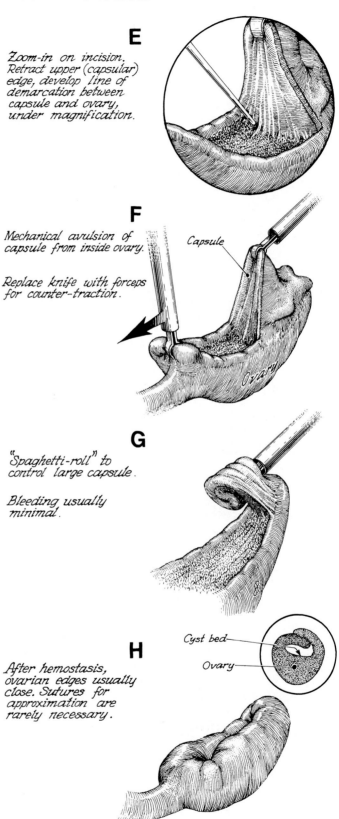

FIGURE 17–4 A–C, Probes for cul-de-sac dissection

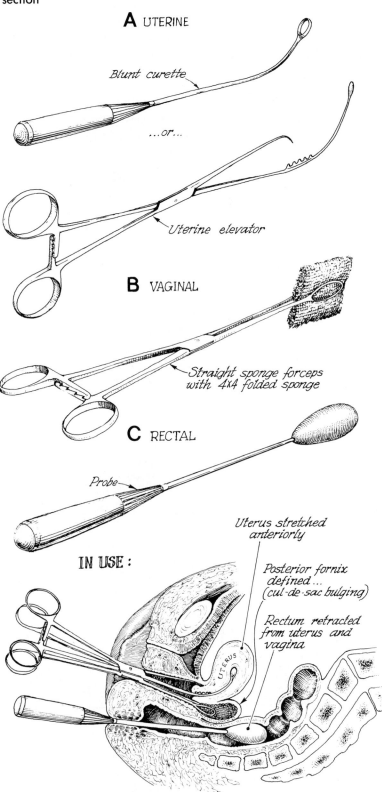

A UTERINE

Blunt curette

...or...

Uterine elevator

B VAGINAL

*Straight sponge forceps
with 4x4 folded sponge*

C RECTAL

Probe

IN USE :

*Uterus stretched
anteriorly*

*Posterior fornix
defined...
(cul-de-sac bulging)*

*Rectum retracted
from uterus and
vagina*

PARTIAL AND COMPLETE CUL-DE-SAC OBLITERATION

Cul-de-sac obliteration implies the presence of retrocervical deep fibrotic endometriosis. Partial cul-de-sac obliteration means that deep fibrotic endometriosis beneath the peritoneum is present and severe enough to alter the course of the rectum. The deep fibrotic endometriosis is usually located on the upper vagina, on the superficial anterior rectum, in the rectovaginal space, in the space between the upper vagina and the cervix (cervicovaginal angle), or in one or both uterosacral ligaments. With deep cul-de-sac obliteration, fibrotic endometriosis or adhesions involve the entire area between the cervicovaginal junction (and sometimes above) and the rectovaginal septum; often one area predominates.

Diagnosis

Careful inspection of the cul-de-sac is necessary to evaluate the extent of upward tenting of the rectum. To determine if cul-de-sac obliteration is partial or complete, a sponge on a ring forceps is inserted into the posterior vaginal fornix (and a rectal probe is inserted in the rectum [Fig. 17–4]).

1. *Normal* cul-de-sac will show a portion of the vaginal wall between the cervix and the rectum as a distinct and separate bulge (Fig. 17–5). The uterosacral ligaments will be clear of this and lateral.

2. *Partial* cul-de-sac obliteration occurs where rectal tenting is visible, but a protrusion from the sponge in the posterior vaginal fornix is noted between the rectum and the inverted U of the uterosacral ligaments (see Fig. 17–5).

3. *Complete* cul-de-sac obliteration implies that the outline of the posterior fornix cannot be visualized initially through the laparoscope—the rectum or fibrotic endometriosis nodules completely obscure the identification of the deep cul-de-sac (see Fig. 17–5).

Surgery

In contrast to the procedure performed for superficial peritoneal endometriosis, deep fibrotic nodular endometriosis involving the cul-de-sac—often with invasion into posterior vagina, rectum, or posterior cervix—is a much more difficult problem and should be attempted only by the most expert laparoscopist. The technique for this advanced procedure appears in Chapter 23.

FURTHER READINGS

Cook AS and Rock JA: The role of laparoscopy in the treatment of endometriosis. Fertil Steril 55:663–680, 1991.

Luciano AA, Lowney J, and Jacobs SL: Endoscopic treatment of endometriosis-associated infertility: Therapeutic, economic and social benefits. J Reprod Med 37:573–576, 1992.

Peterson HB, Hulka JF, and Phillips JM: American Association of Gynecologic Laparoscopists' 1988 membership survey on operative laparoscopy. J Reprod Med 35:587–589, 1990.

Reich H and McGlynn F: Treatment of ovarian endometriomas using laparoscopic surgical techniques. J Reprod Med 31:577–584, 1986.

Reich H, McGlynn F, and Salvat J: Laparoscopic treatment of cul-de-sac obliteration secondary to retrocervical deep fibriotic endometriosis. J Reprod Med 36:516–522, 1991.

Schenken RS: Endometriosis: Contemporary Concepts in Clinical Management. Philadelphia, JB Lippincott, 1989.

FIGURE 17–5 Staging of cul-de-sac obliteration

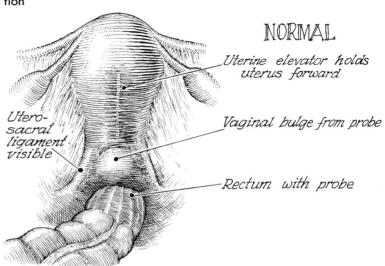

NORMAL

Uterine elevator holds uterus forward

Utero-sacral ligament visible

Vaginal bulge from probe

Rectum with probe

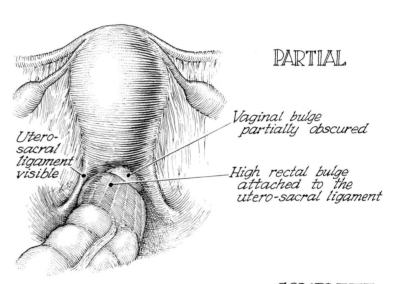

PARTIAL

Utero-sacral ligament visible

Vaginal bulge partially obscured

High rectal bulge attached to the utero-sacral ligament

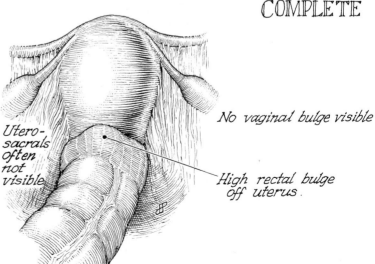

COMPLETE

Utero-sacrals often not visible

No vaginal bulge visible

High rectal bulge off uterus.

Adnexal Surgery

Most adnexal surgery, including oophorectomy, can be performed with the laparoscope, perhaps with less postoperative adhesion formation. In this chapter we present techniques for performing the more common adnexal procedures. Removal of endometriomas is presented in Chapter 17; the management of ectopic pregnancies is presented in Chapter 19; and the controversy concerning laparoscopic oophorectomy is fully reviewed in Chapter 21.

LAPAROSCOPIC OOPHORECTOMY

In 1980 Semm and Mettler reported 37 laparoscopic oophorectomies using a loop ligature and a tissue punch morcellator. Reich and McGlynn (1986) developed a technique for replacing the ligature with bipolar electrosurgical desiccation and eliminating the need to morcellate by tissue removal through culdotomy or extended umbilical incisions. Reich published the results of 44 postmenopausal patients with palpable ovaries managed laparoscopically (Mann and Reich, 1992).

The indications for laparoscopic oophorectomy (or salpingo-oophorectomy) include pelvic pain secondary to ovarian adhesions from previous hysterectomy, pain from ovarian adhesions unresponsive to laparoscopic lysis, pelvic mass secondary to hydrosalpinx from pelvic inflammatory disease (PID), previous surgery, or a benign neoplasm (dermoid, cyst adenoma, or endometrioma), postmenopausal palpable

ovary (PMPO), and first-degree relatives (e.g., mother and sister) with ovarian malignancy.

In women who do not desire future fertility, oophorectomy should be considered for pain or for a mass arising from ovarian endometrioma, hemorrhagic corpus luteum cyst, or dermoid cyst when the contralateral ovary is normal, especially if the lesion is on the left as the left ovary frequently heals adhered to the rectosigmoid. The acronym PMPO is used for the palpation of an ovary that, in a premenopausal woman, would be interpreted as having a normal size—3 to 4 cm in its largest dimension (Barber and Graber, 1971). Such ovaries can almost always be removed intact through a culdotomy incision. Women in families with two or more first-degree relatives with ovarian cancer may have a 50% chance of developing this disease and should consider undergoing early prophylactic oophorectomy, at age 35 if childbearing has been completed. Women without a family history of ovarian cancer have a 1:70 risk of developing this disease.

Preoperatively, endovaginal ultrasound is done to evaluate the ovaries in cases involving a pelvic mass, retrocervical nodules, or fibroids. If the patient is postmenopausal, a CA 125 assay is obtained. (The specificity of this test is low in premenopausal women due to endometriosis.) Intravenous pyelograms are rarely necessary preoperatively but are ordered frequently postoperatively if abdominal pain persists following surgery on or near the

FIGURE 18–1 Identification of the ureter

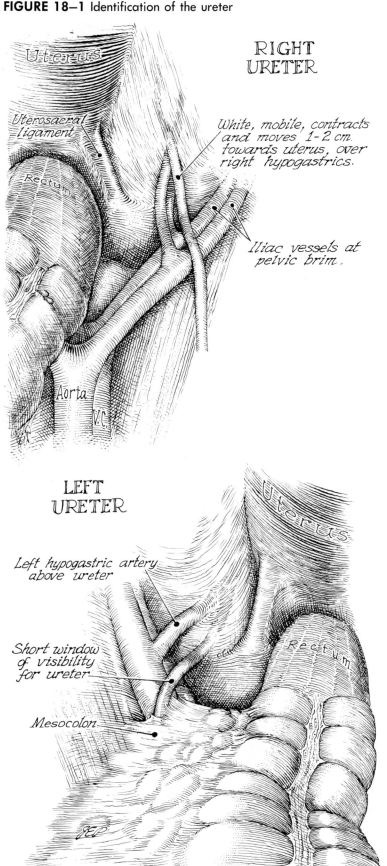

ureter. Presently, there is no indication for a computed tomography (CT) scan or magnetic resonance imaging (MRI) prior to laparoscopic ovarian surgery.

For oophorectomy, the three standard operative incisions are: 10 mm umbilical, 5 mm right, and 5 mm left lower quadrant. The patient is placed in a steep Trendelenburg position (20 to 30 degrees). A Valtchev uterine mobilizer or controlling tenaculum is inserted to antevert the uterus and delineate the posterior vagina. In all cases careful inspection of the pelvis and abdomen is undertaken. The ovaries are evaluated for visual evidence of malignancy. Washings are taken if indicated.

Prior to starting oophorectomy, it is imperative that the surgeon visualize the course of the ureter (Fig. 18–1). It crosses the external iliac artery near the bifurcation of the common iliac artery at the pelvic brim and is usually lower on the left, where its entrance into the pelvis is covered by the inverted V-shaped root of the sigmoid mesocolon. If necessary, the peritoneum above the ureter can be opened with sharp scissors, laser, or cutting current electrosurgery. Thereafter, the space can be further developed by flushing irrigant under pressure from an aquadissector into the space. Smooth grasping forceps are then opened parallel and perpendicular to the retroperitoneal structures until the ureter is identified and grasped. Scissors, laser, or aquadissector can be used to dissect the ureter throughout much of its course along the pelvic sidewall. See Chapter 20 for a more detailed presentation of this technique.

Prior to removal, the ovary must be released from all pelvic sidewall and bowel adhesions using a combination of aquadissection, scissors, electrodissection, and laser dissection. When the ovary or ovarian remnant is fused to or within the pelvic sidewall peritoneum, a retroperitoneal approach for oophorectomy may be considered (again, see Chapter 20). Adhesions are divided, and ovarian endometriomas are drained, if present. The fallopian tube is grasped and pulled medially to stretch out the infundibulopelvic ligament containing the ovarian vessels. Kleppinger bipolar forceps are used to compress and desiccate the infundibulopelvic ligament, the broad ligament (mesovarium and mesosalpinx), the fallopian tube isthmus, and the utero-ovarian ligament (Reich and McGlynn, 1986a; Reich, 1987a). These large blood vessels are compressed, and bipolar *cutting* current is passed until complete desiccation is achieved—the current depletes tissue fluid and electrolytes until it ceases to flow between the forceps as determined by an ammeter or current flowmeter (endpoint monitor: Electroscope EPM-1). In most cases, three contiguous areas are desiccated. Laparoscopic scissors are then used to divide the pedicle. In some cases the mesovarium alone can be desiccated and divided (Fig. 18–2). Alternatively, the ENDO GIA stapler or a suture may be applied, with comparable results as far as operative time and hemostasis are concerned (Daniell et al, 1992). Medial retraction with grasping forceps is helpful while the adnexa is being freed from the pelvic sidewall. The free ovary is then removed through the umbilicus or cul-de-sac as previously described.

FIGURE 18–2 Excision of organs

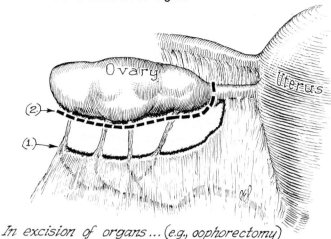

In excision of organs... (e.g., oophorectomy)

(1.) Compress and desiccate ("clamp and ligate") the vessel pedicles.

(2.) Cut close to the specimen, leaving desiccated pedicle for hemostasis.

When the ovary or ovarian remnant is fused to or within the pelvic sidewall peritoneum, a retroperitoneal approach for oophorectomy may be considered. Scissors or CO_2 laser is used to incise the peritoneum lateral to the infundibulopelvic ligament, progressing parallel to the tube and ovary up to the uterine end of the round ligament. With traction on the tube, ovary, or peritoneum, the retroperitoneal space is entered and its loose areolar tissue is dissected with scissors or aquadissection. This dissection is continued downward until the ureter is identified. At this time, the ovarian vessels can be desiccated just caudad to where they cross over the iliac vessels. Following division of the infundibulopelvic ligament, it is placed on traction and the procedure continues caudad with division of the peritoneum just below its ovarian attachments and lateral to its rectosigmoid attachments. Finally, the utero-ovarian ligament and proximal fallopian tube are desiccated and divided, freeing the specimen. Bipolar desiccation of these ligaments is done most safely by inserting the forceps from the opposite side of the pelvis. The peritoneal sidewall defect is left alone.

Bipolar desiccation of ovarian and utero-ovarian vessels has been a safe method of ligation in my (H.R.) experience. Postoperative pain is less than following suture ligation, because electrosurgical desiccation eliminates later distal ischemic necrosis. There have been no late bleeding episodes in more than 400 oophorectomies performed in this manner.

PELVIC ADHESIOLYSIS

The surgical management of extensive pelvic adhesions, including hydrosalpinx, is one of the most difficult problems facing gynecologic surgeons today. While most pelvic reconstructive surgery can be performed laparoscopically with results similar to those obtained with microsurgery (Gomel, 1977), studies are necessary to delineate the role of laparoscopy, microsurgery, and in vitro fertilization in the treatment of pelvic adhesions.

Adhesions involving the anterior abdominal wall peritoneum are often encountered first. If they extend above the umbilicus, a subcostal trocar entry (see Chapter 14) for an operating laparoscope will give a panoramic view of the entire peritoneal cavity, and adhesions can be freed down to and below the umbilicus working from above downward onto the adhesions. The abdominal wall must be cleared of adherent bowel. Bowel injury is avoided by visualizing the entry sites of the lower quadrant sleeves.

The next step is to free all bowel loops in the pelvis. Small bowel attached to the vesicouterine peritoneal fold, uterus, or vaginal cuff, and the rectum is divided as described in Chapter 15. Much of the deep pelvic dissection is done with scissors, aquadissection, suction-traction, and CO_2 laser. Small bowel is grasped with atraumatic grasping forceps or the suction tip of an aquadissector and put on traction. When adhesive interfaces are obvious, scissors are used. When these adhesive aggregates blend into each other, the initial incision is made very superficially with a laser; aquadissection is used to distend the layers of the adhesions and facilitate identification of the involved structures; and further division is continued with laser. The aquadissector is used as a backstop behind adhesive bands that are divided with the CO_2 laser. Injected fluid from the aquadissector also serves as a backstop for this laser.

Ovariolysis

Ovarian adhesions to the pelvic sidewall can be filmy or fused. The object of adhesiolysis is to preserve as much peritoneum as possible while freeing the ovarian surface. Dissection begins by using the aquadissector to develop potential spaces among the adhesions. Thereafter, laparoscopic scissors are used to divide the adhesions, usually taking very small bites and dissecting using blunt scissors to stay close to the ovary. Dissection continues until the ovary is free to its hilum. CO_2 laser can occasionally be used to aid in this dissection, especially if ureteral location is in doubt, because this laser causes minimal thermal damage deep to the operative site.

The rectosigmoid can be adhered to the left adnexa, thus obscuring visualization of the left pelvic sidewall. Dissection starts well out of the pelvis in the left iliac fossa. Scissors are used to develop the space between the sigmoid colon and the psoas muscle to the iliac vessels, and the rectosigmoid is reflected toward the midline. Thereafter, with the rectosigmoid placed on traction, rectosigmoid and rectal adhesions to the left adnexa and pelvic sidewall are divided starting cephalad and continuing caudad.

Salpingo-Ovariolysis Including Salpingostomy

The surgical procedures performed for tubal adhesions are salpingo-ovariolysis, fimbrioplasty, or salpingostomy. Small or large bowel enterolysis often accompanies these procedures. When both tubes are open and the fimbriae of the tube are not involved in the adhesion process, the procedure is called salpingo-ovariolysis. When the distal tube is completely blocked, as documented by no flow of dye after tubal lavage, the surgical procedure is called salpingostomy. When the fimbriae are adhered to the ovary or the distal tube is partially occluded, the procedure is termed fimbrioplasty. In actuality, there is much overlap between these procedures. In performing salpingo-ovariolysis when the tube is completely blocked with its distal end stuck to the ovary, freeing this end from the ovary frequently results in a salpingostomy. (The salpingostomy was performed while doing the salpingo-ovariolysis.) This is a very important point, because if the surgeon makes a tubal incision in these cases before dissecting the distal tube off the ovary (i.e., in the most dilated portion of what looks like the end of the tube), the opening will seal just like a salpingotomy does after ectopic pregnancy surgery. In other words, linear incisions along the length of the tube seal; incisions at what was once the true tubal distal ostium stay open, if opened widely. Salpingo-ovariolysis for a retroperitoneal ovary or a fused tubo-ovarian complex is more difficult than a "pure" terminal salpingostomy with a free ovary, caused by tubes sealing at their distal end before extensive outpouring of purulent material occurs.

During adnexal surgery, scissors constitute the primary instrument used to cut, and microbipolar forceps are used to coagulate. In many cases on the left side, the rectosigmoid must be reflected from its attachments to the left iliac fossa to improve visualization of the left infundibulopelvic ligament and the cephalad portion of the left tube and ovary. The ovary is manipulated with an ovarian forceps on the utero-ovarian ligament when possible. Twisting this forceps places the adhesions between the ovary and the pelvic sidewall on tension. Thereafter, scissors can be used along with aquadissection to help develop tissue planes and preserve the pelvic sidewall peritoneum and ovarian cortex where they have been attached. In cases in which adhesive bands are thicker, use of a well-tuned CO_2 laser can be considered.

Laparoscopic tubal surgery must be done as meticulously as surgery performed by laparotomy. Tubo-ovarian adhesions are placed on traction and divided with scissors. Microbipolar forceps with irrigant are reserved for hemostasis after bleeding occurs. Laser should be avoided during this dissection to prevent adhesions from thermal necrosis. The ability of laser to dissect with hemostasis makes it ideal for separating vascular fused tubo-ovarian complexes. In these cases it is not possible to easily identify dissection planes with traction. Frequent tubal lavage distends the tube to aid in its identification. Aquadissection and CO_2 laser are used to complete the dissection.

FIGURE 18–3 Salpingostomy

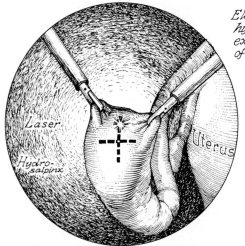

Elevate and twist the hydrosalpinx, to expose puckered scar of invaginated fimbria.

laser a cruciate incision.

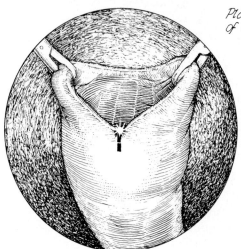

Place forceps on edge of incision,...pull apart.

laser divides only avascular areas, while 300med-in for magnification

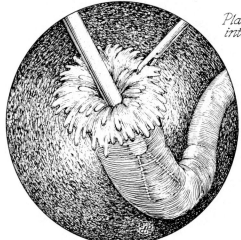

Place forceps deep into ampulla...

...open forceps, and...

slowly withdraw forceps to separate intra-ampullary and fimbrial adhesions.

SALPINGOSTOMY FOR HYDROSALPINX

Gomel described laparoscopic salpingostomy in 1977, but only recently has this approach become more widely used. We have presented our current indications in Chapter 9, and here present the technique.

A preoperative hysterosalpingogram to evaluate the proximal tube for salpingitis isthmica nodosa is helpful. This portion of the tube also requires careful intraoperative inspection.

Chronic PID with hydrosalpinx can almost always be treated laparoscopically. Dissection using scissors should be attempted on the most favorable side, with laser or electrosurgery reserved for the other side (Reich, 1987b). With hydrosalpinx, the distal end of the tube is often fused to the ovary and is opened by dividing all adhesions between the distal tube and the ovarian surface. Difficult surgical decisions must be made when dissecting the distal tube from the ovary, because bleeding often ensues in the tubo-ovarian ligament or fimbria ovarica and can compromise fimbrial ostial blood supply. During mobilization of the distal tube, the hydrosalpinx is often opened if it resulted from agglutination between the tubal fimbria and the ovary. Otherwise, the distal dilated tube is opened with laser, electrosurgery, or scissors. Microscissors are inserted into the phimotic ostium and spread (Fig. 18–3). Avascular areas are divided. Grasping forceps are then inserted and spread, and the ostium is stretched. Avascular areas are again divided. Finally, smooth grasping forceps are inserted and spread, and again avascular areas are divided, which usually results in a wide-open ostium with fimbrial epithelium protruding from it.

Laser eversion is avoided if possible, because its thermal effect frequently causes phimosis or adhesions. More physiologic eversion can often be obtained by cutting bands of fibrous tissue surrounding the tubal ostium and occasionally by performing a suture eversion with 4–0 polydioxanone (PDS) or 5–0 Vicryl. With a large sactosalpinx, laser eversion at a power setting of 1 to 3 W is followed by a suture approximating osteal epithelium to tube serosa effectively covering most of the thermally damaged serosa.

McComb's intussusception salpingostomy method (McComb and Paleologou, 1991) is a good technique in selected cases to avoid thermal damage to the ciliated tubal epithelium from CO_2 laser or electrosurgery. All adhesions among the adnexa, rectosigmoid, and pelvic sidewall are divided with scissors. On occasion, a CO_2 laser can be used instead of scissors when the tube is firmly fused to the ovary. Dilute indigo carmine dye is instilled transcervically to distend the distal tube and to delineate the point of occlusion. Scissors are used to incise the thinned out distal tubal serosa over this punctum, which is the result of agglutination caused by either external purulent fluid or a pyosalpinx. A relatively short incision in the hydrosalpinx is made along the axis of the fimbria ovarica toward the antimesenteric border of the tube. Both scissors and grasping forceps are then inserted into the lumen, which is gently stretched to increase its diameter to approximately 12 mm. The lateral margin of the ostium is grasped with forceps, and the blunt end of the scissors is used to prolapse ampullary epithelium and serosa through the ostium in an intussusception-like fashion. The borders of the incision act as a restrictive collar to maintain the mucosa in this newly everted configuration. In some cases, the ostial margin is sutured to the ampullary serosa with a 6–0 polypropylene suture.

CYSTECTOMY

Ovarian cysts are discovered during a gynecologic pelvic examination or by ultrasonography. If persistent, these cysts should be surgically evaluated because of the small risk of malignancy. Laparotomy with cyst excision is inappropriate because of the increased risk of ovarian adhesions (Eddy et al, 1980).

Laparoscopic inspection of a suspected ovarian cyst often reveals a parovarian cyst, hydrosalpinx, or inflammatory peritoneal pseudocyst. Visual evidence of a malignancy is sought. Cysts with a translucent thin wall are usually functional; most organic cysts have thick walls. All cysts should be smooth-walled and without excrescence. All except the most benign-appearing cysts are removed intact, if possible through the cul-de-sac to avoid the potential risk of metastasis to the anterior abdominal wall. Parovarian cysts are excised if large enough to disrupt ovum pickup, and pseudocysts require excision of pelvic adhesions.

All cysts opened during laparoscopic surgery, either intentionally or during mobilization of the ovary, require a careful examination of their inner walls. Cystectomy is preferable to puncture with biopsy to avoid a recurrence of both functional and organic cysts.

Ovarian cystectomy for functional cysts (e.g., simple cysts, follicle cysts, or corpus luteum cysts) is not a common laparoscopic procedure, and laparoscopic excision should be considered only when persistence of the cyst or pain is documented. Even an actively bleeding hemorrhagic corpus luteum cyst can be totally excised laparoscopically with minimal bleeding. Hemostasis without excision of a bleeding corpus luteum can be obtained using electrosurgical fulguration with an electrode or the argon beam coagulator. Suture repair is sometimes indicated. Oophorectomy for a ruptured hemorrhagic corpus luteum is rarely indicated.

Simple cysts are aspirated with a needle attached to a syringe after cul-de-sac washings have been obtained. It must be emphasized that drainage with a needle does not prevent spill and is done for only the most benign-appearing cysts. After documentation of clear or hemosiderin-filled fluid, the ovarian cortex is opened at its most dependent portion with a knife electrode at a 70-W cutting current. The ovarian cortex is grasped with one biopsy forceps, and the cyst wall is grasped with another. Using traction, a dissection plane is obtained between the cyst wall and the ovarian tissue. Aquadissection helps to mobilize the cyst wall atraumatically from inside the ovary. During dissection of the ovarian cyst from the cortex, much repositioning of the traction forceps is necessary close to the cleavage plane. Either a cyst or ovarian cortex is peeled depending on which is easier. With careful dissection the entire cyst wall is excised. These cysts are removed through the 10-mm umbilical trocar sleeve. Hemostasis inside the ovary is secured by identifying individual bleeders using irrigation through an irrigating channel and coagulating them with microbipolar forceps. The ovary is usually closed with a pursestring stitch using a straight needle applied close to the utero-ovarian ligament in one direction and the infundibulopelvic ligament in the other. Alternately, a curved needle with 5–0 suture enters the lateral ovary near the infundibulopelvic ligament, exits it near the utero-ovarian ligament, re-enters the medial ovary near the utero-ovarian ligament, and, finally, exits cephalad; the curved needle can often be held stationary while ovarian cortex is picked up and placed on the needle.

Enlarged ovaries containing cysts are either free in the peritoneal cavity or attached to the pelvic sidewall, uterosacral ligament, or cul-de-sac. Frequently, a cyst attached to the sidewall proves to be an endometrioma. During mobilization of the cyst from the pelvic sidewall, "chocolate"-like hemosiderin-filled fluid spills from the ovary. When this occurs, the ovary is completely mobilized to its hilum using aquadissection and careful blunt dissection to avoid unnecessary pelvic sidewall peritoneal damage. The endometrioma cyst wall is then excised (see Fig. 17–2) (Reich and McGlynn, 1986b). The cyst wall is most firmly attached to the ovarian cortex in the area of rupture during dissection or avulsion, that is, on the portion adhered to the pelvic sidewall or uterosacral ligament. A knife electrode at a 70- to 100-W cutting current is used at the junction of ovarian cortex and endometrioma cyst wall to develop a dissection plane in this firmly attached area. If possible, this incision is extended through the visible 360-degree circumference of the opening. The cutting current destroys endometriosis at the ovarian cortex-endometrioma junction while making a divot of separation between the two structures. Thereafter, biopsy forceps are placed on the ovarian cortex and the endometrioma cyst wall, and traction is exerted to peel the endometrioma cyst wall from the ovary. Minimal bleeding accompanies this type of procedure and usually stops spontaneously. When the defect is large, the ovary is suture repaired, usually with one pursestring suture.

When a dermoid cyst is suspected, drainage is avoided and an attempt is made to excise the cyst without spillage. If a dermoid cyst is encountered during syringe aspiration, cyst excision should be accomplished with as little spillage as possible (see later).

If the ovary is free of the pelvic sidewall and other structures (even if the patient has a history of endometriosis), a dermoid cyst or other benign neoplasm may be present. Instead of puncturing the cyst at the start of the procedure, a very superficial longitudinal incision is made in the cortex with a CO_2 laser. The incision is extended with scissors and undermined with a combination of scissors and aquadissection. If the cyst is neoplastic, it will rarely rupture. If it is a functional cyst (follicle cyst or corpus luteum), its thin wall will usually rupture spontaneously. After rupture, the cyst is enucleated completely. If rupture does not occur, cystectomy without spillage is accomplished as described in the dermoid cyst section.

If the cyst could represent an ovarian cancer, sterile H_2O is left in the peritoneal cavity to lyse cells; otherwise, Ringer's lactate is used.

DERMOID CYSTS

Benign cystic teratoma (dermoid cyst) is the single most common ovarian neoplasm (44%) according to a 10-year retrospective review of 861 women with a postoperative diagnosis of ovarian neoplasm (Koonings et al, 1989). It is also the most frequently occurring teratoma with the highest prevalence found in ovulating women (Gerald, 1975). Both ovaries are involved in 10 to 15% of cases (Doss et al, 1977). Traditionally, dermoid cysts were managed by cystectomy or oophorectomy at laparotomy. Oophorectomy with culdotomy extraction can be considered for previously diagnosed or intraoperatively discovered dermoid cysts in women who have no desire for future child bearing and who have a normal contralateral ovary. Spillage is rare and can be directed through the culdotomy incision (Reich, 1987a).

Should laparoscopic cyst excision with associated intentional spillage be considered? Kistner (1952) described the aftermath of intraperitoneal rupture of benign cystic teratomas. The intraperitoneal spillage of dermoid contents sets up a granulomatous reaction in the peritoneum that, when viewed grossly, may be confused with tuberculosis or carcinomatosis.

In 1986, at a national meeting, Semm described the treatment of more than 70 dermoid cysts using laparoscopic surgical techniques. The cysts were drained into the cul-de-sac and then stripped from surrounding normal ovarian tissue. No adverse effects occurred. Reich (1989b), Reich and McGlynn (1986b), and Reich and associates (1989, 1992), and Nezhat and associates (1989) reported dermoid cystectomies with no complications from spillage. Bruhat's group in France has had a similar experience (Bruhat et al, 1992). Shelling out a dermoid from inside an ovary following drainage is usually much easier than endo-metrioma cyst wall excision. Vigorous peritoneal cavity irrigation with at least 10 liters of Ringer's lactate and underwater examination with direct suctioning of fatty and epidermal elements is recommended to prevent a chronic granulomatous reaction.

In most cases bilateral involvement, if present, will be evident on clinical examination. A normal opposite ovary with no identifiable tumor may be either left alone or cystic areas may be drained with the knife electrode as described in the section on polycystic ovaries (Doss et al, 1977). Synchronous covert bilaterality of mature teratomas is not common, and a visually normal contralateral ovary should not be routinely bivalved or wedge resected.

The literature is replete with reports of malignant elements found in ovarian teratomas (Shirley et al, 1971) with late sequelae including gliomatosis peritonei (Shefren et al, 1991). Thus, since January 1989, this author (H. R.) has attempted to remove dermoid cysts intact and still preserve the ovary. In all cases careful inspection of the pelvis and abdomen is undertaken. The ovaries are evaluated for visual evidence of malignancy. All cysts should be smooth-walled and should have no excrescence. Cystectomy without spillage is accomplished by using the CO_2 laser at 10 to 20 W in the superpulse or ultrapulse mode to vaporize a superficial incision through the ovarian cortex, avoiding rupture of the underlying cyst wall. Rupture could not be avoided when electrosurgical microelectrodes were used. After locating the cleavage plane between the cyst wall and the ovarian cortex, scissors are inserted and the opening is extended. Forceps traction and aquadissection are used to separate the dermoid cyst from surrounding ovarian tissue. Laser and scissors are used to separate fibrous adherences and vessels near the hilum. Caution is constantly exercised to prevent puncturing the cyst wall. Following excision of the intact cyst from inside the ovary, electrosurgical fulguration is used, if necessary, inside the ovary to obtain complete hemostasis. Usually the edges reapproximate, and suturing is not required; large ovarian defects are suture repaired.

FIGURE 18–4 Large ovarian cyst removed through a cul-de-sac

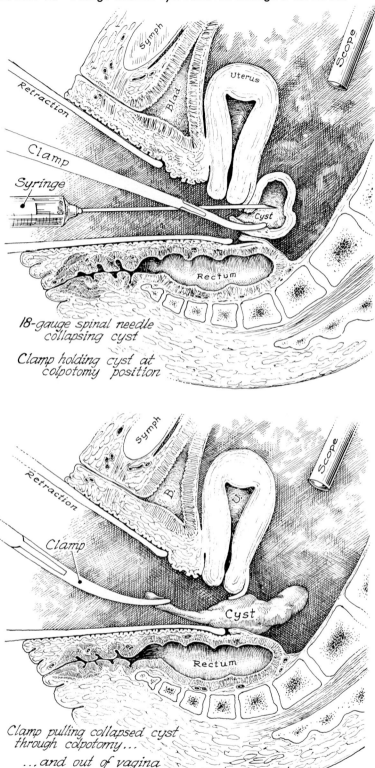

18-gauge spinal needle collapsing cyst

Clamp holding cyst at colpotomy position

Clamp pulling collapsed cyst through colpotomy...

...and out of vagina

The cyst is removed through the cul-de-sac using the previously described laparoscopic culdotomy incision (Fig. 18–4), which is made with the CO_2 laser at high power with resultant large spot size (3 to 4 mm) for hemostatic cutting.

The intact cyst is pushed deep into the cul-de-sac, where it is aspirated vaginally using a 14-gauge needle on a needle extender attached to a 50-ml syringe until it is small enough to pop out of the culdotomy incision. Thereafter the laser culdotomy incision is closed, vaginally or laparoscopically, with a 2–0 Vicryl suture on a curved needle. When the laparoscopic approach is employed, pneumoperitoneum is maintained by placing a No. 26 French Foley catheter with a 30-ml balloon into the vagina, a curved needle is inserted through a 5-mm trocar incision, and the suture is tied extracorporeally using the Clarke knot pusher. Two to three sutures usually result in a watertight closure of the cuff. Underwater examination is performed at the close of each procedure, and complete hemostasis is obtained. Two liters of Ringer's lactate solution are left in the peritoneal cavity. The umbilical incision is closed with a 4–0 Vicryl suture, and the lower quadrant incisions are closed with collodion.

Presently, following laser culdotomy, an impermeable sac (LapSac: Cook OB/ GYN) is inserted into the peritoneal cavity through the vagina. This 5 × 8 in. nylon bag has a polyurethane inner coating and a nylon drawstring. It is impermeable to water and dye. The free intact specimen is placed in the bag, which is closed by pulling the drawstring. The drawstring is delivered through the posterior vagina; the bag is opened; and the intact specimen is visually identified, decompressed, and removed.

When spillage occurs, vigorous peritoneal cavity irrigation and suction are repeated during underwater examination, which is performed by replacing the CO_2 pneumoperitoneum with lactated Ringer's solution. Direct suctioning of fatty and epidermal elements is performed until the effluent is clear of fat globules and blood products, usually after 10 to 20 liters of solution, to prevent a chronic granulomatous reaction.

POLYCYSTIC OVARIES

Polycystic ovaries can be drilled laparoscopically using electrosurgery or laser (Daniell and Miller, 1989; Gjönnaess, 1984). Polycystic or sclerocystic ovaries are usually enlarged with a smooth, thickened capsule and have no evidence of ovulatory stigma. Numerous 2- to 6-mm subcapsular follicular cysts are present with surrounding hyperplasia of the theca interna (stromal hyperthecosis). Following diagnosis by endocrinologic studies and vaginal ultrasound, women desiring present fertility should be treated with clomiphene citrate, alone or in combination with dexamethasone, and if resistant, clomiphene citrate–hCG. When clomiphene citrate does not work, the patient should be given the option of treatment with gonadotropin (Pergonal) or laparoscopic multiple cyst puncture. Laparotomy ovarian wedge resection should be avoided because of the high incidence of adnexal adhesions (25%) resulting from this procedure (Toaff et al, 1976).

At laparoscopy, multiple, symmetrically placed holes are drilled over subcapsular follicle cysts and into the stroma. Small polycystic ovarian cysts do not bleed like physiologic follicle cysts following incision. Although studies have not been performed to determine the actual depth of penetration into the stroma using the various energy sources, cutting current electrosurgery at 30 to 60 W makes a precise focal incision extending into the stroma, and more than 30 such incisions can be placed in each ovary. When using CO_2 or contact tip lasers, the surface puncture is much larger, limiting the number of cysts that can be actually drained and increasing the chances of later adhesion formation. Depth of penetration may be important in this procedure to destroy functioning theca surrounding the small ovarian follicles. Cutting current electrosurgery penetrates well on its way back to the indifferent dispersing electrode. On the other hand, CO_2 laser energy vaporizes extremely superficially and may not be the best energy source for this procedure.

Laparoscopic drilling of polycystic ovaries is, at best, a temporary solution. Normal ovulatory cycles may result for a short time. Concern remains regarding the possibility of ovarian adhesions or premature menopause from extensive ovarian damage by electrosurgery or laser. Care should be taken to avoid ovarian disruption close to the tubo-ovarian ligament to preserve tubal fimbrial freedom. Minor adhesions following this procedure were reported in 2 of 10 ovaries at second-look laparoscopy (Dabirashrafi et al, 1991), and presentations at meetings have revealed that more serious adhesions are possible.

ACUTE ADNEXAL TORSION

Adnexal torsion is a rare cause of acute pelvic pain. Although torsion occurs most frequently if there is an adnexal lesion, healthy organs can twist (Hibbard, 1985). The event can occur in the gravid or nongravid woman. Classically, management has been by laparotomy with excision of the afflicted organ without untwisting the pedicle. The reason for this approach was to avoid the risk of embolization from the occluded ovarian venous plexus (Jeffcoate, 1975).

Adnexal torsion usually occurs in young women in whom preservation of ovarian function is of paramount importance. Early laparoscopy is recommended for early diagnosis to reduce irreparable adnexal ischemia (Hibbard, 1985). Early laparoscopic evaluation also serves to exclude those patients in whom no organic lesion exists and permits immediate management of most other causes of acute pelvic pain. In Hibbard's series of 102 patients (1985), the adnexa were salvaged in only nine cases.

It has been suggested that ovarian preservation can be achieved if early diagnosis is made and the pedicle is simply untwisted. Laparoscopic unwinding was performed in 32 of 35 cases. It was possible to preserve 27 adnexa. No cases of thromboembolism occurred (Mage et al, 1989).

In my (H. R.) limited experience with acute adnexal torsion (nine cases), early laparoscopic intervention permitted diagnosis and immediate conservative management with organ preservation and reduced hospital stay. Two of nine women were pregnant (10 to 12 weeks) and delivered at term. All patients presented with acute unilateral, lower quadrant pain with onset within 72 hours of treatment. In four patients, a palpable mass was evident. All of the patients were free of pain postoperatively. There were no immediate postoperative complications.

The torsed adnexa are untwisted using a blunt probe or aquadissector and grasping forceps. Following complete unraveling of the tube and ovary, often involving multiple turns, the affected adnexa are observed to ensure viability of the involved structures usually while additional surgical procedures are performed. No special precautions are taken in pregnant patients other than avoiding the placement of an intrauterine manipulator (Reich et al, 1992).

Adnexal torsion will be seen more frequently because ovaries that have been stimulated with exogenous gonadotropins are more susceptible to this condition (Mashiach et al, 1990). It would appear that early recourse to laparoscopy permits accurate diagnosis, and effective, safe ovarian conservation while limiting hospital stay and therefore cost.

PAROVARIAN CYSTS

Parovarian cysts are often found dangling from the serosa surrounding the tubal fimbriae. Excision demonstrates the route that electric current follows as it passes to the patient return electrode. Usually a hooked electrode is placed adjacent to the cyst and its pedicle stretched. Care is taken to ensure that the cyst is not touching any surrounding viscus. Approximately 50 W of cutting current is applied for 0.5 second. A white desiccated area results adjacent to the tube where the pedicle enters but does not appear next to or beneath the electrode adjacent to the cyst. The current travels from the cyst along the pedicle to the tube with the area of desiccation occurring at the narrow segment of the pedicle before the current is dispersed in the wide tube on its way back to the return electrode. After desiccation adjacent to the tube, the pedicle is divided and the parovarian cyst is removed through 5- or 10-mm trocar sleeves.

In many cases the parovarian cysts are large and intermingled in the serosa surrounding the fimbriae. In these cases, the peritoneum is opened very carefully. Aquadissection is used to help dissect tissue planes and separate the cyst from the serosa and to protect the cyst from inadvertent rupture. Using scissors or laser, the cyst is extirpated from inside the serosa. When encountered, the cyst pedicle requires bipolar desiccation. After extraction, the tubal serosa is usually left alone but in some cases is opposed with a suture. Large cysts require aspiration before they are removed through a 5- or 10-mm trocar sleeve. Culdotomy is not necessary because these cysts are rarely malignant.

REFERENCES

Barber HR and Graber EA: The PMPO syndrome (postmenopausal palpable ovary syndrome). Obstet Gynecol *38*:921–923, 1971.

Bruhat MA, Mage G, Pouly JL, et al: Salpingostomy. *In* Operative Laparoscopy. New York, McGraw-Hill, 1992, pp 95–108.

Dabirashrafi H, Mohamad K, Behjatnia Y, and Moghadami-Tabrizi N: Adhesion formation after ovarian electrocauterization on patients with polycystic ovarian syndrome. Fertil Steril *55*:1200–1201, 1991.

Daniell JF and Miller W: Polycystic ovaries treated by laparoscopic laser vaporization. Fertil Steril *51*:232–236, 1989.

Daniell JF, Kurtz BR, and Lee J-Y: Laparoscopic oophorectomy: Comparative study of ligatures, bipolar coagulation, and automatic stapling devices. Obstet Gynecol *80*:325–328, 1992.

Doss N, Forney JP, Vellios F, and Nalick R: Covert bilaterality of mature ovarian teratomas. Obstet Gynecol *50*:651–653, 1977.

Eddy CA, Asch RH, and Balmaceda JP: Pelvic adhesions following microsurgical and macrosurgical wedge resection of the ovaries. Fertil Steril *33*:557–561, 1980.

Gerald PS: Origin of teratomas. N Engl J Med *292*:103–104, 1975.

Gjönnaess H: Polycystic ovarian syndrome treated by ovarian electrocautery through the laparoscope. Fertil Steril *41*:20–25, 1984.

Gomel V: Salpingostomy by laparoscopy. J Reprod Med *18*:265–268, 1977.

Hibbard LT: Adnexal torsion. Am J Obstet Gynecol *152*:456–461, 1985.

Jeffcoate TNA: Torsion of the pelvic organs. *In* Principles of Gynaecology, 4th ed. London, Butterworths, 1975, pp 280–282.

Kistner RW: Intraperitoneal rupture of benign cystic teratomas: Review of the literature with a report of two cases. Obstet Gynecol Surv *7*:603–617, 1952.

Koonings PP, Campbell K, Mishell DR Jr, and Grimes DA: Relative frequency of primary ovarian neoplasms: A 10-year review. Obstet Gynecol *74*:921–926, 1989.

Mage G, Canis M, Mahnes H, et al: Laparoscopic management of adnexal torsion: A review of 35 cases. J Reprod Med *34*:520–524, 1989.

Mann W and Reich H: Laparoscopic adnexectomy in postmenopausal women. J Reprod Med *37*:254–256, 1992.

Mashiach S, Bider D, Moran O, et al: Adnexal torsion of hyperstimulated ovaries in pregnancies after gonadotropin therapy. Fertil Steril *53*:76–80, 1990.

McComb PF and Paleologou A: The intussusception salpingostomy technique for the therapy of distal oviductal occlusion at laparoscopy. Obstet Gynecol *78*:443–447, 1991.

Nezhat C, Winer WK, and Nezhat F: Laparoscopic removal of dermoid cysts. Obstet Gynecol *73*:278–281, 1989.

Reich H: Laparoscopic oophorectomy and salpingo-oophorectomy in the treatment of benign tubo-ovarian disease. Int J Fertil *32*:233–236, 1987a.

Reich H: Laparoscopic oophorectomy without ligature or morcellation. Contemp Obstet/Gynecol *9*:34–46, 1989a.

Reich H: Laparoscopic treatment of extensive pelvic adhesions, including hydrosalpinx. J Reprod Med *32*:736–742, 1987b.

Reich H: New techniques in advanced laparoscopic surgery. Baillieres Clin Obstet Gynaecol *3*:655–681, 1989b.

Reich H, DeCaprio J, McGlynn F, and Taylor PJ: Laparoscopic diagnosis and management of acute adnexal torsion. Gynaecol Endosc *2*:37–38, 1992.

Reich H, DeCaprio J, McGlynn F, et al: Peritoneal trophoblastic tissue implants after laparoscopic treatment of tubal ectopic pregnancy. Fertil Steril *52*:337–339, 1989.

Reich H and McGlynn F: Laparoscopic oophorectomy and salpingo-oophorectomy in the treatment of benign tuboovarian disease (Abstract). J Reprod Med *31*:609, 1986a.

Reich H and McGlynn F: Treatment of ovarian endometriomas using laparoscopic surgical techniques. J Reprod Med *31*:577–584, 1986b.

Reich H, McGlynn F, Sekel L, and Taylor P: Laparoscopic management of ovarian dermoid cysts. J Reprod Med *37*:640–644, 1992.

Semm K and Mettler L: Technical progress in pelvic surgery via operative laparoscopy. Am J Obstet Gynecol *138*:121–127, 1980.

Shefren G, Collin J, and Soriero O: Gliomatosis peritonei with malignant transformation: A case report and review of the literature. Am J Obstet Gynecol *164*:1617–1620, 1991.

Shirley RL, Piro AJ, and Crocker DW: Malignant neural elements in a benign cystic teratoma: A case report. Obstet Gynecol *37*:402–407, 1971.

Toaff R, Toaff ME, and Peyser MR: Infertility following wedge resection of the ovaries. Am J Obstet Gynecol *124*:92–96, 1976.

FURTHER READINGS

OOPHORECTOMY

Levine RL: Pelviscopic surgery in women over 40. J Reprod Med 35:597–600, 1990.

Parker WH and Berek JS: Management of selected cystic adnexal masses in postmenopausal women by operative laparoscopy: A pilot study. Am J Obstet Gynecol 163:1574–1577, 1990.

Price FV, Edwards R, and Buchsbaum HJ: Ovarian remnant syndrome: Difficulties in diagnosis and management. Obstet Gynecol Surv 45:151–156, 1990.

Reich H and McGlynn F: Short self-retaining trocar sleeves. Am J Obstet Gynecol 162:453–454, 1990.

Reich H, McGlynn F, and Wilkie W: Laparoscopic management of Stage I ovarian cancer. J Reprod Med 35:601–605, 1990.

Reich H, McGlynn F, and Wilkie W: Laparoscopic management of stage I ovarian cancer. Obstet Gynecol Surv 45:772–773, 1990.

HYDROSALPINX

Reich H: Laparoscopic adhesiolysis techniques. The Female Patient 15:85–91, 1990.

Reich H: Laparoscopic treatment of extensive pelvic adhesions, including hydrosalpinx. J Reprod Med 32(10):736–742, 1987.

POLYCYSTIC OVARY

Armar NA, McGarrigle HHG, Honour J, et al: Laparoscopic ovarian diathermy in the management of anovulatory infertility in women with polycystic ovaries: Endocrine changes and clinical outcome. Fertil Steril 53:45–49, 1990.

Dabirashrafi H: Complications of laparoscopic ovarian cauterization. Fertil Steril 52:878, 1989.

Greenblatt E and Casper RF: Endocrine changes after laparoscopic ovarian cautery in polycystic ovarian syndrome. Am J Obstet Gynecol 156:279–285, 1987.

Hutchinson-Williams KA and DeCherney AH: Pathogenesis and treatment of polycystic ovary disease. Int J Fertil 32:421–430, 1987.

Ectopic Pregnancy

One in 66 pregnancies in the United States is an ectopic pregnancy. This complex yet increasingly common condition can occur in a variety of locations and under a diverse set of circumstances that can be appropriately managed using minimally invasive techniques with emphasis on tubal preservation. Pregnancy rates subsequent to laparoscopic management are the same as those obtained by laparotomy (Koninckx et al, 1991; Lundorff et al, 1992; Murphy et al, 1992; Sultana et al, 1992). Advantages of laparoscopic treatment over conventional surgical management include minimal cosmetically placed incisions, short hospital stay, significant reduction in recuperation time (Vermesh et al, 1989; Zouves et al, 1992), and fewer postoperative adhesions (Lundorff et al, 1991). Laparoscopic advantages over medical management include accurate assessment of pregnancy status and location, ability to lyse tubo-ovarian adhesions and evaluate the contralateral tube, confirmation by direct visualization of adequate treatment and complete hemostasis, and evacuation of all blood clots at the close of the procedure. For these reasons, laparoscopic management is emerging as the standard of care for early, unruptured pregnancies.

GENERAL CONSIDERATIONS

Considering the diversity and complexity of the problem, it is not surprising that controversy exists regarding the best way to preserve the tube in an early unruptured tubal pregnancy. The contenders are:

- Primary laparoscopic salpingotomy with or without closure
- Medical treatment with methotrexate
- Transvaginal injection of the ectopic pregnancy under sonographic guidance with prostaglandin, hypertonic glucose, potassium chloride (KCl), methotrexate
- Expectant management to let most of the contents absorb spontaneously

To address this controversy, multiple studies with long-term follow-up are necessary to determine tubal patency, fertility outcome, and subsequent recurrence of ectopic pregnancies following each of these treatment modalities. These studies must include better documentation regarding the location of the ectopic pregnancy, including whether it has penetrated the muscularis, an accurate description of its viability, and whether surrounding blood or clot is present. This documentation may not be obtainable using medical treatment, which is also unlikely to remove the underlying tubal cause. Intensely sclerosing agents like methotrexate may actually increase tubal adhesions when injected into the tubal lumen. A blood clot left to organize in the tube may do the same.

Large tubal diameter should not be considered a contraindication to laparoscopic treatment. Ipsilateral and contralateral adhesions are usually treated during the same laparoscopic procedure. At least 2 liters of lactated Ringer's solution are left in the peritoneal cavity at the close of the procedure. Postoperatively, Rh immunoglobulin (Ig) is administered to unsensitized Rh-negative patients with an ectopic pregnancy (50 μg of Rh Ig is usually adequate to prevent sensitization). As blood transfusion is rare in the stable patient, blood products are not typed and cross-matched preoperatively. Antibiotics are administered only in cases that last for more than 2 hours. Patients are followed postoperatively with β-hCG titers obtained on a weekly basis until undetectable.

EVACUATION OF HEMOPERITONEUM

A 5-mm aquadissector is usually sufficient to evacuate the hemoperitoneum, including large clots requiring much manipulation to disrupt them. In cases of tubal rupture, when the patient may be unstable and hemoperitoneum with clots may be excessive, an 11-mm trocar is inserted directly into the pelvis, and wall suction tubing is threaded through it (seamless surgical connecting tubing with an internal diameter of 0.25 in.) after cutting a 1-cm air hole 25 cm from the tubing tip to prevent bowel entrapment.

ANATOMY

An ectopic pregnancy can be tubal (ampullary, isthmic, or infundibular [Fig. 19–1]), interstitial, ovarian, cervical, or abdominal and can be present in more than one location or with an associated intrauterine pregnancy. Ectopic pregnancy is usually located within the lumen of the ampullary tube (67%) or in its extraluminal space between the serosa and the muscularis. The ectopic pregnancy may be leaking small or large amounts of blood through the distal tubal ostium; it may be in the process of rupturing; or it may be frankly ruptured with varying degrees of intravascular volume compromise. Distal tubal abortion may be in progress or completed. The ectopic pregnancy may be viable with fetal movement noted on ultrasound or dead with surrounding blood clot in various stages of organization.

SALPINGECTOMY

Laparoscopic salpingectomy is the method of choice when future fertility is not desired or in cases of rupture. Other indications are

- Ectopic pregnancy following sterilization failure
- In a blind-ending distal tubal segment following partial salpingectomy
- In a previously reconstructed tube
- In a woman requesting sterilization
- With continuing hemorrhage following salpingotomy
- Chronic tubal pregnancy

FIGURE 19–1 Anatomy of an ectopic tubal pregnancy

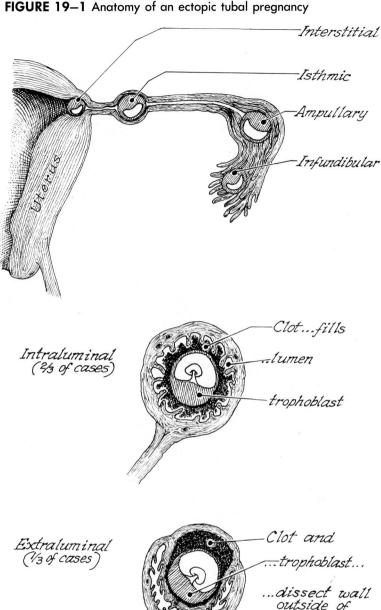

Interstitial

Isthmic

Ampullary

Infundibular

Uterus

Intraluminal (⅔ of cases)

Clot...fills ..lumen

trophoblast

Extraluminal (⅓ of cases)

Clot and ...trophoblast... ...dissect wall outside of ...lumen

FIGURE 19–2 Salpingectomy

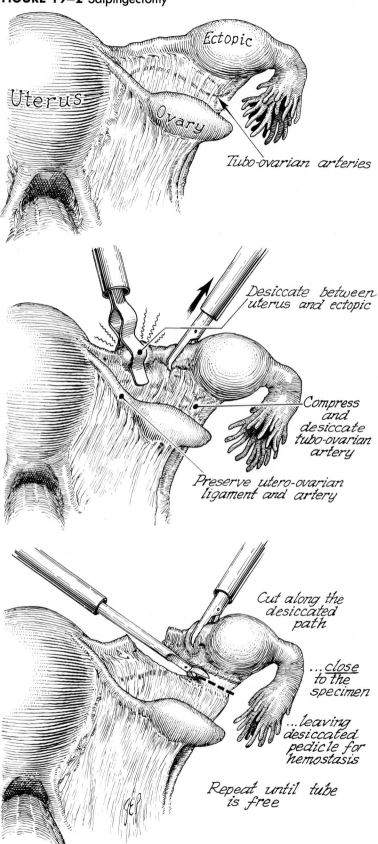

Ectopic

Uterus

Ovary

Tubo-ovarian arteries

Desiccate between uterus and ectopic

Compress and desiccate tubo-ovarian artery

Preserve utero-ovarian ligament and artery

Cut along the desiccated path

...close to the specimen

...leaving desiccated pedicle for hemostasis

Repeat until tube is free

Following evacuation of hemoperitoneum, Kleppinger bipolar forceps and laparoscopic scissors are introduced successively to desiccate and cut the tube and its mesosalpinx (Fig. 19–2). Bipolar continuous sinusoidal wave current (cutting) at 25 W should be used. An endpoint monitor is essential to indicate cessation of current flow representing the completion of desiccation and to reduce char sticking to the forceps as carbonization occurs thereafter. An Endoloop ligature (Ethicon) can also be used around the distended tube to perform a salpingectomy safely.

The segment of tube with its enclosed ectopic pregnancy is then removed from the peritoneal cavity through the 11-mm umbilical trocar sleeve, using forceps placed through the operating port of a right-angled operating laparoscope, as described previously. The laparoscope and sleeve are reinserted, and a final inspection is performed. Removal of a tube in this manner may result in a "milking" process in which products of conception, which are extruded from the tube as it is being pulled through the trocar sleeve, remain in the peritoneal cavity from where they can be removed with the aquadissector or biopsy forceps. Salpingotomy (ampullotomy) with aspiration of the products of conception can be considered to reduce its volume before extracting the tube through the umbilical trocar sleeve to prevent the milking effect.

The umbilical extension technique described in Chapter 14 is our present method of choice for removal of tubes containing products of conception from the peritoneal cavity. The products of conception can also be removed through a lower quadrant 5- or 11-mm trocar sleeve and rarely by culdotomy as described previously. Large tubal pregnancies can be pushed through the culdotomy incision from above, or they can be pulled through from below with ring forceps inserted vaginally under direct visualization.

SALPINGOTOMY

Tubal preservation should be attempted in all cases of ectopic pregnancy surgery in which future fertility may be desired, vital signs are stable, and gross rupture is not evident. Following evacuation of hemoperitoneum, the tube-ovary complex is mobilized usually with the aid of the aquadissector. In many cases a "phlegmon" of tube-ovary exists that should be separated using the aquadissector.

The mesosalpinx can be *infiltrated* with a dilute vasopressin solution as first described and popularized by Pouly and associates (1986) (Fig. 19–3; see preventive hemostasis in this figure). Dilute vasopressin solution (Pitressin, Parke Davis) combines 20 international units (1 ampule) diluted with 50 ml of physiologic solution. More dilute or more concentrated solutions may be used (20 to 100 ml). Either a 3-mm or 5-mm injection and puncture cannula with a 22-gauge sharp, beveled tip can be used through the lower quadrant trocar sleeves. Alternatively, the Veress needle shaft (disassembled) can be inserted directly through the skin at the pubic hairline level, lateral to the deep inferior epigastric vessels, and can act as a convenient guide for a 22-gauge spinal needle. Care must be taken at initial insertion into the mesosalpinx to avoid laceration of the blood vessels. The serosa should be gently punctured prior to the start of infiltration of solution (see Atlas, Plate 19). Thereafter, 10 to 20 ml of the solution (4 to 8 units) can be infiltrated causing a grossly visible swelling in the mesosalpinx. The effect persists for approximately 2 hours, allowing physiologic hemostasis to occur.

Because intravascular injection can cause arterial hypertension, a gentle touch is necessary during penetration of the mesosalpingeal peritoneum. Extravascular injection itself can induce a moderate increase in the arterial blood pressure or a moderate bradycardia. Because vasopressin is a coronary artery vasoconstrictor, its use is contraindicated in patients with ischemic heart disease and it should be monitored continuously for 2 hours. To date, no short- or long-term complications with its use have

FIGURE 19–3 Pitressin hemostasis for salpingotomy

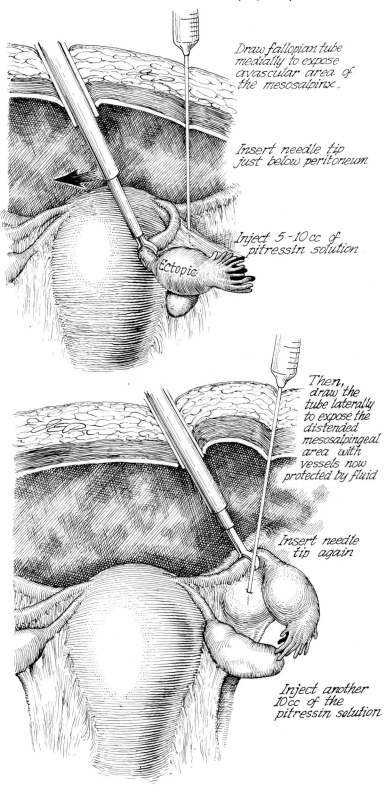

Draw fallopian tube medially to expose avascular area of the mesosalpinx.

Insert needle tip just below peritoneum

Inject 5-10 cc of pitressin solution.

Ectopic

Then, draw the tube laterally to expose the distended mesosalpingeal area with vessels now protected by fluid

Insert needle tip again

Inject another 10 cc of the pitressin solution

FIGURE 19–4 Salpingotomy

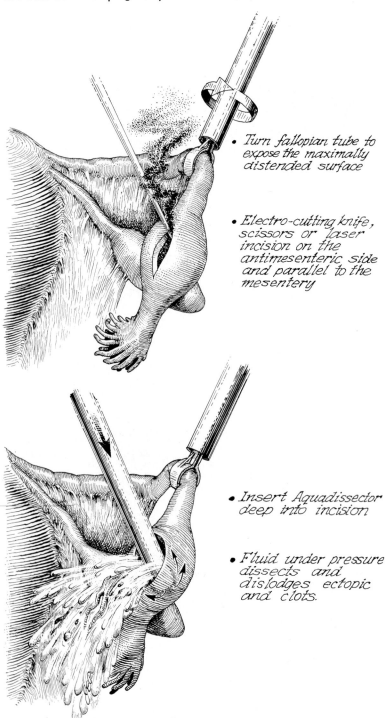

- Turn fallopian tube to expose the maximally distended surface

- Electro-cutting knife, scissors or laser incision on the antimesenteric side and parallel to the mesentery

- Insert Aquadissector deep into incision

- Fluid under pressure dissects and dislodges ectopic and clots.

been reported in the United States. Synthetic vasoconstrictor injection during surgical procedures has been abandoned in France. While complications secondary to its use during laparoscopic procedures have not been reported, deaths have occurred during laparotomy, myomectomy, and cervical procedures, perhaps because of the intravascular injection of this medication.

Trophoblast has a high metabolic requirement for oxygen, and these cells do not tolerate anoxia. As a result, it is very possible that vasopressin, by depriving the ectopic tissue of oxygen for 1 hour, may kill all nonremoved trophoblast and reduce the 5 to 15% risk of persistent ectopic pregnancy seen with conservative salpingotomy. These benefits outweigh the rare risk of cardiovascular reactions to vasopressin inadvertently given intravenously.

A knife electrode, introduced through a 5-mm second-puncture sleeve, is used to make a 1- to 2-cm tubal incision in the antimesenteric border over the point of maximal tubal dilatation, using cutting or blended current (20 to 70 W) (Fig. 19–4; see also Atlas, Plate 20). There is no evidence that any presently available laser offers an advantage over unipolar cutting current for making the salpingotomy incision. Tubal layers can often be identified: serosa followed by stretched out muscularis-mucosa prior to entering the tubal lumen. On occasion, a blood clot can be expressed from the extraluminal space prior to opening the muscularis-mucosa separately. In other cases, trophoblastic tissue is encountered following serosal incision, in the extraluminal space; in these cases, the true tubal lumen is rarely entered.

Following division of the tubal serosa over the point of maximal dilatation, blood clot should be evacuated. If products of conception are not evident, and the muscularis-mucosa is intact, it should then be divided to enter the tubal lumen. When the pregnancy is viable, it is often extremely friable and can be suction-evacuated using mainly the suction from an aquadissector. In most cases, however, the pregnancy is nonviable and surrounded by a blood clot in varying degrees of organization. Frequently, this blood clot surrounding the products of conception can be flushed out of the salpingotomy incision using pressurized irrigation from the aquadissector.

In other cases, the blood clot may have to be mobilized using smooth grasping forceps or pulled out with biopsy forceps. It is rare for the products of conception to extrude themselves. Thereafter, the placental bed and salpingotomy incision are well irrigated. With intraluminal tubal pregnancy, the irrigant will be seen to flow freely from the fimbrial end of the tube, and retrograde irrigation through the fimbriae will result in a jet of fluid from the salpingotomy incision. Transcervical tubal lavage using indigo carmine dye often demonstrates tubal patency. If the ectopic pregnancy is located in the extraluminal space, flushing through the salpingotomy incision results in distention of the tubal serosa with no flow of fluid from the fimbrial end of the tube. It is important to remember that large viable, friable, intraluminal ectopic pregnancies can often be more easily evacuated through a smaller incision than can nonviable intraluminal ectopic pregnancies. However, viable extraluminal pregnancies are extremely difficult to excise because their margins infiltrate the muscularis.

In these situations in which further dissection of possible trophoblast may damage the tubes or lead to uncontrollable hemorrhage, use of Pitressin will result in prolonged anoxia of the suspicious area. This treatment may devitalize residual trophoblast sufficiently to prevent persistent growth postoperatively. Anoxia rather than surgery would eliminate trophoblast and leave the tube minimally damaged.

An umbilical extension technique (see Chapter 14) is preferred to remove products of conception with or without enclosed tube from the peritoneal cavity. Following the evacuation of the products of conception from the tube, they can be removed from the peritoneal cavity through the 11-mm umbilical sleeve, usually using an operating laparoscope with its enclosed biopsy forceps. In other cases, the products of conception are reduced to smaller pieces using biopsy forceps and the aquadissector.

The tube is then irrigated distally with the aquadissector and proximally through a cervical Cohen-Eder cannula (Eder Instrument Co.). The salpingotomy is usually left open. If the defect is large, or marked eversion of mucosa occurs, a seromuscular suture can be placed. However, in second-look laparoscopies performed in Kiel, Germany, where suturing was routinely used, adhesion formation has been noted (Mecke et al, 1989).

If bleeding from the tubal edge or implantation site is present following evacuation of the products of conception, pressure with a grasping forceps should be attempted before resorting to electrosurgical coagulation, laser, or a suture. Frequently, 5 minutes of compression at the salpingotomy edge will result in complete hemostasis. Lifting the tube-ovary above the pelvic brim, in effect kinking the mesosalpingeal vessels, gives a similar result.

Arterial bleeding can be identified after evacuating surrounding clot and is best treated with pinpoint bipolar desiccation made possible by irrigating over the bleeding site through one incision and applying microbipolar electrodes through the other. Diffuse venous bleeding, especially in the extraluminal space following evacuation of trophoblastic tissue invading the muscularis, is best treated with electrosurgical fulguration. A spark or arc is generated using coagulation current at 25 to 50 W through an electrode in noncontact mode, which rapidly chars and carbonizes the underlying tissue until hemostasis is complete. The large amount of superficial char in the extraluminal space will not impede healing of the tubal epithelium, which has been compressed by the extraluminal tubal pregnancy.

If uncontrollable hemorrhage occurs during the evacuation of the ampulla, it can be compressed with an Endoloop (Ethicon). After 5 to 10 minutes, during which time the cul-de-sac and the subphrenic space are irrigated and evacuated, the ligature is released. In most cases, the bleeding subsides or can be accurately located and coagulated; if not, one can try to control bleeding by selecting an appropriate area to suture-ligate mesosalpingeal vessels.

FIGURE 19–5 Partial salpingectomy

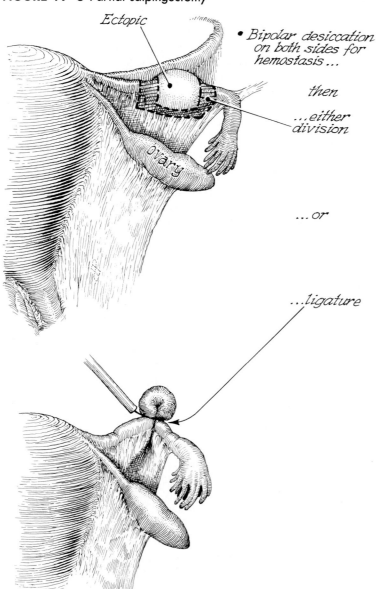

Ectopic

• *Bipolar desiccation on both sides for hemostasis...*

then

...either division

...or

...ligature

ovary

PARTIAL SALPINGECTOMY (MIDTUBE RESECTION)

Laparoscopic partial salpingectomy can be attempted to preserve the tube if salpingotomy fails, for ruptured tubal pregnancy, isthmic ectopic pregnancy (DeCherney and Boyers, 1985), distal interstitial ectopic pregnancy, and ipsilateral recurrent tubal pregnancy (Fig. 19–5). Kleppinger bipolar forceps are used to desiccate the tube on each side of the distention made by the tubal pregnancy. The resultant desiccated areas are then divided with laparoscopic scissors. The mesosalpinx supplying the involved tubal segment is next coagulated and divided, and the tube segment is removed from the peritoneal cavity through the 11-mm umbilical trocar sleeve or by laparoscopic laser culdotomy.

Alternatively, to eliminate thermal necrosis (but not ischemic necrosis), an Endoloop ligature (Ethicon) can be placed around the tube segment with its enclosed ectopic pregnancy. Again the tube and its mesosalpinx are divided with laparoscopic scissors. If the Endoloop ligature slips, the pedicles can be regrasped and either another Endoloop ligature can be placed or complete hemostasis can be obtained using bipolar forceps.

FIMBRIAL EVACUATION OF TUBAL PREGNANCY

Fimbrial evacuation, tubal aspiration without salpingotomy, and tubal abortion without salpingotomy all refer to the technique of removing products of conception at or near the fimbrial end of the tube using either suction or grasping forceps, and on occasion, using grasping forceps gently to push the products of conception toward the fimbrial end. In some cases, tubal abortion is already in progress.

Concern regarding incomplete removal of trophoblast and increased tubal damage has resulted in fimbrial evacuation of tubal pregnancy being condemned using either laparoscopic or laparotomy technique, especially following the study of Budowick and associates (1980) implying that most tubal pregnancies occur in the extraluminal space. The findings of Sherman and colleagues (1987) of excellent reproductive outcome after fimbrial expression may encourage the laparoscopic surgeon to reconsider this method.

If most ampullary tubal pregnancies rapidly invade the tubal wall and grow in the loose connective tissue between mucosa and serosa, milking the ectopic pregnancy out of the fimbriae would cause further tubal destruction. However, most ampullary or fimbrial pregnancies are intraluminal and can be treated gently with aqua expression (Fig. 19–6). With this technique, in selected cases of nonviable intraluminal ampullary ectopic pregnancy, the tip of the aquadissector is inserted through the open end of the affected tube into the ampulla and fluid under pressure is used to dislodge and expel the intraluminal products of conception with surrounding blood clot (a tubal cast) without a salpingotomy incision. They can then be aspirated from the peritoneal cavity. In eight cases in which we performed surgery, there were no intraoperative or postoperative complications, and β-hCG titers were in the nonpregnant range 2 weeks after surgery in all cases (Reich, 1990).

FIGURE 19–6 Fimbrial aqua expression

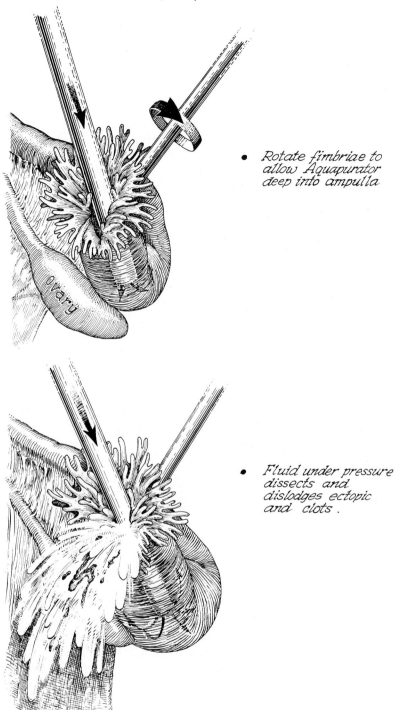

• *Rotate fimbriae to allow Aquapurator deep into ampulla*

• *Fluid under pressure dissects and dislodges ectopic and clots.*

EXTRALUMINAL TUBAL PREGNANCY

In 1980, Budowick and associates concluded from a series of 20 dissections of tubal pregnancies that the growing gestation rapidly penetrates the wall of the tube and subsequently most of its growth occurs in an extratubal location between the tubal serosa and its muscularis. Stock (1985) reviewed the histopathology of 110 cases of tubal gestation and concluded that the developing tubal pregnancy was intraluminal, within the muscularis of the tube, in all except one case. Pauerstein and associates (1986), following a systematic gross and histopathologic study of 25 consecutive ectopic pregnancies, concluded that an intraluminal location was present in 67%. This evolving understanding of the pathophysiology of ectopic tubal pregnancy has significant clinical implications regarding management decisions.

In most cases of extraluminal ectopic pregnancy, on opening the tubal serosa over the most distended portion of the tube, products of conception will be evident and often extrude themselves. Thereafter, irrigation with the aquadissector will produce distention of the tube without any flow of irrigant out of the fimbrial end. If bleeding is present, the surgeon can err by trying to open the tube further.

Rarely will the surgeon enter the true tubal lumen. Occasionally, the blood clot or products of conception will envelope the space between the serosa and the muscularis through 360 degrees. After removal of the bulk of the products of conception and obtaining hemostasis with pressure, electrosurgical fulguration, or laser, the surgeon should end the procedure and follow the patient carefully with β-hCG titers. Adjuvant therapy with methotrexate may be considered.

INTERSTITIAL ECTOPIC PREGNANCY

Interstitial ectopic pregnancies can be treated laparoscopically by electrosurgical cornual wedge resection resulting in preservation of most of the distal portion of the tube but destruction of much interstitium,

making a future anastomosis unlikely to succeed. Bipolar desiccation of both the ascending uterine and utero-ovarian arteries may be necessary to gain hemostasis. To avoid postoperative hemorrhage as constricted arterioles relax, vasopressin is not used (Reich et al, 1990).

The same techniques employed during laparotomy can be applied to laparoscopic resection of an interstitial pregnancy—segmental resection of the cornua using cutting- or blended-current electrosurgery. The principles involved are very similar to those gained from removing fibroids from the myometrium during laparoscopic surgery. Large vessel hemostasis can be obtained with bipolar forceps, and dissection planes can be developed with the aquadissector. Alternatively, following vasopressin infiltration, an incision can be made with the knife electrode or laser down to the gestational sac, which can then be aspirated with an aquadissector.

Methotrexate may prove to be a useful adjuvant for interstitial pregnancy. Tanaka and associates (1982) and Brandes and colleagues (1986) have documented its successful use.

RUPTURED TUBAL PREGNANCY

Ruptured tubal pregnancy has been considered a contraindication to a laparoscopic approach. However, many ruptured tubes can be easily and safely removed with bipolar desiccation.

In a series of 109 consecutive tubal pregnancies (Reich et al, 1988), there were 16 cases of ruptured tubal pregnancy. Salpingectomy or partial salpingectomy was performed in 13 of these cases, and salpingotomy was done in three cases. Subsequently two women have had intrauterine pregnancies. Another woman in this group, who underwent salpingectomy, has since had two pregnancies in her remaining tube, both treated by laparoscopic salpingotomy.

According to Pouly and associates (1986), of 118 women still desiring fertility who had tubal pregnancies treated by laparoscopic salpingotomy, a ruptured tube was present in 47 cases. Intrauterine pregnancies were later recorded in 27 of these women (57.4%), and recurrent ectopic pregnancy was recorded in 9 (19%). A ruptured tube was present in 32 of the 100 cases of laparoscopic salpingectomy that Dubuisson and associates (1987) reported.

Little controversy exists when tubal rupture with unstable vital signs occurs. The bleeding must be stopped, and the tube is usually removed as quickly as possible. Most gynecologists will be more comfortable with a direct laparotomy in this situation. Laparoscopic bipolar desiccation works rapidly to seal even large uterine and ovarian vessels permanently following the expulsion and disruption of fluids, electrolytes, and the fibromuscular matrix of which they are composed. Alternately, suture ligature with an Endoloop (Ethicon) can be considered. Following cessation of all bleeding, the tube or tubal segment can easily be removed in a similar manner. Ruptured interstitial pregnancy can also be treated with bipolar desiccation of the uterine and ovarian vessels. However, concern remains regarding weakness in the wall of the uterus should a subsequent pregnancy occur.

OVARIAN PREGNANCY

Ovarian ectopic pregnancy, when recognized, can be treated much like any other ovarian cyst of unknown etiology—it can be shelled out, often intact through a small superficial ovarian cortex incision. Usually ovarian function is not disrupted. Ovarian pregnancy should be suspected in women with β-hCG titers above 6000, empty uterus by ultrasound, and no evidence of a tubal pregnancy at laparoscopy. The knife electrode at 20- to 30-W cutting current is used to bivalve the ovary perpendicular to its longest axis, starting at its most dependent part where the cystic area meets the solid area. Thereafter, the cortex over the cystic area can be lifted with grasping forceps, and the aquadissector can be inserted to aquadissect the gestational sac gently from surrounding ovarian tissue. An intact sac can often be removed from inside the ovary with little accompanying ovarian bleeding. The ovary usually falls together without a suture thereafter.

PERSISTENT TROPHOBLASTIC TISSUE

Successful conservative treatment of tubal pregnancy is documented by declining quantitative β-hCG levels. Persistent trophoblastic tissue has been described and implies trophoblast's surviving either within the tube or in the peritoneal cavity following conservative surgery. It should be suspected if serum levels of the β subunit of human chorionic gonadotropin are detectable 2 weeks after surgery. Thereafter titers should be followed, and a tentative diagnosis should be made if they plateau or rise. A second laparoscopy should be performed to confirm the diagnosis and institute treatment.

Stock (1991) described histologic findings in eight cases. After the obvious distal clots had been removed by salpingotomy or fimbrial expression, trophoblast tissue remained in the medial portion of the conserved tubes. He suggested the use of vasopressin in the mesosalpinx to deprive trophoblast of oxygen and to reduce the incidence of persistent disease.

In our series of 56 consecutive tubal pregnancies treated laparoscopically, one persistent ectopic pregnancy occurred and was treated with a second laparoscopic salpingotomy procedure 4 weeks later. Two other women had persistent β-hCG titers: laparoscopy 4 weeks later revealed ectopic trophoblastic tissue on the pelvic sidewall and cul-de-sac peritoneum. Treatment consisted of excision with laparoscopic biopsy forceps or laser vaporization (Reich et al, 1989).

Persistent trophoblastic tissue has been successfully treated with methotrexate without a laparoscopic procedure. However, laparoscopy has the advantage of documenting the location of the tissue. If the trophoblastic tissue is in the form of peritoneal implants, patency can be confirmed in the salpingotomized tube. Conversely, if methotrexate therapy can be instituted without laparoscopic diagnosis, future hysterosalpingography revealing patent tubes should not be misconstrued as evidence supporting the benefits of methotrexate therapy.

REFERENCES

Brandes MC, Youngs DD, Goldstein DP, and Parmley TH: Treatment of cornual pregnancy with methotrexate: Case report. Am J Obstet Gynecol 155:655–57, 1986.

Budowick M, Johnson TRB Jr, Genadry R, et al: The histopathology of the developing tubal ectopic pregnancy. Fertil Steril 34:169–171, 1980.

Dubuisson JB, Aubriot FX, and Cardone V: Laparoscopic salpingectomy for tubal pregnancy. Fertil Steril 47:225–228, 1987.

Koninckx PR, Witters K, Brosens J, et al: Conservative laparoscopic treatment of ectopic pregnancies using the CO_2-laser. Br J Obstet Gynaecol 98:1254–1259, 1991.

Lundorff P, Hahlin M, Källfelt B, et al: Adhesion formation after laparoscopic surgery in tubal pregnancy: A randomized trial versus laparotomy. Fertil Steril 55:911–915, 1991.

Lundorff P, Thorburn J, and Lindblom B: Fertility outcome after conservative surgical treatment of ectopic pregnancy evaluated in a randomized trial. Fertil Steril 57:998–1002, 1992.

Murphy AA, Kettel LM, Nager CW, et al: Operative laparoscopy versus laparotomy for the management of ectopic pregnancy: A prospective trial. Fertil Steril 57:1180–1185, 1992.

Pauerstein CJ, Croxatto HB, Eddy CA, et al: Anatomy and pathology of tubal pregnancy. Obstet Gynecol 67:301–308, 1986.

Pouly JL, Mahnes H, Mage G, et al: Conservative laparoscopic treatment of 321 ectopic pregnancies. Fertil Steril 46:1093–1097, 1986.

Reich H: Aquadissection. In Baggish M (ed): Clinical Practice of Gynecology. Vol 2: Endoscopic Laser Surgery. Amsterdam, Elsevier, 1990, pp 159–185.

Reich H, Johns DA, DeCaprio J, et al: Laparoscopic treatment of 109 consecutive ectopic pregnancies. J Reprod Med 33:885–890, 1988.

Reich H, McGlynn F, Budin R, et al: Laparoscopic treatment of ruptured interstitial pregnancy. J Gynecol Surg 6:135–138, 1990.

Sherman D, Langer R, Herman A, et al: Reproductive outcome after fimbrial evacuation of tubal pregnancy. Fertil Steril 47:420–424, 1987.

Stock RJ: Histopathologic changes in tubal pregnancy. J Reprod Med 30:923–928, 1985.

Stock RJ: Persistent tubal pregnancy. Obstet Gynecol 77:267–270, 1991.

Sultana CJ, Easley K, and Collins RL: Outcome of laparoscopic versus traditional surgery for ectopic pregnancies. Fertil Steril 57:285–289, 1992.

Tanaka T, Hayashi H, Kutsuzawa T, et al: Treatment of interstitial ectopic pregnancy with methotrexate: Report of a successful case. Fertil Steril 37:851–852, 1982.

Vermesh M, Silva P, Rosen G, et al: Management of unruptured ectopic gestation by linear salpingostomy: A prospective randomized clinical trial of laparoscopy versus laparotomy. Obstet Gynecol 73:400–404, 1989.

Zouves C, Urman B, and Gomel V: Laparoscopic surgical treatment of tubal pregnancy: A safe, effective alternative to laparotomy. J Reprod Med 37:205–209, 1992.

FURTHER READINGS

DeCherney AH and Boyers SP: Isthmic ectopic pregnancy: Segmental resection as the treatment of choice. Fertil Steril 44:307–312, 1985.

DeCherney AH, Romero R, and Naftolin F: Surgical management of unruptured ectopic pregnancy. Fertil Steril 35:21–24, 1981.

Mecke H, Semm K, Freys I, et al: Incidence of adhesions in the true pelvis after pelviscopic operative treatment of tubal pregnancy. Gynecol Obstet Invest 28:202–204, 1989.

Reich H, DeCaprio J, McGlynn F, et al: Peritoneal trophoblastic tissue implants after laparoscopic treatment of tubal ectopic pregnancy. Fertil Steril 52:337–339, 1989.

Reich H, Freifeld M, McGlynn F, and Reich E: Laparoscopic treatment of tubal pregnancy. Obstet Gynecol 69:275–279, 1987.

Semm K: Operative Manual for Endoscopic Abdominal Surgery: Operative Pelviscopy: Operative Laparoscopy. Chicago, Year Book Medical Publishers, 1987.

Semm K: Technique of second look pelviscopic surgery: Prevention of recurrent adhesions. Abstract no. 82 in Third World Congress on the Fallopian Tube, July 3 to 6, 1990, Kiel, West Germany.

Pelvic Sidewall Dissection

Locating pelvic retroperitoneal structures should be second nature to surgeons performing advanced gynecologic laparoscopic surgery. When operating near the ureter, it is safer to expose it at an early stage than to check its position repeatedly during the procedure.

Pelvic sidewall dissection refers to:

- The division or excision of pathologic adhesions, lesions, or organs adherent to or invading into the pelvic sidewall peritoneum
- Retroperitoneal dissection either to confirm normal anatomic relationships or to excise pathologic tissue

Laparoscopic access for pelvic sidewall dissection is superior to laparotomy because of increased magnification from the laparoscope and the video monitor, and the ability to stop bleeding and evacuate a blood clot at the close of the procedure by direct visualization. For surgeons without gynecologic oncology training, pelvic sidewall structures are easier to identify with a laparoscope. In this chapter we present the anatomy and technique of dissection.

INSTRUMENT CHOICES AND TECHNIQUES

Aquadissection

To perform intraperitoneal pelvic sidewall dissection, the tip of the aquadissector is placed against the adhesive interface between bowel/adnexa, adnexa/pelvic side-wall, or bowel/pelvic sidewall, and the pressurized fluid gushing from it is used to develop a cleavage plane that can be extended bluntly or with more fluid pressure. Aquadissection is also used to develop and distend the retroperitoneal spaces to aid in their dissection during excision or vaporization of endometriosis on the peritoneal undersurface and for retroperitoneal surgery.

Scissors Dissection

Straight scissors are used to lyse sharply thin and thick adhesions between the tube, ovary, and pelvic sidewall. This is the primary technique used for adhesiolysis in infertile women to diminish the potential for adhesion formation; electrosurgery and laser are often reserved for tubal, ovarian, and pelvic sidewall hemostasis. Spontaneous hemostasis often occurs in sharply divided vessels, but they should be examined at the close of the procedure to detect bleeding from delayed relaxation of vessels in spasm.

Hooked scissors are valuable when the surgeon can get completely around the structure being divided, but they rarely maintain their sharpness. Blunt-tipped 5-mm sawtooth scissors maintain their sharp edge (E8383.46, Wolf; Manhes scissors, Storz). They should be employed whenever possible during separation of the adnexa and rectosigmoid from pelvic sidewall peritoneum, and they should also be used for blunt dissection. Scissors lysis of the attachment of rectosigmoid to the left iliac fossa just above the pelvis followed by its medial reflection is a useful technique to expose the left ureter at the pelvic brim and to gain better access to the left adnexa.

Electrosurgery

To avoid ureteral and venous injury, unipolar electrosurgery should be avoided when working on the pelvic sidewall or retroperitoneal space unless the surgeon is well versed in this modality. The expert laparoscopic surgeon can use unipolar electrosurgery safely to cut or fulgurate tissue, but desiccation (coagulation) of sidewall structures should be performed with bipolar techniques.

Laser Dissection

Use of the CO_2 laser through the operating channel of the laser laparoscope allows the surgeon a panoramic field of vision with the ability to cut or ablate tissue in this field.

In addition, a CO_2 laser with its 0.1-mm depth of penetration and inability to transverse through water allows the surgeon much security when working around the bowel, ureter, and major vessels. Backstops are rarely necessary because of this superficial depth of penetration and wet surgical field, especially when the operator develops the skill to use the tissue to be vaporized as the backstop.

When working around the pelvic sidewall structures, the CO_2 laser is set between 25 and 35 W in superpulse or ultrapulse mode so that very high power is released for brief surges, theoretically allowing tissue to cool between pulses and thus reduce surrounding thermal conduction.

ANATOMY OF THE PELVIC SIDEWALL

Following the bifurcation of the common iliac artery, the external iliac artery passes along the pelvic brim to a point beneath the inguinal ligament, midway between the anterior superior iliac spine and the pubic symphysis (Fig. 20–1). The external iliac vein lies partly beneath and medial to it. The rest of the vessels of the pelvic sidewall are branches of the internal iliac artery and vein. Progressing downward along the pelvic sidewall, the vessels most frequently encountered are the superior vesical artery, hypogastric vein (deeper), obturator artery and vein (deeper), uterine artery and veins, vaginal vessels, inferior vesical vessels, middle rectal vessels, internal pudendal vessels, and the superior rectal artery on the left.

The ureter runs downward and medial from the kidney on the psoas major muscle in the subserous fascia of the peritoneum. It enters the pelvic cavity by crossing either the common iliac or external iliac vessels at their bifurcation. The right ureter lies to the right of the inferior vena cava and is crossed by the right colic and ileocolic vessels, the small bowel mesentery, and the terminal part of the ileum. The left ureter is crossed by the left colic vessels from the inferior mesenteric vessels, and just above the pelvic brim passes behind the sigmoid colon and its mesocolon. In the pelvis, the ureter lies in front of the hypogastric artery and medial to the obturator, uterine, inferior vesical, and middle rectal arteries. The ureter usually forms the posterior boundary of the ovarian fossa and then runs medial and forward on the lateral aspect of the cervix and upper part of the vagina to reach the fundus of the bladder. In this part of its course, it is accompanied for about 2 cm by the uterine artery, which then crosses over the ureter and ascends between the two leaves of the broad ligament.

The adventitia or outer fibrous coat of the ureter is divided into an outer network (ureteric sheath), with unconvoluted vessels that anastomose with each other, and an inner network containing densely convoluted corkscrew arteries. Small arteries run radially from the adventitia to supply the muscle coat and the mucosa. The pelvic portion of the ureter is supplied by the common iliac artery, internal iliac artery, iliolumbar artery, superior gluteal artery, superior and inferior vesical arteries, ovarian artery, and middle rectal artery.

Two avascular spaces filled with fat and areolar connective tissue are present on each pelvic sidewall: the paravesical and the pararectal space. Development of the pararectal space is often important during pelvic sidewall dissection. This space is covered by peritoneum lateral to the uterosacral ligaments, posterior vagina, and rectum. The landmarks for entry into the space are the ureter attached to the medial peritoneum, the internal iliac (hypogastric) artery laterally, the sacrum posteriorly, and the broad ligament anteriorly.

FIGURE 20–1 Laparoscopic view of pelvic sidewall

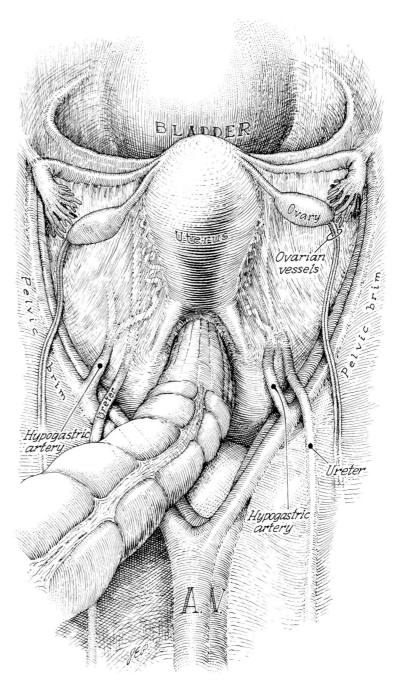

FIGURE 20–2 Identification of the ureter

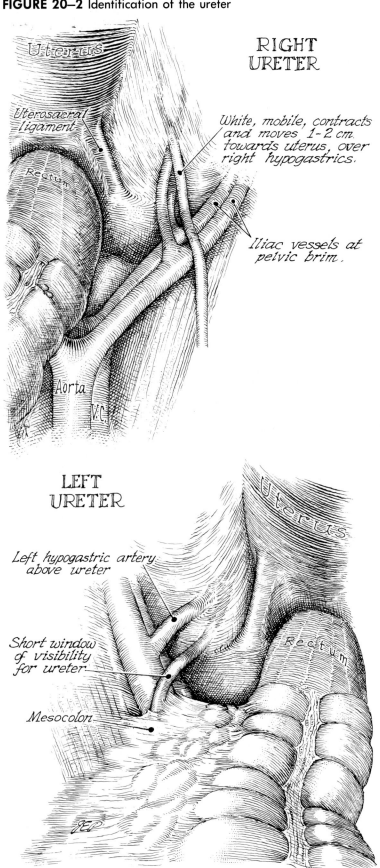

RIGHT URETER

White, mobile, contracts and moves 1-2 cm towards uterus, over right hypogastrics.

Uterus

Uterosacral ligament

Rectum

Iliac vessels at pelvic brim.

Aorta

V.C.

LEFT URETER

Left hypogastric artery above ureter

Short window of visibility for ureter

Mesocolon

Uterus

Rectum

PROCEDURES INVOLVING PELVIC SIDEWALL DISSECTION

Ureteral Dissection

Pelvic structures may be matted down by extensive endometriosis, dense adhesions following infection or previous surgery, cancer, or radiation fibrosis, obliterating most surgical landmarks (Fig. 20–2). Blunt dissection or aquadissection can be attempted initially, but soon thereafter, mobilization of the rectosigmoid and ureteral dissection must be performed. On the left side, the rectosigmoid may obscure all structures including the ovary and ureter. On the right, the cecum and small bowel may act similarly, but in many cases the rectosigmoid is also adhesed there. Dissection should start well out of the pelvis. Initially, the ureters may be visualized above the sacral promontory. On the left, the ureter may be seen crossing the common iliac artery, beneath the branches of the inferior mesenteric vessels. On the right, the ureter is usually further lateral, crossing the right external iliac artery soon after its origin from the common iliac artery. A 30-degree Trendelenburg position facilitates this visualization, as does reflection of the small bowel mesentery superiorly and to the right.

On the left, dissection begins well out of the pelvis where the descending colon becomes the sigmoid colon and the sigmoid colon with its inverted-V shaped mesocolon traverses the psoas muscle. Using blunt-tipped, sawtooth scissors, the lateral reflection of the rectosigmoid in the paracolic gutter and the iliac fossa is divided. Using the blunt tip of the scissors and aquadissection, the sigmoid colon is reflected medially exposing the fossa muscle. Dissection continues until the external iliac artery is exposed. Starting laterally along this vessel, the ovarian vessels are identified and, as medial progress is made, the ureter is visualized, followed by the superior rectal artery. It is safer to expose the ureter starting at the pelvic brim and continuing down into the pelvis at the same time that the rectosigmoid is freed from deep pelvic sidewall structures. Scissors are used to cut the peritoneum overlying the ureter. Fibrotic tissue between the rectosigmoid and the ureter should be excised. As the dissection continues into the deep pelvis, a rectal probe is passed to delineate further its position and facilitate retraction of the rectosigmoid away from pelvic sidewall structures. The ureter is usually lower on the left than on the right.

On the right side, small bowel and appendiceal adhesions are frequently encountered. Both scissors and CO_2 laser through the operating laparoscope are used to divide these adhesions. Once the parietal peritoneum has been incised, aquadissection can be used to develop a plane between the peritoneum and the small bowel serosa. The external iliac artery is exposed, and the ureter is identified crossing it and traced into the pelvis. Dissection continues using CO_2 laser or scissors on top of the ureter. Atraumatic forceps or suction-traction with the aquadissector are used for traction.

Smooth blunt-tipped grasping forceps are used to free the ureter from the surrounding areolar tissue. These forceps are opened parallel and perpendicular to the ureter to free it. The dissection often continues down into the deep pelvis, where the ureter is crossed by the uterine vessels.

Laparoscopic Adhesiolysis

The rectosigmoid can be stuck to the pelvic sidewall, obscuring visualization of the left adnexa. Again, dissection should start well out of the pelvis as just described. Aquadissection is used to distend the space between the sigmoid colon and the common external iliac vessels to identify the junction of the sidewall parietal peritoneum with the sigmoid serosa, and the rectosigmoid is reflected toward the midline. Thereafter, with the rectosigmoid placed on traction toward the midline, rectosigmoid and rectal adhesions to the left pelvic sidewall are divided starting cephalad and continuing caudad.

Small bowel adhesions should be divided, if possible, with scissors alone. The small bowel is grasped with atraumatic grasping forceps or the suction tip of an aquadissector and put on traction. Often, fluid can be injected into the adhesive spaces with the aquadissector to facilitate identification of the involved structures. In other cases, the aquadissector can be used as a backstop behind an adhesive band that is divided with the CO_2 laser. Injected fluid from the aquadissector also serves as a good backstop when operating close to the small bowel with this laser.

Ovarian adhesions to the pelvic sidewall can be filmy or fused. The object of adhesiolysis in these cases is to preserve as much peritoneum as possible while freeing the ovary. Dissection begins by using the aquadissector to develop potential spaces among the adhesions. Thereafter, laparoscopic scissors are used to divide thick adhesions, taking very small bites and using the scissors tips to separate the ovarian cortex bluntly from the parietal peritoneum. Dissection continues until the ovary is free to its hilum. On occasion, a CO_2 laser can be used to aid in this dissection, especially if ureteral location is in doubt, because this laser has very little depth of penetration.

Endometriosis: Peritoneal Implants

Peritoneum close to the lateral or undersurface of the ovary should be preserved, if possible, especially if no adhesions are present at the start of the procedure. Superficial fibrotic or hemorrhagic pelvic sidewall peritoneal endometriosis is vaporized precisely using CO_2 laser at 30-W superpulse, 50-W ultrapulse, or cutting current through a pointed electrode at 30 W. All other endometriosis implants are excised, including fibrotic endometriosis overlying the ureters and uterine vessels, especially on the sides of the uterus. An elliptical incision is made in the normal peritoneum surrounding the lesions; its edge is lifted upward; and the lesion is undermined using aquadissection. This pushes pelvic sidewall structures away so that the undersurface of the lesion can be divided with laser, electrosurgery, or scissors. Following excision, the ureter is checked and superficial endometriosis in this area is excised or vaporized.

Ovarian Remnant

Persistent pelvic pain after total abdominal hysterectomy with bilateral salpingo-oophorectomy may be secondary to an ovarian remnant, especially if the hysterectomy was performed for extensive ovarian adhesions or endometriosis. In this author's (H. R.) experience with 12 patients treated laparoscopically, the ureter was contiguous with the ovarian remnant in all 12 cases. Ten were left-sided and completely covered by the rectosigmoid in a retroperitoneal position. The two right-sided remnants were also retroperitoneal, with the rectosigmoid involved in one case.

Dissection on the left side should start well out of the pelvis, where the descending colon meets the sigmoid colon. The lateral attachments of this junction in the paracolic gutter are divided and the descending colon/rectosigmoid junction is reflected medially. Further dissection and reflection are necessary until the external iliac artery is exposed. Going along this large vessel, the ureter is identified, and in most cases the ovarian vessel pedicle can be lifted just lateral to the ureter as it crosses the external iliac artery. Both are followed into the deep pelvis with careful dissection. The rectosigmoid is carefully reflected from the deeper ureter, and the ovarian vessel pedicle that lies above the ovarian remnant can be identified. Once the rectosigmoid is completely detached from the sidewall, ureteral dissection proceeds deeper into the pelvis, just beyond all the attachments to the remnant. Thereafter the ovarian vessel pedicle is desiccated with bipolar forceps; divided; and put on medial traction to expose further the lateral limits of the ovary attached to retroperitoneal structures, usually the superior vesicle and obturator vessels. Dissection continues until the ovary is completely freed from the pelvic sidewall. Bleeding from neovascularization is controlled with the microbipolar forceps, usually underwater. The ovarian remnant is removed from the peritoneal cavity through the umbilical incision. Underwater examination is used to confirm complete hemostasis on the pelvic sidewall and the rectosigmoid.

FURTHER READING

Price FV, Edwards R, and Buchsbaum HJ: Ovarian remnant syndrome: Difficulties in diagnosis and management. Obstet Gynecol Surv 45:151–156, 1990.

GYNECOLOGIC CONTROVERSIES

Operative laparoscopy is a rapidly developing field in which many innovations are being constantly introduced. In the dynamic process of medical progress, some procedures gain instant acceptance; some raise strong controversy by challenging standard procedures, assumptions, or theories; and some fade away or languish for the medical establishment to rediscover in the future. This textbook has up to now presented procedures that can be considered medically and legally standard accepted practices for the general gynecologist and the advanced gynecologic laparoscopist. We now turn to current controversies.

The authors have selected from the wide assortment of laparoscopic procedures being described those that are currently raising the strongest controversies and are challenging established methods of management. In a few years after this edition is published, the medical establishment will have accepted some of these procedures as superior to standard care and will have rejected others. Rather than predict the outcome of these controversies or pass judgment on the merits of the argument, we introduce the controversies in a "for" and "against" format, presenting as best as we can the rationale and data supporting each position.

The area of management of persistent adnexal masses (see Chapter 21) brings into conflict the laparoscopic inclinations of the reproductive surgeons and the open laparotomy standards of gynecologic oncologists. We have therefore asked a board-certified reproductive endocrinologist, Jouko K. Halme, M.D., to review the current data supporting laparoscopic management, and we have also asked a board-certified gynecologic oncologist, David H. Moore, M.D., to present the current concerns of oncologists regarding ovarian carcinoma and this approach (see Chapter 21). Both are on the faculty of the Department of Obstetrics and Gynecology at the University of North Carolina at Chapel Hill. Nicholas Kadar, M.D., Grad IS, MRCOG, Associate Professor and Director, Division of Pelvic Surgery,

Robert Wood Johnson Medical School, New Brunswick, NJ, joined Harry Reich in writing the chapter on pelvic lymphadenectomy (see Chapter 27) and brings to this textbook the experience of our British colleagues in the use of laparoscopy for gynecologic oncology. Joel M. Childers, M.D., Assistant Professor of Gynecologic Oncology at the University of Arizona in Tucson, has pioneered techniques of laparoscopic lymphadenectomy, both pelvic and aortic, in the United States and adds a discussion of aortic node dissection (see Chapter 28).

Laparoscopic Management of Persistent Ovarian Masses

REASONS FOR

Jouko K. Halme, M.D., Ph.D.

Incidence of Cancer in Ovarian Masses

In women in the childbearing years, and beyond, most ovarian neoplasms are benign. To arrive at an estimate of the frequency of cancer in these neoplasms, I have reviewed and summarized recent data.

Koonings and colleagues (1989) reviewed all persistent ovarian masses operated on at the University of Southern California for a 10-year period. Of 290 patients aged 20 to 29, only 4% of the masses were malignant and 2% were borderline tumors. All functional cysts, endometriomas, and müllerian remnant masses were excluded from the analysis, and therefore the 6% malignancy rate is a great overestimation of the risk of malignancy in a persistent ovarian mass. Even if preoperative sonographic examination had mistakenly diagnosed a parovarian cyst as an ovarian cystic mass, the chance of malignancy is low. Stein and associates (1990) evaluated 168 parovarian tumors and found only three malignancies—all were larger than 8 cm in diameter and had internal papillary projections. It appears unlikely that one could miss such tumors on preoperative or laparoscopic evaluation. Another piece of information that helps us to estimate the likelihood of a neoplasm, either malignant or benign, among persistent benign-appearing ovarian masses, is the article by Ayers and colleagues (1990). They report on sonographic evaluation of 120 patients younger than 45 with persistent ovarian masses. Of these, five masses did not meet the criteria of unilocularity, hypoechogenicity, and absence of ascites, and the patients were subjected to laparotomy. All five were benign neoplasms. The remaining 115 masses were subjected to sonographically guided aspiration; 33 were found to be endometriomas; and 82 were found to be dysfunctional cysts.

Taking all these data together, one would estimate that approximately 5% of all ovarian unilocular masses are neoplasms and that only approximately 5% of ovarian neoplasms are malignant. Thus, the absolute risk of malignancy in an ovarian mass that appears unilocular on preoperative ultrasound is 0.25% or 2.5:1000.

This estimate agrees quite well with published experience to date in laparoscopic management of ovarian masses. The 1988 American Association of Gynecologic Laparoscopists' survey of operative laparoscopy yielded 3 (0.06%) cases of spillage of malignant cysts in 5075 ovarian masses (Peterson et al, 1990). Hasson (1990) found no malignancies among 83 laparoscopically managed persistent ovarian masses. Parker and Berek (1990) resorted to laparotomy in 3 (12%) of 25 patients for laparoscopic management of postmenopausal ovarian cysts. In Kiel, Germany, where essentially all ovarian masses are subjected to initial laparoscopy, Lehmann-Willenbrock and colleagues reported on 969 patients of all ages (Lehmann-Willenbrock et al, 1990a and 1990b). Mainly because of other pathology or suspected malignancy on inspection, 187 (18%) were subjected to laparotomy; 782 patients were managed laparoscopically only, and among them, two invasive carcinomas (0.2%) were not recognized during the procedure and were inadvertently managed through the laparoscope. In the 1990 American Association of Gynecological Laparoscopists' (AAGL) survey of laparoscopic management of ovarian masses (Hulka et al, 1992), approximately 15% of laparoscopies were converted to laparotomies after gross inspection. Of those patients managed by laparoscopy alone, about 0.4% proved to have stage I cancer that was not diagnosed at the time of surgery. These survey findings are highly consistent with the individual series cited earlier.

Prognosis after Rupture of Cyst with Ovarian Carcinoma

What is the risk of rupture of a malignant mass and possible spillage of tumor cells into the peritoneal cavity? Although an older series (Webb et al, 1973) from the Mayo Clinic did suggest a deleterious effect of tumor rupture on survival, newer data from careful multivariate analysis by Dembo and associates (1990) clearly indicate that tumor rupture is not a significant predictor of 5-year disease-free survival. This holds true even if corrected for grade, presence of ascites, or major tumor adherence. These data and other similar results have

prompted the International Federation of Gynecology and Obstetrics (FIGO) to consider removing stage 1c from the classification of stage 1 ovarian cancer. It appears that tumor rupture may not be as detrimental as was previously thought.

Preoperative and Operative Diagnosis

On the basis of the foregoing, I would recommend the following management of persistent ovarian masses. Premenopausal ovarian cysts do not appear to respond to hormone suppression therapy even when "functional" (Steinkampf et al, 1990); thus a trial of suppression is no longer warranted. Ultrasound-guided cyst aspiration to rule out malignancy has also not been warranted, in large part because of the poor negative predictive value (77%) of the cytology of cystic aspirates (Granberg et al, 1991). An endoscopist and an oncologist, Parker and Berek (1990), have suggested preoperative ultrasonic criteria for management of postmenopausal cystic masses:

- Less than 10 cm in diameter
- Distinct borders
- No irregular or solid parts
- No thick septa
- No ascites
- No matted bowel
- Normal CA 125

A diagnostic laparoscopy is then performed in which the pelvis is carefully inspected and evaluated. The surface of the tumor and the presence or absence of adhesions and ascites are evaluated and assessed; contents of the cystic mass are identified by aspiration; and the cyst fluid is evaluated by inspection or cytology. Then a representative tissue biopsy of the mass is sent for histology on frozen section. Finally, the cyst cavity is carefully evaluated.

These criteria for laparoscopic management are consistent with those proposed as a "risk of malignancy index" (RMI) by Jacobs and associates (1990). Their index consists of multiplying three variables: (1) CA 125 value, (2) menopausal status (pre = 1, post = 3), (3) abdominal ultrasound findings (none = 0; one = 1; two to five = 3) of the following:

- Multilocular cyst
- Solid areas
- Metastases
- Ascites
- Bilateral lesions

Treatment

Laparoscopic treatment of a mass should follow immediately after the diagnostic part of the procedure has revealed no evidence of malignancy. Most cystic masses can be managed with drainage and fenestration. If an endometrioma is encountered, removal of the cyst wall is preferable. In some cases when the ovary is not deemed to be salvageable, an oophorectomy or salpingo-oophorectomy can be performed laparoscopically. Finally, extensive irrigation of the pelvis will be performed to minimize the chances that malignant or irritating cellular material would have been present and disseminated.

Benefit-Risk of the Approach

The advantage of laparoscopic surgery is its being an outpatient procedure with shorter recovery time and lower cost. From the Kiel data, supported by Parker and Berek (1990), and the AAGL survey it appears that of 1000 patients with adnexal masses, approximately 20% will require laparotomy for size, known carcinoma, or other pathology, but 800 women can avoid major surgery for a benign asymptomatic condition. Since spillage at the time of surgery does not affect outcome, the laparoscopies will not worsen the prognosis of the two patients found to have unsuspected ovarian cancer.

REASONS AGAINST

David H. Moore, M.D.

Gynecologists are frequently confronted with the problem of a persistent ovarian cyst. Physical findings (e.g., bilaterality, size, liver enlargement, ascites, metastases) and abdominal symptoms (e.g., bloating, cramping, nausea or vomiting, constipation) strongly suggest a malignant etiology. In the absence of these signs and symptoms the diagnosis is often unclear, and the appropriate medical or surgical approach is undefined.

Operative laparoscopy is being increasingly used for the treatment of a variety of pelvic maladies, and it was inevitable that the laparoscopist expand the horizons of endoscopic pelvic surgery to include the removal of ovarian cysts. Proponents of laparoscopic surgery cite lower morbidity, shorter hospital stay, and reduced cost as advantages over laparotomy. The question is: Does the capability define the indication? To address this question, it is essential that we contemplate two other pertinent questions:

1. How accurately can we exclude the presence of ovarian malignancy through preoperative evaluation?

2. What are the possible consequences of laparoscopic removal of a malignant ovarian neoplasm?

Accuracy of Preoperative Evaluation

Conventional management of the cystic ovarian mass is illustrated by the study that Spanos (1973) presented at the 1972 Pacific Coast Obstetrical and Gynecological Society meeting. After excluding patients with possible ovarian malignancy, 286 premenopausal women were treated for 6 weeks with an estrogen/progestin combination; 81 patients underwent surgical exploration for mass persistence. No functional cysts were found, and 6.8% of cysts proved to be malignant. This study is dated by the complete reliance on the pelvic examination as a diagnostic tool, which is unheard of in modern gynecology. Nonetheless, it proves

that the incidence of malignancy in a persistent ovarian mass is not zero, even among premenopausal women. Several series would suggest that the incidence of malignancy is probably less than 1%, perhaps as much a testimony to our recent ability to detect benign ovarian cysts as it is a demonstration of the overall infrequency of ovarian cancer.

Finkler and colleagues (1988) used a pelvic examination, CA 125 analysis, and ultrasonography in 131 consecutive women about to undergo exploratory laparotomy for an adnexal mass. Single test specificities for excluding the presence of malignant disease ranged from 69 to 96% in premenopausal women and 85 to 92% in postmenopausal women. By combining all three tests, negative predictive values were unchanged in premenopausal women but improved from 41 to 80% in postmenopausal women. The absence of ovarian cancer was not reliably confirmed by preoperative evaluation.

Jacobs and associates (1990) similarly found a simple combination of CA 125 value, premenopausal versus postmenopausal status, and abdominal ultrasound findings could be expressed as a risk of malignancy index (RMI). In their study, an RMI of greater than 200 had 42 times the background risk of cancer; an RMI of lower than 200 had 0.15 times the background risk.

Reports using color Doppler to detect decreased capillary resistance in malignant ovarian neoplasms from Yugoslavia (Kurjak et al, 1991 and 1992), Japan (Kawai et al, 1992), and Israel (Weiner et al, 1992) hold promise for a specific and sensitive preoperative predictor of malignancy, although color Doppler may not be more useful than combinations of ultrasound, MRI, and CA 125 (Hata et al, 1992). Perhaps the development of other imaging techniques such as computed tomography, endovaginal probe ultrasound, magnetic resonance imaging, or serologic testing for other tumor-associated markers will also enable the clinician to eliminate cancer from the preoperative differential diagnosis. Otherwise, when determining the surgical approach, the possibility for ovarian cancer must always be recognized.

Consequences of Laparoscopic Removal of Ovarian Cancer

The diagnosis of ovarian cancer is established on histopathologic grounds. Although uncommon, several benign conditions can give rise to the appearance of "metastases" or ascites. The presence of an ovarian malignancy is suspected with the discovery of an enlarged, multilobulated ovary with external excrescences and is confirmed with the microscope.

Techniques of laparoscopic cyst removal are well described in the medical literature. Large cysts are virtually impossible to remove intact; therefore, needle aspiration of cyst contents or cyst wall fenestration is usually necessary (Hasson, 1990). What are the implications of cyst rupture in the event of ovarian malignancy? Two studies contradict the assumption of worsened prognosis with cyst rupture (Dembo et al, 1990; Sevelda et al, 1989). However, most patients in these series received adjuvant therapy, and implications of cyst rupture in untreated patients were not addressed. Laparoscopic tumor dissemination has been reported with metastases developing at trocar insertion sites (Hsiu et al, 1986). Results from Gynecologic Oncology Group protocols no. 7601/7602 have identified a subset of patients with ovarian cancer without need of adjuvant treatment (Young et al, 1990). This subset does not include patients with cyst rupture; consequently, many women are exposed unnecessarily to chemotherapy or radiation therapy through inadequate operative technique.

Despite statements to the contrary (Reich et al, 1990), laparoscopy is not yet accepted as a surgical approach to suspected ovarian malignancy. The incidence of retroperitoneal lymph node metastases exceeds 30% in apparent early ovarian cancer (Burghardt et al, 1986; Young et al, 1983). The ability to assess adequately the retroperitoneum with the laparoscope is questionable. Furthermore, laparoscopy can miss tumor deposits within the abdominal cavity as much as 50% of the time (Berek et al, 1981; Ozols et al, 1981). Finally, the size of disease residual is a significant prognostic factor, and tumor debulking via the laparoscope is not possible.

CONCLUSIONS

Operative laparoscopy is a welcome, exciting, developing addition to the armamentarium of the gynecologic surgeon. Like all clinical tools, it has the potential for misuse. It must be responsibly applied in appropriately selected circumstances.

The inability to detect or exclude the presence of ovarian malignancy accurately is a clinical dilemma for all gynecologists and oncologists. Any ovarian mass requiring surgical definition must be considered malignant until proved otherwise. A laparotomy incision of size sufficient to permit removal without capsular rupture remains the treatment of choice and the standard for future comparison.

Ultrasound has undoubtedly increased the detection of ovarian cysts, many of which might otherwise resolve without surgical therapy. Detection of functional and benign ovarian cysts with various imaging studies may explain the relative rarity of invasive cancer compared with the older gynecologic literature. Indications for surgical intervention are not clear in many published series. It is equally important that gynecologists determine the natural history of thin-walled, unilocular, ovarian cysts that are less than 6 cm, because they determine the role of operative laparoscopy in the surgical management of all ovarian cysts.

REFERENCES

Ayers JWT, Peterson EP, Knight L, and Peterson S: Transvaginal sonographic assessment and aspiration of ovarian cysts—"organ preserving" therapy for the persistent adnexal mass. Presented at the 46th annual meeting of the American Fertility Society, Washington, DC. Abstract O–116, 1990.

Berek JS, Griffiths CT, and Leventhal JM: Laparoscopy for second-look evaluation in ovarian cancer. Obstet Gynecol *58*:192–198, 1981.

Burghardt E, Pickel H, Lahousen M, and Stettner H: Pelvic lymphadenectomy in operative treatment of ovarian cancer. Am J Obstet Gynecol *155*:315–319, 1986.

Dembo AJ, Davy M, Stenwig AE, et al: Prognostic factors in patients with stage I epithelial ovarian cancer. Obstet Gynecol *75*:263–273, 1990.

Finkler NJ, Benacerraf B, Lavin PT, et al: Comparison of serum CA125, clinical impression, and ultrasound in the preoperative evaluation of ovarian masses. Obstet Gynecol *72*:659–664, 1988.

Granberg S, Norstrom W, and Wikland M: Comparison of endovaginal ultrasound and cytological evaluation of cystic ovarian tumors. J Ultrasound Med *10*:9–14, 1991.

Hasson HM: Laparoscopic management of ovarian cysts. J Reprod Med 35:863–867, 1990.

Hata K, Hata T, Manabe A, et al: A critical evaluation of transvaginal Doppler studies, transvaginal sonography, magnetic resonance imaging, and CA 125 in detecting ovarian cancer. Obstet Gynecol 80:922–926, 1992.

Hsiu J-G, Given FT, and Kemp GM: Tumor implantation after diagnostic laparoscopic biopsy of serous ovarian tumors of low malignant potential. Obstet Gynecol 68:90s–93s, 1986.

Hulka JF, Parker WH, Surrey MW, and Phillips JM: Management of ovarian masses. AAGL 1990 Survey. J Reprod Med 37:599–602, 1992.

Jacobs I, Oram D, Fairbanks J, et al: A risk of malignancy index incorporating CA 125, ultrasound and menopausal status for the accurate preoperative diagnosis of ovarian cancer. Br J Obstet Gynaecol 97:922–929, 1990.

Kawai M, Kano T, Kikkawa F, et al: Transvaginal Doppler ultrasound with color flow imaging in the diagnosis of ovarian cancer. Obstet Gynecol 79:163–167, 1992.

Koonings PP, Campbell K, Mishell DR Jr, and Grimes DA: Relative frequency of primary ovarian neoplasms: A 10-year review. Obstet Gynecol 74:921–926, 1989.

Kurjak A, Schulman H, Sosic A, et al: Transvaginal ultrasound, color flow, and Doppler waveform of the postmenopausal adnexal mass. Obstet Gynecol 80:917–921, 1992.

Kurjak A, Zalud I, and Alfirevic Z: Evaluation of adnexal masses with transvaginal color ultrasound. J Ultrasound Med 10:295–297, 1991.

Lehmann-Willenbrock E, Meck H, and Semm K: Preoperative assessment of tumor dignity: A retrospective analysis of 1016 ovarian tumors. VII World Congress of Human Reproduction, Helsinki, Finland, June 26 to July 1, 1990a, Abstract 58.

Lehmann-Willenbrock E, Meck H, and Semm K: The treatment of ovarian cysts by operative pelviscopy: A retrospective study of 969 cases. VII World Congress of Human Reproduction, Helsinki, Finland, June 26 to July 1, 1990b, Abstract 57.

Ozols RF, Fisher RI, Anderson T, et al: Peritoneoscopy in the management of ovarian cancer. Am J Obstet Gynecol 140:611–619, 1981.

Parker WH and Berek JS: Management of selected cystic adnexal masses in postmenopausal women by operative laparoscopy: A pilot study. Am J Obstet Gynecol 163:1574–1577, 1990.

Peterson HB, Hulka JF, and Phillips JM: American Association of Gynecologic Laparoscopists' 1988 membership survey on operative laparoscopy. J Reprod Med 35:587–589, 1990.

Reich H, McGlynn F, and Wilkie W: Laparoscopic management of stage I ovarian cancer: A case report. J Reprod Med 35:601–605, 1990.

Sevelda P, Dittrich C, and Salzer H: Prognostic value of the rupture of the capsule in stage I epithelial ovarian carcinoma. Gynecol Oncol 35:321–322, 1989.

Spanos WJ: Preoperative hormonal therapy of cystic adnexal masses. Am J Obstet Gynecol 116:551–556, 1973.

Stein AL, Koonings PP, Schlaerth JB, et al: Relative frequency of malignant parovarian tumors: Should parovarian tumors be aspirated? Obstet Gynecol 75:1029–1031, 1990.

Steinkampf MP, Hammond KR, and Blackwell RE: Hormonal treatment of functional ovarian cysts: A randomized, prospective study. Fertil Steril 54:775–777, 1990.

Webb MJ, Decker DG, Mussey E, and Williams TJ: Factors influencing survival in Stage I ovarian cancer. Am J Obstet Gynecol 116:222–228, 1973.

Weiner Z, Thaler I, Beck D, et al: Differentiating malignant from benign ovarian tumors with transvaginal color flow imaging. Obstet Gynecol 79:159–62, 1992.

Young RC, Decker DG, Wharton JT, et al: Staging laparotomy in early ovarian cancer. JAMA 250:3072–3076, 1983.

Young RC, Walton LA, Ellenberg SS, et al: Adjuvant therapy in stage I and II epithelial ovarian cancer. Results of two prospective randomized trials. N Engl J Med 322:1021–1027, 1990.

Laparoscopic Hysterectomy

Hysterectomy is the third most common abdominal surgical procedure in the United States (after cesarean section and cholecystectomy). Approximately 600,000 hysterectomies are performed annually. In the United States, about one in every three women has had a hysterectomy by the time that she is 60 years of age. In women under 65 years of age, 70% of hysterectomies are performed using an abdominal approach (Bachmann, 1990).

Laparoscopic hysterectomy can be considered a substitute for abdominal hysterectomy (but not for vaginal hysterectomy). Most hysterectomies that currently require an abdominal approach can be performed with laparoscopic dissection of part or all of the abdominal portion followed by removal through the vagina.

DEFINITIONS

Laparoscopic hysterectomy was first performed in January 1988 (Reich et al, 1989). The sine qua non for laparoscopic hysterectomy is the laparoscopic ligation of the uterine vessels either by electrosurgical desiccation, suture ligature, or staples.

Although hysterectomy is not the most difficult laparoscopic procedure, it can be long and tedious because four very well defined vascular pedicles must be ligated.

Laparoscopic Hysterectomy Classification

The laparoscope can be used for *diagnostic* purposes, when indications for a vaginal

approach are equivocal, to determine if *vaginal hysterectomy* is possible (Kovac et al, 1990). After hysterectomy, the vaginal cuff and pedicles can be inspected for hemostasis, and clot evacuated.

Laparoscopically assisted vaginal hysterectomy (LAVH) implies a surgical procedure performed laparoscopically after which vaginal hysterectomy is done. In these procedures, adhesions are lysed; endometriosis is excised; or oophorectomy is performed (Maher et al, 1992; Minelli et al, 1991; Summitt et al, 1992).

Laparoscopic hysterectomy (LH) denotes laparoscopic ligation of the uterine arteries. All maneuvers after uterine vessel ligation can be done vaginally or laparoscopically including anterior and posterior vaginal entry, cardinal and uterosacral ligament division, uterine removal intact or by morcellation, and vertical or transverse vaginal closure (Liu, 1992; Reich et al, 1989).

Total laparoscopic hysterectomy (TLH) is a laparoscopically assisted abdominal hysterectomy. Laparoscopic dissection continues until the uterus lies free of all attachments in the peritoneal cavity.

Laparoscopic supracervical hysterectomy has regained advocates after Kilkku and associates (1983) from Finland reported reduction in orgasms after hysterectomy compared with supravaginal amputation. The uterus can be removed by morcellation from above or below.

REASONS FOR

A major benefit of laparoscopic and vaginal hysterectomy is the avoidance of an abdominal incision that typically requires a longer hospitalization (5 days) and recuperation time (4 to 6 weeks). This reduction of time away from work and family is increasingly important to today's woman. The major intraoperative advantages of a laparoscopic approach to hysterectomy include ureteral identification and the ability to achieve complete hemostasis and evacuate all blood clots. Liberal lavage to remove bacteria introduced vaginally may reduce the postoperative infections associated with vaginal hysterectomy, further decreasing postoperative hospitalization and recovery time. Ileus is rare after extensive laparoscopic surgery.

In the United States, 75% of hysterectomies are done with an abdominal approach. If laparoscopic hysterectomy is added to our surgical armamentarium, most hysterectomies will be done without an abdominal incision over the next few years, with great economic benefit to women who are able to return to their normal activities earlier.

Finally, the true objective is for the patient to avoid an abdominal wall incision without jeopardizing her safety. The surgeon must remember that if vaginal hysterectomy is possible after ligating the utero-ovarian ligaments, it should be done. Laparoscopic inspection at the end of the procedure still allows the surgeon to control any bleeding and evacuate a clot. Unnecessary operations should not be done because of the gynecologist's preoccupation with the development of surgical skills and operative technique or by those who are not knowledgeable in reproductive anatomy, physiology, and the clinical manifestations of pelvic disease.

REASONS AGAINST

The first, and most obvious, line of questioning regarding this procedure is why? Many experienced surgeons have had satisfactory experience with vaginal hysterectomy as a fairly rapid procedure with low morbidity. In the hands of vaginal surgeons, the addition of procedures such as laparoscopic coagulation and division of the

ovaries and ligaments attaching to the uterus may not be worthwhile. This was the conclusion of a prospective, randomly assigned study comparing standard vaginal hysterectomy with one assisted by laparoscopy (Stovall et al, 1992).

The combination of laparoscopy and vaginal hysterectomy to substitute for an abdominal hysterectomy assumes that the abdominal incision is the cause of postoperative morbidity. In fact, a good argument can be made that the more extensive pathology leading surgeons to require an abdominal approach (large fibroids or adnexal masses) causes the observed morbidity, not the abdominal incision.

Some residencies produce physicians who are more comfortable with laparoscopic dissection than in the past because of the incorporation of laparoscopic management of ectopic pregnancy into standard practice. To these physicians, perhaps more skilled in laparoscopy than in vaginal surgery, this approach may be appealing.

As Pitkin (1992) points out in an editorial, however, prospective, randomly assigned comparisons between the morbidity and cost of abdominal hysterectomy compared with laparoscopically assisted hysterectomy are needed to justify this approach. It may well be that in the hands of recent resident trainees, laparoscopically coagulated and divided tubes, ligaments, and even uterine vessels would result in more secure hemostasis and less anatomic distortion. To justify using this approach, the operating room time, blood loss, and recovery time should be compared between abdominal hysterectomy and laparoscopically assisted vaginal hysterectomy. Such comparisons have been made between laparotomy and laparoscopy for ectopic pregnancy (Lundorff et al, 1991) with results favorable for laparoscopy. Results of such comparisons for laparoscopically assisted hysterectomy should resolve this current controversy soon.

INDICATIONS

The indications for laparoscopic hysterectomy include benign pathology usually requiring the selection of an abdominal approach to hysterectomy: fibroids, endometriosis, adnexal masses, and adhesions from endometriosis, inflammatory disease, or previous surgery. Laparoscopic hysterectomy may also be considered for stage I endometrial, ovarian, and cervical cancer (Canis et al, 1990; Querleu et al, 1991; Reich et al, 1990).

PREOPERATIVE PREPARATION

Gonadotropin-releasing hormone (GnRH) analogs may reduce the total uterine volume in patients with uterine leiomyomata from 35 to 50%. This reduction in uterine volume is more pronounced in the nonmyoma portion of the uterus (Schlaff et al, 1989). Because intramuscular (IM) leuprolide acetate for depot suspension (Lupron-Depot), once monthly, reduces uterine volume and the size of the vessels supplying the fibroid, and may shrink leiomyomas, women who choose hysterectomy for large myomas should be pretreated for at least 3 months (despite the expense), because shrinking the size of the myoma should make laparoscopic or vaginal hysterectomy easier (Stovall et al, 1991). During treatment with Lupron-Depot at a dose of 3.75 mg IM once per month, for 3 to 6 months, anemia secondary to hypermenorrhea resolves, and autologous blood donation can be considered prior to laparoscopic hysterectomy. Packed red blood cells obtained in this manner have a shelf life of 35 days if stored at 1 to 6°C.

Lupron-Depot is often administered after ovulation in the cycle preceding surgery to avoid operating on ovaries that contain a corpus luteum. Patients are encouraged to hydrate and eat lightly for 24 hours before admission to the hospital on the day of surgery. When extensive cul-de-sac involvement with endometriosis is suspected, either clinically or from another physician's operative record, a mechanical bowel preparation is advised (e.g., polyethylene glycol-based isosmotic solution: GOLYTELY or Colyte). Lower abdominal, pubic, or perineal hair is *not* shaved. A Foley catheter is inserted during surgery to distend the bladder with indigo carmine solution, thus aiding in its identification,

and is removed the next morning. Antibiotics (usually cefoxitin) are administered in all cases lasting for longer than 2 hours, at the 2-hour mark.

TECHNIQUE

My current technique (H. R.) has evolved from that published in 1989 (Reich et al, 1989). The standard three laparoscopic puncture sites including the umbilicus are used: 10-mm umbilical, 5-mm right, and 5-mm left lower quadrant. Placement of the lower quadrant trocar sleeves just above the pubic hairline and lateral to the deep epigastric vessels (and thus, the rectus abdominis muscle) is preferred. When the ENDO GIA 30 clamp is used, the 5-mm right lower quadrant incision is increased with a 12-mm trocar sleeve, or the clamp is inserted through the umbilical incision and the procedure is viewed through a 5-mm laparoscope in one of the 5-mm lower quadrant sites.

A Valtchev uterine mobilizer with a 100-mm–long, 10-mm–thick obturator is inserted to antevert the uterus and delineate the posterior vagina. When this device is in the anteverted position, the cervix sits on a wide acorn, making the cervicovaginal junction readily visible between the uterosacral ligaments when the cul-de-sac is inspected laparoscopically.

Ureteral Dissection

Immediately after exploration of the upper abdomen and pelvis, each ureter is isolated deep in the pelvis, if possible. This is done early in the operation before the pelvic sidewall peritoneum becomes edematous or opaque from irritation by the CO_2 pneumoperitoneum or aquadissection and before ureteral peristalsis is inhibited by surgical stress, pressure, or the Trendelenburg position. The ureter and its overlying peritoneum are grasped deep in the pelvis on the left to avoid division of the lateral rectosigmoid attachments required for high identification. An atraumatic grasping forceps is used from a right-sided cannula to grab the ureter and its overlying peritoneum on the left pelvic sidewall below and caudal to the left ovary, lateral to the left uterosacral ligament. Scissors are used to divide the peritoneum overlying the ureter and are then inserted into the defect that has been created and spread. Thereafter, one blade of the scissors is placed on top of the ureter; the buried blade of the scissors is visualized through the peritoneum: and the peritoneum is divided (see Atlas, Plate 23). This is continued into the deep pelvis where the uterine vessels cross the ureter. Connective tissue between the ureter and the vessels is sharply divided with scissors. Bleeding is controlled with microbipolar forceps.

Abdominal and adnexal adhesions, if present, are lysed to mobilize the specimen to be removed.

Bladder Mobilization

The left round ligament is divided with minimal bleeding at its mid-portion using a spoon electrode at 150-W cutting current. Persistent bleeding is controlled with unipolar fulguration at 80-W coagulation current or bipolar desiccation at 30-W cutting current. Thereafter scissors are used to divide the vesicouterine peritoneal fold, starting at the left side and continuing across the midline to the right round ligament. The right round ligament is divided (as was the left) with unipolar electrosurgery. The bladder is mobilized off the uterus and upper vagina using scissors (see Atlas, Plate 24).

Upper Uterine Blood Supply

When ovarian preservation is desired, the utero-ovarian ligament and fallopian tube are divided adjacent to the uterus with the ENDO GIA. For this portion of the procedure, a 5-mm laparoscope is inserted through the left 5-mm cannula. The ENDO GIA is then inserted through the umbilical incision, either through a 12-mm cannula or directly with no cannula. The ENDO GIA is applied to the pedicle and is fired. Often two ENDO GIAs are necessary on each side for this part of the procedure. When ovarian preservation is not desired, the infundibulopelvic ligaments and broad ligaments are coagulated until desiccated and then divided.

Uterine Vessel Ligation

The broad ligament on each side is skeletonized down to the uterine vessels. Each uterine vessel pedicle is suture-ligated with 0 Vicryl on a CT-1 needle or 0 POLYSORB on a GS-21 needle (27 in.). The needles are introduced into the peritoneal cavity by pulling them through a 5-mm incision (Reich et al, 1992). The curved needle is inserted on top of the unroofed ureter, where it turns medially toward the previously mobilized bladder (see Atlas, Plate 25). A short rotary movement of the Cook oblique curved needle holder brings the needle around the uterine vessel pedicle. Sutures are tied extracorporeally using a Clarke knot pusher. A single suture placed in this manner on each side serves as a "sentinel stitch," identifying and watching over the ureter for the rest of the case.

In my experience, one ureteral injury occurred with bipolar desiccation, and I have come close to it with the ENDO GIA. In 1988, a right ureterovaginal fistula occurred that was treated successfully with a stent. In that case, the injury was secondary either to bipolar desiccation of the right uterine vessels or to the performance of the vaginal portion of the procedure with the hip joints extended. On multiple occasions when using the ENDO GIA, inspection of the ureter after putting the ENDO GIA into position, but before firing it, revealed entrapment of the ureter. It is important to realize that the ENDO GIA is a straight device without staples in its distal 1-cm end and is much wider than a Kelly clamp. Two other ureteral injuries associated with the ENDO GIA have recently been reported (Woodland, 1992). In addition, during laparoscopic application, the uterine fundus is usually not put on upward traction.

Circumferential Culdotomy (Division of Cervicovaginal Attachments)

The cardinal ligaments on each side are divided with the CO_2 laser at high power or the spoon electrode at 150-W cutting current. Control of bleeding is often necessary using bipolar forceps. The vagina is entered posteriorly over the Valtchev retractor, which identifies the junction of cervix with vagina (see Atlas, Plate 26). Continuing toward the left, the vaginal fornix is divided. Thereafter it is possible to insert the Aqua-Purator into the anterior vagina above the cervix tenaculum on the anterior cervical lip. Following insertion of the Aqua-Purator tip or application of a ring forceps, and using it as a backstop, the anterior fornix is divided. The Aqua-Purator is inserted from posterior to anterior to delineate the right vaginal fornix, which is divided. The uterus can then be pulled out of the vagina. Alternately, a 4-cm–diameter operative colonoscope (Wolf Corp.) is used to outline circumferentially the cervicovaginal junction; it also serves as a backstop for laser work.

Laparoscopic Vaginal Vault Closure and Suspension with McCall Culdoplasty

Vaginal repair is accomplished after packing the vagina. The left uterosacral ligament and posterolateral vagina are first elevated. A suture is placed through this uterosacral ligament and into the vagina; it exits the vagina including posterior vaginal tissue near the midline on the left, and re-enters just adjacent to this spot on the right. Finally, an opposite-sided oblique Cook needle holder is used to fixate the right posterolateral vagina to the right uterosacral ligament. This suture is tied extracorporeally and gives excellent support to the vaginal cuff apex, elevating it superiorly and back toward the hollow of the sacrum. The rest of the vagina and overlying pubocervical fascia are closed vertically with a figure-of-eight suture.

Laparoscopy is then used to inspect the operative sites (particularly the vaginal vault area) for blood clots or continued bleeding. Hemostasis is achieved with bipolar compression and desiccation. Complete hemostasis is confirmed by underwater inspection of the operative site in a reverse Trendelenburg position (Reich, 1989). To reduce vaginally introduced bacteria, the pelvis is liberally lavaged with lactated Ringer's solution and clots are evacuated. Leaving 2 liters in the abdominal cavity may decrease postoperative infection associated with vaginal hysterectomy, further decreasing postoperative hospitalization and recovery time. The laparoscopic

instruments are removed, and the abdominal punctures are closed. All incisions over 7 mm require precise identification and closure of the deep fascia to prevent incisional hernias.

SPECIAL PROBLEMS

Many problems are encountered during division of the lateral cervix from the vagina because of ascending vaginal vessels and thick cardinal and uterosacral ligaments. It is very difficult to maintain CO_2 pneumoperitoneum once the vagina has been opened anteriorly and posteriorly. The vagina is packed, but the levers of the Valtchev retractor make an airtight closure impossible. In these situations, it is often best to remove the Valtchev retractor and the single-toothed tenaculum from the vagina and then pack the vagina with a wet pack or with a pack inside a surgical glove. Thereafter, division of the cervix from its junction with the vagina is accomplished by lifting the anterior vaginotomy to put the cervicovaginal junction on tension and dividing this junction with scissors through 360 degrees until the uterus is free in the peritoneal cavity. Scissors with an electrosurgical capability can reduce cuff bleeding. The scissors are used to grasp the junction; cutting current is applied; and the cervicovaginal tissue is divided.

After completely freeing the cervix, it is grasped with the tenaculum and the uterus is pulled into the vagina. If the uterus is too large for this maneuver, the surgeon reverts to a vaginal approach to morcellate the uterus. Otherwise, the uterus is pulled into the vagina, and its fundus is left there to occlude the vagina and maintain the pneumoperitoneum. The vaginal cuff is further inspected for bleeding. Arteriolar and venous bleeding on the vaginal cuff is fulgurated with unipolar coagulation current, the argon beam coagulator, or bipolar desiccation. The cuff is then closed with three sutures of 0 Vicryl on a CT-1 needle. The first suture apposes the uterosacral ligaments across the midline. The second suture brings the cardinal ligaments and underlying vagina across the midline. The third suture closes the anterior vagina and its pubocervicovesicular fascia.

RESULTS

Between April 1983 and September 1991, 94 women underwent either laparoscopic hysterectomy or laparoscopically assisted vaginal hysterectomy. Their average age at time of surgery was 46, and the age range was 30 to 79 years. The most common reason for surgery was a symptomatic fibroid uterus. The average operation lasted fewer than 3 hours. The average length of hospital stay was fewer than 2 days, and recuperation was rapid. There was one conversion to laparotomy following extensive adhesiolysis with incidental enterotomies.

REFERENCES

Bachmann GA: Hysterectomy: A critical review. J Reprod Med 35:839–862, 1990.

Canis M, Mage G, Wattiez A, et al: Does endoscopic surgery have a role in radical surgery of cancer of the cervix uteri (Letter)? J Gynecol Obstet Biol Reprod [Paris] 19:921, 1990.

Kilkku P, Grönroos M, Hirvonen T, and Rauramo L: Supravaginal uterine amputation vs. hysterectomy: Effects on libido and orgasm. Acta Obstet Gynecol Scand 62:147–152, 1983.

Kovac SR, Cruikshank SH, and Retto HF: Laparoscopy-assisted vaginal hysterectomy. J Gynecol Surg 6:185–189, 1990.

Liu CY: Laparoscopic hysterectomy: Report of 215 cases. Gynaecol Endoscopy 1:73–77, 1992.

Lundorff P, Hahlin M, Källfelt B, et al: Adhesion formation after laparoscopic surgery in tubal pregnancy: A randomized trial versus laparotomy. Fertil Steril 55:911–915, 1991.

Maher PJ, Wood EC, Hill DJ, and Lolatgis NA: Laparoscopically assisted hysterectomy. Med J Aust 156:316–318, 1992.

Minelli L, Angiolillo M, Caione C, and Palmara V: Laparoscopically-assisted vaginal hysterectomy. Endoscopy 23:64–66, 1991.

Pitkin RM: Editorial. Operative laparoscopy: Surgical advance or technical gimmick? Obstet Gynecol 79:441–442, 1992.

Querleu D, Leblanc E, and Castelain B: Laparoscopic pelvic lymphadenectomy in the staging of early carcinoma of the cervix. Am J Obstet Gynecol 164:579–581, 1991.

Reich H: New techniques in advanced laparoscopic surgery. Baillieres Clin Obstet Gynecol 3:655–681, 1989.

Reich H, Clarke HC, and Sekel L: A simple method for ligating with straight and curved needles in operative laparoscopy. Obstet Gynecol 79:143–147, 1992.

Reich H, DeCaprio J, and McGlynn F: Laparoscopic hysterectomy. J Gynecol Surg 5: 213–216, 1989.

Reich H, McGlynn F, and Wilkie W: Laparoscopic management of stage I ovarian cancer: A case report. J Reprod Med 35:601–605, 1990.

Schlaff WD, Zerhouni EA, Huth JA, et al: A placebo-controlled trial of a depot gonadotropin-releasing hormone analogue (leuprolide) in the treatment of uterine leiomyomata. Obstet Gynecol 74:856–862, 1989.

Stovall TG, Ling FW, Henry LC, and Woodruff MR: A randomized trial evaluating leuprolide acetate before hysterectomy as treatment for leiomyomas. Am J Obstet Gynecol 164:1420–1425, 1991.

Stovall TG, Summitt RL Jr, Bran DF, and Ling FW: Outpatient vaginal hysterectomy: A pilot study. Obstet Gynecol 80:145–149, 1992.

Summitt RL Jr, Stovall TG, Lipscomb GH, and Ling FW: Randomized comparison of laparoscopy-assisted vaginal hysterectomy with standard vaginal hysterectomy in an outpatient setting. Obstet Gynecol 80:895–901, 1992.

Woodland MB: Ureter injury during laparoscopy-assisted vaginal hysterectomy with the endoscopic linear stapler. Am J Obstet Gynecol 167:756–757, 1992.

FURTHER READINGS

Clarke HC: Laparoscopy: New instruments for suturing and ligation. Fertil Steril 23:274–277, 1972.

Dicker RC, Scally MJ, Greenspan JR, et al: Hysterectomy among women of reproductive age: Trends in the United States, 1970–1978. JAMA 248:323–327, 1982.

Doering DL, Barnhill DR, Weiser EB, et al: Intraoperative evaluation of depth of myometrial invasion in stage I endometrial adenocarcinoma. Obstet Gynecol 74: 930–933, 1989.

Liu CY: Laparoscopic hysterectomy: A review of 72 cases. J Reprod Med 37:351–354, 1992.

Reich H: Laparoscopic hysterectomy. Surg Laparosc Endosc 2:85–88, 1992.

Reich H: Laparoscopic lymphadenectomy. Surg Laparosc Endosc 2:61–63, 1992.

Reich H and McGlynn F: Short self-retaining trocar sleeves for laparoscopic surgery. Am J Obstet Gynecol 162:453–454, 1990.

Reich H, McGlynn F, and Salvat J: Laparoscopic treatment of cul-de-sac obliteration secondary to retrocervical deep fibrotic endometriosis. J Reprod Med 36:516–522, 1991.

Laparoscopic Management of Cul-de-Sac Endometriosis

REASONS FOR

Better Visualization

Endometriosis involving the rectum presents as partial or complete cul-de-sac obliteration. As explained in Chapter 17, these dissections can involve lesions infiltrating deep into the rectum or vagina, as well as difficult dissection of adhesions near the ureter and rectal wall. Pain is the initiation for surgery of cul-de-sac endometriosis, and the excision, rather than superficial ablation, of deeply infiltrating lesions is important for effective treatment of this condition (Koninckx et al, 1991). Although many surgeons would prefer to undertake these risks at open laparotomy, we believe that the skills in anatomic definition, dissection, and excision of pathology can be practiced equally efficaciously by laparoscopy, in which much superior visualization compensates for restricted surgical maneuverability. Nodules can be palpated by the surgeon's finger rectally during laparoscopy, and good tactile sense is also available through a laparoscopic probe. The limits of laparoscopic management of rectal endometriosis thus become those of the surgeon's skill and experience, as well as the comparative time required for adequate management.

Operative Advantages

The operative advantages of a laparoscopic approach to cul-de-sac obliteration include easy intraoperative access to the rectum and vagina, a magnification source that is easier to manipulate than an operating microscope, and the ability to perform an underwater examination at the end of the procedure during which all blood clot is evacuated and complete hemostasis is obtained. The general advantages of laparoscopy include same-day diagnosis and treatment, short hospitalization, rapid recuperation because of the rarity of ileus, superior cosmetics, excellent patient acceptance, cost-effectiveness, and results at least equal to those with laparotomy.

In our experience, obliteration of the cul-de-sac secondary to endometriosis can be effectively treated laparoscopically by cul-de-sac dissection with excision of deep fibrotic endometriosis and restoration of cul-de-sac anatomy resulting in resolution of infertility, pelvic pain, and hypermenorrhea in most cases. Patient benefits include avoidance of major abdominal surgery with its related morbidity or ovarian suppressive therapy that prohibits fertility during administration and does not appear to penetrate deep, infiltrating endometriotic lesions. The laparoscopic approach can be lengthy, and the persistent nature of the disease may dictate more than one application. Therefore, significant determining factors in achieving the desired outcome may be a combination of surgical skill and tenacity and patient persistence.

Excision

Extensive endometriosis of the cul-de-sac can be controlled laparoscopically if the surgeon is willing to spend the time. Koninckx and colleagues (1991) presented good evidence that pain is associated with infiltrating endometriosis. They point out that even the current American Fertility Society (AFS) system of describing endometriosis does not describe or grade depth of infiltration. If endometriosis is the sole cause of pain, laparoscopic removal often results in relief of pain, regardless of the severity of the endometriosis. Danazol rarely relieves pain when ovarian endometriomas or retrocervical deep fibrotic endometriosis exist (Telimaa, 1988). Surgical skill and tenacity are the keys to successful treatment of infiltrating endometriosis. Rather than concentrating on excision of the nodular mass, attention is first directed to complete dissection of the anterior rectum throughout its area of involvement.

REASONS AGAINST

Inadequate Treatment

Endometriosis is occasionally a deeply penetrating disease that is not limited to superficial tissue. When this happens with the rectum, the laparoscopist might be tempted to perform a superficial ablation to consider the disease visually cured. This condition requires palpation, which is always possible at laparoscopy but seldom performed, to appreciate the full depth of the involvement of glands and scar in the rectum. Thus many surgeons may treat the disease superficially, leaving the deeper (and more symptomatic) portions of the disease behind and necessitating eventual laparotomy.

Time and Skill Required

Assuming that the laparoscopist is skilled in defining the extent and depth of the disease and is able to perform the excision of the lesion, the disease may penetrate the bowel all the way to the mucosa. Repair of the defect left after excision would require suturing. Although these techniques exist and are described in this book, they may be well beyond the average laparoscopist in skill and time required. Thus in many hands

it may be wiser to abandon the laparoscopic approach in favor of the more rapid and secure technique of open laparotomy and excision of rectal lesions.

HISTORY

In 1921, Sampson defined cul-de-sac obliteration as "extensive adhesions in the cul-de-sac obliterating its lower portion and uniting the cervix or the lower portion of the uterus to the rectum; with adenoma of the endometrial type invading the cervical and the uterine tissues and probably also (but to a lesser degree) the anterior wall of the rectum." Cul-de-sac obliteration secondary to endometriosis implies the presence of retrocervical deep fibrotic endometriosis beneath the peritoneum. This endometriosis is located on or invades into the anterior rectum, posterior vagina, posterior cervix, rectovaginal septum, and the uterosacral ligaments. Partial cul-de-sac obliteration (PCDSO) means that deep fibrotic endometriosis is severe enough to alter the course of the rectum (see Fig. 17–5). With complete cul-de-sac obliteration (CCDSO), fibrotic endometriosis or adhesions involve the entire cul-de-sac: the cervix, vagina, and rectum.

Treatment options for pain or infertility secondary to cul-de-sac obliteration include ovarian suppressive therapy with danazol or gonadotrophin-releasing hormone agonists, or surgery. In our clinical experience, and that of others (Fayez et al, 1988; O'Shea and Jones, 1985; Telimaa, 1988), danazol therapy never cures endometriosis when ovarian endometriomas or deep fibrotic endometriosis exists and may make surgical procedures more difficult. Metzgar and associates (1988) reported that the hormonal responsiveness of endometrial implants is unpredictable and inconsistent. Cornillie and colleagues (1990) found that deep (>5-mm infiltration) endometriotic lesions were histologically different and more active than were intermediate (2 to 4 mm) or superficial (<1 mm) infiltration. In their study, deep endometriosis was limited to areas within fibromuscular tissue such as the cul-de-sac, uterosacral ligament, and the vesicouterine peritoneal fold, and a strong correlation was found between deep, infiltrating endometriosis and pelvic pain. There is also a significant correlation between excision of extensive cul-de-sac endometriosis and fertility (Reich, 1991b).

In 1973 Gray reported on 179 cases of bowel endometriosis selected from a series of approximately 1500 women with surgical endometriosis of which only 10 required end-to-end anastomosis and 27 had full-thickness excision of the anterior wall. In no case was the mucosa perforated or rectal bleeding noted. Weed and Ray (1987) reviewed 163 bowel endometriosis cases and found that suspected bowel lesions can be completely excised, requiring opening of the bowel mucosa in only 15% of implant resections. Kelly and Diamond (1989), reporting on 68 women who underwent laparotomy for endometriosis, found that it was rarely necessary to penetrate the bowel lumen to excise endometriosis; colon endometriosis was vaporized down to normal tissue as documented by palpation and viewing with magnification. Coronado and associates (1990), reporting on 77 women with bowel endometriosis treated by full-thickness excision, found that preoperative proctosigmoidoscopy documented invasion into the lumen of the bowel in only two cases proved by biopsy, although 16 women did have a change of bowel appearance. These authors did not report histologic evidence as to depth of invasion and extent of surgical margins for any of the 77 cases. Bowel resection surgery required an average 7.4-day length of stay (range of 5 to 20 days). An attempt by Martin and associates (1989) to resect bowel infiltration laparoscopically in five women led to five failures with two undergoing immediate laparotomy, two delayed laparotomy for persistent pain, and the last considering a second procedure.

OBJECTIVES OF SURGERY

For infertility or the preservation of fertility, reconstructive surgery can be considered either by laparotomy microsurgery or by laparoscopy, depending on the skill and experience of the surgeon. For pain, when future fertility is not desired, excision of endometriotic tissue should be considered, as it is easier to excise this tissue from the bladder, vagina, and rectum if the uterus has not been removed. However, hysterectomy with bilateral salpingo-oophorectomy is commonly performed. A problem with this approach is that the hysterectomy is usually done with an intrafascial technique, leaving fibrotic endometriosis on the vagina and rectum, assuming that it will resolve following castration; future surgical procedures may be necessary to relieve pain from vaginal cuff or rectal endometriosis (Coronado et al, 1990; Gray, 1973).

TeLinde and Scott defined the objectives of surgical treatment of endometriosis in 1952: "one should excise or fulgurate all evident endometriosis." The surgical objectives of laparoscopic treatment are similar—to remove all evident endometriosis by excising large superficial and deep lesions and by vaporizing smaller deposits. In my (H. R.) approach, first the anterior rectum is freed by dissecting through fibrotic tissue while identifying the rectal outline with use of a blunt probe inside the rectum; this is possible even when anterior rectal infiltration is present. In most cases, following the initial documentation of rectal involvement, dissection to the loose areolar tissue of the rectovaginal septum revealed that the bulk of the fibrotic lesion was on the posterior vagina (Reich et al, 1991b). With a laparotomy approach, retrocervical deep fibrotic endometriosis has commonly been managed by bowel resection, assuming that the major portion of the lesion infiltrates the anterior rectum. In these cases the deep fibrotic lesion is mobilized, starting on the posterior uterus and progressing downward to the rectum where it appears to be attached.

In 1922 Sampson suggested that operative treatment for extensive bowel endometriosis was an unsettled question. Almost 70 years later, the question of what kind of operative therapy for bowel endometriosis still remains unsettled. Differentiation of the portion of a fibrotic lesion that is endometriosis from fibrotic tissue caused by endometriosis is presently not possible. A comprehensive laparoscopic procedure, although not eradicating all endometriosis, may result in considerable pain relief or a desired pregnancy. While we recognize that bowel resection by laparotomy or laparoscopy may be necessary in rare cases, it seems prudent to curtail rather than encourage the widespread use of an aggressive, potentially morbid procedure.

INDICATIONS

The major indication for cul-de-sac dissection is pelvic pain from partial or complete cul-de-sac obliteration. Less frequently encountered symptomatology includes hypermenorrhea and asymptomatic pelvic mass. The diagnosis is made either at a primary laparoscopic procedure or is known from another surgeon's operative report. Unfortunately, this diagnosis is sometimes missed at diagnostic laparoscopy. The index of suspicion for cul-de-sac or bowel endometriosis should be high when the patient reports deep dyspareunia, pain with bowel movements, rectal spasm, or rectal bleeding with menses. A rectovaginal examination is diagnostic when deep cul-de-sac and rectovaginal septum nodularity can be palpated and specific tenderness is elicited in these nodules. On occasion endometriosis is visualized penetrating the full thickness of the vagina posterior to the cervix.

CONTRAINDICATIONS

Contraindications are few for cul-de-sac dissection. Even women who have a history of multiple prior abdominal surgeries have been treated laparoscopically without incident. When extensive endometriosis and pelvic adhesions coexist, the most prudent approach may be a two-stage intervention, limiting each procedure to approximately 4 hours. It is critical in these cases that women undergo extensive preoperative counseling including discussion of currently available options. In some cases, a laparoscopic excisional operation with cul-de-sac dissection should be considered prior to laparoscopic or vaginal hysterectomy at a later date.

The major contraindication is inexperience of the surgeon. Surgeons who are equipped, physically and mentally, to perform cul-de-sac dissection with excision of fibrotic endometriosis by laparoscopy or laparotomy are few. Surgeons advocating vaporization of endometriosis should avoid this operation and make an appropriate referral. This surgery can be more demanding than radical hysterectomy or ovarian cancer operations.

PREOPERATIVE EVALUATION

Whenever extensive cul-de-sac involvement with endometriosis is suspected preoperatively, a mechanical bowel preparation (GOLYTELY or Colyte) is administered orally on the afternoon before surgery to induce brisk, self-limiting diarrhea that rapidly cleanses the bowel without disrupting the electrolyte balance. Basically, there are no exclusion criteria.

No preoperative or postoperative medical treatment is used. Cul-de-sac dissection procedures are performed between menstrual cycle days 5 and 12 (before ovulation). When scheduling conflicts with the proliferative phase of a natural cycle, ovulation is delayed using norethindrone acetate (10 mg) from the first day of the last menstrual period to the day before surgery or depoleuprolide (Depo-Lupron) (3.75 mg IM premenstrually during the month before surgery).

Transvaginal scanning has proved to be helpful in documenting the status of the ovaries, which frequently cannot be palpated because of tenderness during pelvic examination and pelvic induration and adhesions. Ovarian endometriomas are suspected when ovarian cysts are found.

INSTRUMENTATION

For dissection we use a combination of scissors, ultrapulse or superpulse CO_2 laser, electrosurgery with knife or spatula electrodes, and aquadissection. To define the rectum and posterior vagina and to open the posterior vagina (culdotomy), a sponge on a ring forceps is inserted into the posterior vaginal fornix and a No. 81 French rectal probe is placed in the rectum (Fig. 23–1). In addition, a No. 3 or 4 Sims curette or Hulka uterine elevator is placed in the endometrial cavity to antevert the uterus markedly and stretch out the cul-de-sac to aid in this position. If available, a Valtchev uterine mobilizer (Conkin Surgical Instruments) with a 100-mm long, 10-m thick obturator is the best available single instrument to antevert the uterus and delineate the posterior vagina throughout complicated cases.

INTRAOPERATIVE STAGING

To determine if cul-de-sac obliteration is partial or complete, a sponge on a ring forceps is inserted into the posterior vaginal fornix. Complete cul-de-sac obliteration is diagnosed when the outline of the posterior fornix cannot be seen through the laparoscope. Partial cul-de-sac obliteration is determined when rectal tenting is visible but some protrusion of the sponge in the posterior vaginal fornix is identified between the rectum and the inverted U shape of the uterosacral ligaments (see Fig. 17–4).

FIGURE 23–1 A–C, Probes for cul-de-sac dissection

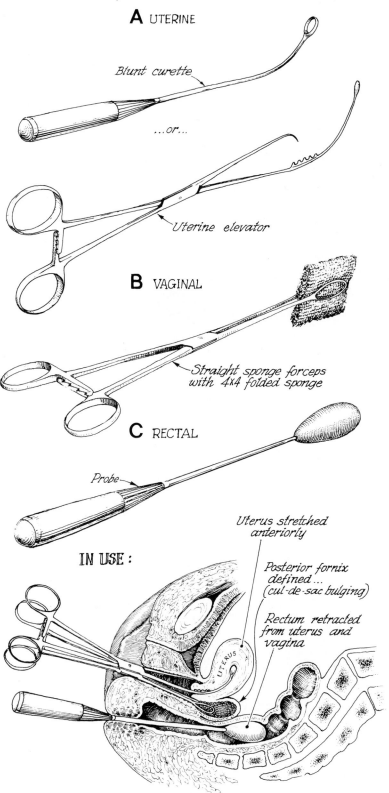

A UTERINE

Blunt curette

...or...

Uterine elevator

B VAGINAL

Straight sponge forceps with 4×4 folded sponge

C RECTAL

Probe

IN USE:

Uterus stretched anteriorly

Posterior fornix defined... (cul-de-sac bulging)

Rectum retracted from uterus and vagina

UTERUS

FIGURE 23–2 *A* and *B*, Cul-de-sac endometriosis dissection and excision

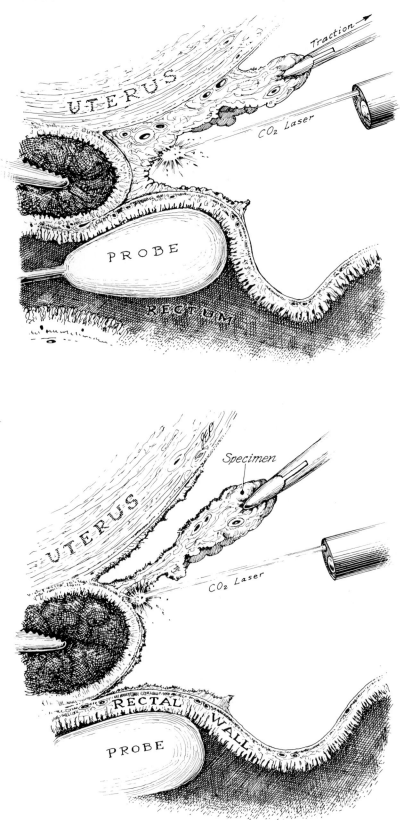

TECHNIQUE

All laparoscopic procedures for extensive endometriosis are performed using general anesthesia with arm, shoulder, and leg supports as described in Chapter 13. Ovarian endometriomas up to 15 cm are excised (Reich and McGlynn, 1986).

Deep fibrotic nodular endometriosis involving the cul-de-sac requires excision of nodular fibrotic tissue from the uterosacral ligaments, posterior cervix, posterior vagina, and the rectum. Attention is first directed to complete dissection of the anterior rectum throughout its area of involvement until loose areolar tissue of the rectovaginal space is reached. Using the rectal probe as a guide, the rectal interface with the cul-de-sac lesion is identified and opened at this junction with CO_2 laser or scissors. Careful blunt dissection then ensues, using the aquadissector for aquadissection and suction-traction. Laser or scissors are used for sharp dissection until the rectum, with or without fibrotic endometriosis, is separated from the posterior uterus and upper vagina and is identifiable below the lesion (Fig. 23–2A). Loose areolar tissue of the rectovaginal space should be reached. Excision of the fibrotic endometriosis from the posterior vagina, uterosacral ligaments, and rectum should be attempted only after the rectum is mobilized.

When a ureter is close to the lesion, its course is traced starting at the pelvic brim, and on occasion the peritoneum overlying the ureter is opened to confirm ureteral position deep in the pelvis. Bipolar forceps are used to control arterial and venous bleeding.

After separation of the rectum from the back of the uterus and the upper posterior vagina, deep fibrotic, often nodular, endometriotic lesions are excised from the uterosacral ligaments, the upper posterior vagina (the location of which is continually confirmed by the sponge in the posterior fornix), and the posterior cervix (see Fig. 23–2B). The dissection on the outside of the vaginal wall proceeds using laser, aquadissection, electrosurgery, or scissors. Usually an endopelvic fascial layer, infiltrated with endometriosis, is identified, and after this layer is excised, soft pliable upper posterior vaginal wall is uncovered. It is frequently difficult to distinguish fibrotic endometriosis accurately from the posterior cervix at the cervicovaginal junction, deep beneath the inverted U found between the insertion of the uterosacral ligaments into the cervix. Frequent palpation using rectovaginal examinations helps to identify occult lesions. On occasion, the lesion infiltrates deep into or completely penetrates the vaginal wall. Dissection is then performed accordingly with removal of all visible endometriosis. Lesions extending totally through the vagina are treated with an "en bloc" laparoscopic resection from the cul-de-sac to the posterior vaginal wall; pneumoperitoneum is maintained with a 30-ml Foley catheter in the vagina. The posterior vaginal wall is closed either vaginally or laparoscopically, depending on the surgeon's preference.

Endometriotic nodules infiltrating the anterior rectal muscularis are excised, partially or totally, usually with the surgeon's or the assistant's finger in the rectum just beneath the lesion. In some cases, the anterior rectum is reperitonealized by plicating the uterosacral ligaments and lateral rectal peritoneum across the midline using a 3–0 or 4–0 suture. The suture is applied using curved needles with a curved needle driver (Cook Ob Gyn). The suture is then tied outside the peritoneal cavity and is pushed downward with the Clarke knot pusher (Marlow Surgical). Deep rectal muscularis defects are always closed with suture.

At the close of each procedure, complete hemostasis is documented by using an underwater examination to detect bleeding from vessels tamponaded during the procedure by the increased intraperitoneal pressure of the CO_2 pneumoperitoneum. The CO_2 pneumoperitoneum is replaced with Ringer's lactate solution, and the peritoneal cavity is vigorously irrigated with this solution until the effluent is clear of blood products, usually after 10 to 20 liters. Underwater inspection of the pelvis is performed to detect any further bleeding, which is controlled using microbipolar forceps. A final copious lavage with Ringer's lactate solution is undertaken, and all clot is directly aspirated; at least 2 liters of Ringer's lactate solution is left in the abdomen to separate raw surfaces during early healing. No other antiadhesive agents are employed.

CLINICAL EXPERIENCE

In my clinical experience, more than 400 women have undergone laparoscopic cul-de-sac dissection for deep fibrotic endometriosis. Statistical information was tabulated for the first 100 cases only: 48 women had partial obliteration, and 52 women had complete obliteration; 52 women had a prior history of medical or surgical therapy. Surgical techniques included aquadissection and electrosurgery (44 cases) and a combination of laser, electrosurgery, and scissors dissection (56 cases). Cul-de-sac disease post hysterectomy was not included.

The goal of laparoscopic surgery was to excise all macroscopic fibrotic endometriosis and to restore normal anatomic relationships. Indications were pain (46 cases), infertility (46 cases), hypermenorrhea (7 cases), and mass (1 case). Cases were staged using the AFS classification: 6%, stage II; 30%, stage III; and 64%, stage IV. A total of 136 laparoscopies were performed, including second- and third-look procedures.

Operating room time and hospital stay were calculated for the most extensive procedures only. The average operating time was 3 hours with a range from 1 to 9 hours. Average operating time was 2 hours for partial obliteration and almost 4 hours for complete obliteration.

Approximately 25% of these women had more than one laparoscopic surgical procedure. At second laparoscopy, persistent endometriosis was found in more than half of the women. There was less adhesion formation than at initial laparoscopy in all except one case. Pregnancy was achieved in 74% (34 of 46) of the women desiring children, including 5 of 11 couples with male factor infertility. Most women (89% or 41 of 46) who underwent laparoscopy for pelvic pain noted significant relief 6 months after laparoscopy (two of these women conceived). Of the seven women who had an initial complaint of hypermenorrhea, 86% (6 of 7 women) reported significant relief 1 year after laparoscopy. The one asymptomatic woman who presented with pelvic mass remained asymptomatic 1 year after surgery.

Following their first operative procedure, 72 women were discharged on the operative day and 28 women were discharged on the next morning. All the women were back to full activity within 1 week. No hysterectomies or laparotomies were necessary. Results for partial and complete obliteration were similar in all categories, confirming our impression that we were dealing with the same disease process—deep fibrotic endometriosis.

COMPLICATIONS

Laparotomies were not performed on any of the over 400 women. No laparoscopies were converted intraoperatively to laparotomy. The rectum or rectosigmoid was entered in four cases and repaired with laparoscopic sutures (Reich et al, 1991a). One delayed rectal perforation occurred from devascularized bowel after deep rectal muscularis endometriosis excision; laparoscopic suture repair was accomplished on unprepared bowel 14 days postoperatively, after evacuating a 1000-ml pelvic abscess. One low anterior rectosigmoid resection was done laparoscopically with the anastomosis 5 cm from the anal verge. Other postoperative complications included anemia, corneal abrasion, and transient unilateral brachial plexus injury. There were no problems with fluid overload. One case of adult respiratory distress syndrome (ARDS) occurred and required a 1-month hospitalization. No other late complications were encountered.

REFERENCES

Cornillie FJ, Oosterlynck D, Lauweryns JM, and Koninckx PR: Deeply infiltrating pelvic endometriosis: Histology and clinical significance. Fertil Steril 53:978–983, 1990.

Coronado C, Franklin R, Lotze E, et al: Surgical treatment of symptomatic colorectal endometriosis. Fertil Steril 53:411–416, 1990.

Fayez JA, Collazo LM, and Vernon C: Comparison of different modalities of treatment for minimal and mild endometriosis. Am J Obstet Gynecol 159:927–932, 1988.

Gray LA: Endometriosis of the bowel; role of bowel resection, superficial excision and oophorectomy treatment. Ann Surg 177:580–587, 1973.

Kelly R and Diamond MP: Laparotomy in infertility patients with endometriosis: Use of the CO_2 laser. J Reprod Med 34:25–28, 1989.

Koninckx PR, Meuleman C, Demeyere S, et al: Suggestive evidence that pelvic endometriosis is a progressive disease, whereas deeply infiltrating endometriosis is associated with pelvic pain. Fertil Steril 55:759–765, 1991.

Martin DC, Hubert GD, and Levy BS: Depth of infiltration of endometriosis. J Gynecol Surg 5:55–60, 1989.

Metzgar DA, Olive DL, and Haney AF: Limited hormonal responsiveness of ectopic endometrium: Histologic correlation with intrauterine endometrium. Hum Pathol 19:1417–1424, 1988.

O'Shea RT and Jones WR: Danazol: Objective assessment in the treatment of endometriosis. Clin Reprod Fertil 3:205–206, 1985.

Reich H and McGlynn F: Treatment of ovarian endometriomas using laparoscopic surgical techniques. J Reprod Med 31:577–584, 1986.

Reich H, McGlynn F, and Budin R: Laparoscopic repair of full-thickness bowel injury. J Laparoendosc Surg 1:119–122, 1991a.

Reich H, McGlynn F, and Salvat J: Laparoscopic treatment of cul-de-sac obliteration secondary to retrocervical deep fibrotic endometriosis. J Reprod Med 36:516–522, 1991b.

Sampson JA: Intestinal adenomas of endometrial type. Arch Surg 5:217–280, 1922.

Sampson JA: Perforating hemorrhagic (chocolate) cysts of ovary. Arch Surg 3:245–323, 1921.

Telimaa S: Danazol and medroxyprogesterone acetate inefficacious in the treatment of infertility in endometriosis. Fertil Steril 50:872–875, 1988.

TeLinde RW and Scott RB: Diagnosis and treatment of endometriosis. Gen Pract 5:61–65, 1952.

Weed J and Ray J: Endometriosis of the bowel. Obstet Gynecol 69:727–730, 1987.

FURTHER READINGS

Donnez J: CO_2 laser laparoscopy in infertile women with endometriosis and women with adnexal adhesions. Fertil Steril 48:390–394, 1987.

Martin DC: Laparoscopic and vaginal colpotomy for the excision of infiltrating cul-de-sac endometriosis. J Reprod Med 33:806–808, 1988.

Martin DC: Laparoscopic treatment of endometriosis. In Azziz R, Murphy A (eds): Practical Manual of Operative Laparoscopy and Hysteroscopy. New York, Springer Verlag, 1992, pp 101–109.

Redwine DB: Conservative laparoscopic excision of endometriosis by sharp dissection: Life table analysis of reoperation and persistent or recurrent disease. Fertil Steril 56:628–634, 1991.

Redwine DB: Laparoscopic en bloc resection for treatment of the obliterated cul-de-sac in endometriosis. J Reprod Med 37:695–698, 1992.

Redwine DB and Sharpe DR: Laparoscopic segmental resection of the sigmoid colon for endometriosis. J Laparoendosc Surg 1:217–220, 1991.

Reich H: New techniques in advanced laparoscopic surgery. Baillieres Clin Obstet Gynecol 3:655–681, 1989.

Reich H, Clarke HC, and Sekel L: A simple method for ligating with straight and curved needles in operative laparoscopy. Obstet Gynecol 79:143–147, 1992.

Laparoscopic Management of Tubo-Ovarian and Pelvic Abscess

REASONS FOR

A *pelvic abscess* is a localized collection of a large number of organisms, inflammatory exudate, and necrotic debris that is often separated from surrounding tissue by a fibrous capsule. Some tubo-ovarian abscesses (TOAs) lack a classic abscess wall and are made up of an agglutination of tube and ovary to adjacent pelvic and abdominal structures following a reaction to purulent exudate from the inflamed tube as a tubo-ovarian complex. True pelvic abscesses with classic abscess wall can occur in the ovary and following rupture of a diverticulum. Whatever the terminology, purulent material exists in a collection within the pelvis.

Abscess is the result of an acute or subacute infection that often begins with an initial peritonitis stage in which aerobic bacteria predominate, followed by the development of an intra-abdominal abscess with emergence of anaerobic bacteria as the predominant flora. Abscesses contain a large number of organisms in high concentration, but not in a rapid growth phase, making them less susceptible to antimicrobial agents requiring actively growing organisms for efficacy. In addition, the fibrous capsule that the host makes in an attempt to control the infection may inhibit adequate levels of antimicrobial agents from entering the abscess. The anaerobic milieu itself may hinder host defense mechanisms, reducing the ability of neutrophils to phagocytize and kill bacteria. Thus, therapy for abscesses must include some technique of adequate drainage along with appropriate antimicrobial agents.

Until the early 1970s, clinicians who suspected a pelvic abcess or TOA considered extirpative surgery (e.g., total abdominal hysterectomy or bilateral salpingo-oophorectomy). More recently, an unruptured abscess is treated with intravenous antibiotics, and surgery is reserved for women who respond poorly to that therapy. Although this approach avoids immediate operation, prolonged contact between necrotic and inflamed tissue often causes dense fibrous adhesions that impair reproductive potential. In an effort to avoid this problem, some gynecologists advocate the use of laparoscopy with early lysis of acute adhesions as an alternative to antibiotic therapy alone.

The commonly accepted belief that surgical intervention during acute pelvic infection would result in greater injury than waiting for the infection to subside began with a New York City study by Simpson (1909), suggesting that early surgery is associated with increased technical difficulty. This opinion prevailed until recently, even though the risks associated with surgical intervention had changed drastically since the early part of this century.

In reality, it is much easier to operate on acute adhesions than it is to deal with dense adherences between structures that obliterate normal anatomic relationships and have, by their chronicity, developed neovascularization. For example, second-look laparoscopic adhesiolysis soon after infertility surgical procedures is much easier than the original operation (Jansen, 1988). Electrosurgery, laser surgery, and sharp scissors dissection—all useful for chronic pelvic inflammatory disease (PID)—have no place in the treatment of acute adhesions. Simply stated, the laparoscopic treatment of acute PID with or without abscess does not require the high level of technical skill necessary to excise endometrioma, open a hydrosalpinx, or remove an ectopic pregnancy under laparoscopic control. It is essentially an exercise in careful blunt dissection using a probe, or aquadissection with a suction-irrigation device, and can be performed by gynecologists experienced in operative laparoscopy using equipment available in most hospitals (see Atlas, Plate 17).

Why Laparoscopic Treatment Works

Peritoneal defense mechanisms that protect the host from invading bacteria include absorption of the microbes from the peritoneal cavity by the lymphatic system, phagocytosis by macrophages and polymorphonuclear leukocytes, complement effects, and fibrin trapping (Skau et al, 1986). Fibrin trapping and sequestration of the bacterial inoculum by the omentum and intestine and the formation of a tubo-ovarian complex act to contain the infection initially, although abscesses may form eventually. Although the deposition of fibrin indeed traps bacteria and decreases the frequency of septicemic death, thick fibrin deposits ultimately represent a barrier to in situ killing by neutrophils, with resultant abscess formation. Once formed, the abscess walls inhibit the effectiveness of antibiotics and the ability of the host to resolve the infection naturally.

Ahrenholz and Simmons (1980) studied the role of purified fibrin in the pathogenesis of experimental intraperitoneal infection. Their conclusion was that fibrin delays the onset of systemic sepsis, but the entrapped bacteria cannot be eliminated easily by normal intraperitoneal bactericidal mechanisms and, as a result, abscesses can form. They also believed that radical peritoneal débridement or anticoagulation may reduce the septic complications of peritonitis. Stated another way, procedures that decrease fibrin deposition or facilitate its removal, either enzymatically or surgically, decrease the frequency of intraperitoneal abscess formation, and thus the rationale

for extensive peritoneal lavage and radical excision of inflammatory exudate in patients with TOA. Our success with laparoscopic versus laparotomy treatment of TOA (Reich and McGlynn, 1987) and that of others (Henry-Suchet et al, 1984; Hudspeth, 1975; Rivlin and Hunt, 1986) substantiates the laboratory work of Ahrenholz and Simmons. Laparoscopic drainage of a pelvic abscess followed by lysis of all peritoneal cavity adhesions and excision of necrotic inflammatory exudate allows host defenses effectively to control the infection.

Laparotomy Compared with Laparoscopy

Most reports on operative technique for treatment of TOA by laparotomy emphasize that the tissues are edematous, congested, friable, and tear easily. Moreover, they note that capillary and venus oozing can be profuse. Hemostasis is often judged less than ideal in such cases, and blood loss requiring transfusion is common. These reports also suggest that meticulous dissection is virtually impossible and caution that the bowel is particularly vulnerable to injury when it is being separated from the pelvic viscera.

In contrast, laparoscopic adhesiolysis using the aquadissector is rarely bloody. Capillary oozing does occur, but it ceases spontaneously as the procedure progresses. In my (H. R.) experience, blood loss is rarely greater than 100 ml, and blood transfusion has not been reported following laparoscopic treatment of a pelvic abscess.

Complications of treatment of pelvic abscess by laparotomy include superficial or deep wound infection, wound dehiscence, bowel injury including delayed perforation secondary to unrecognized injury, bowel obstruction, persistent undrained collections of pus, thrombophlebitis, pulmonary embolism, septic shock, and subdiaphragmatic abscesses. In contrast neither wound disruption nor dehiscence is possible using a laparoscopic approach, and the other possible complications have not been reported.

I have treated 40 pelvic abscesses using laparoscopic surgical techniques from 1976 to 1989. One patient required total abdominal hysterectomy, bilateral salpingo-oophorectomy in 1977 for a recurrence 1 month postoperatively. All others demonstrated long-term resolution of their TOA. Ten second-look laparoscopies documented minimal filmy adhesions (see Atlas, Plate 18).

The goals in management of acute tubo-ovarian abscess are prevention of the chronic sequelae of infection, including infertility and pelvic pain, both of which often lead to further surgical intervention. Laparoscopic treatment is effective and economical. It offers the gynecologist 100% accuracy in diagnosis while simultaneously accomplishing definitive treatment with a low complication rate (Henry-Suchet et al, 1984; Reich and McGlynn, 1987).

REASONS AGAINST

Infrequent Opportunity in Normal Practice

Henry-Suchet and associates (1984) and Reich and McGlynn (1987) present an impressive argument for the immediate and long-term results of management of pelvic abscess by laparoscopic lysis and drainage. There were about two to three cases each year in these referral practices—a very low incidence to develop these techniques and skills. Incidence is perhaps the most practical argument against the universal recommendation of this method for management. With PID and abscesses diminishing in view of today's more conservative sexual conduct and awareness of sexually transmitted disease, the standard gynecologic practice may never have sufficient experience with lysis and drainage of these abscesses to gain sufficient confidence to make this approach a standard of care.

Why Add Surgery to the Risks?

The standard of care for acute PID with abscess remains a conservative antibiotic approach with bed rest (Droegemueller et al, 1987; Landers and Sweet, 1983). Results of this approach are acceptable, and the gynecologist-laparoscopist is not faced with the fear of making a medically manageable situation surgically complicated. Modern choice of antibiotics would be imipenem with cilastatin sodium given intravenously. This antibiotic has a broad spectrum, including anaerobes and gram-negative bacteria, and has good abcess penetration. If laparoscopy is contemplated, the antibiotic should be started before surgery since these abcesses are polymicrobial infections and culture at surgery is of little practical use.

Laparoscopy for Diagnosis?

There is a very good argument for the laparoscopic *diagnosis* of PID with abscess. All of Henry-Suchet's cases were extensions of the diagnostic laparoscopy routinely used in France to diagnose PID. The classic studies of Weström (Jacobson, 1980), which were confirmed in Canada (Sellors et al, 1991), indicate that PID is misdiagnosed 30 to 50% of the time. Even abscess symptoms and ultrasonographic findings have appeared with acute or ruptured endometriomas of the pelvis and ruptured appendix. Thus, use of the laparoscope to *diagnose* PID in young women has been advocated for years outside the United States. If more liberal use of laparoscopy diagnoses PID with abscess, perhaps the techniques that Henry-Suchet describes could then be incorporated to accelerate recovery of the patients who are already at laparoscopy. Until the United States adapts laparoscopy as a standard for diagnosing PID, however, the techniques described for *management* of PID abscess by laparoscopy may remain a documented method whose opportunities for implementation will be infrequent in the United States.

TECHNIQUE

Preoperative Considerations

Women with lower abdominal pain in association with a palpable or questionable pelvic mass should undergo laparoscopy to determine the true diagnosis as even "obvious TOA" may prove to be endometriomas, hemorrhagic corpus luteum cysts, or an abscess surrounding a ruptured appendix. The worldwide average rate of misdiagnosis of PID is 35% when laparoscopy has been used for confirmation.

The diagnosis of TOA should be suspected in women with a recent or past history of PID who have persistent pain and pelvic tenderness on examination. Fever and leukocytosis may or may not be present. Ultrasound frequently documents a tubo-ovarian complex and findings that appear to be consistent with the image of an abscess. After a presumptive diagnosis of TOA is made, hospitalization should be arranged for the patient for laparoscopic diagnosis and treatment soon thereafter.

In patients suspected of having TOA, intravenous antibiotics should be initiated on admission to the hospital, usually 2 to 24 hours prior to laparoscopy. Adequate and sustained blood levels of antibiotics are required to combat transperitoneal absorption of bacteria during the operative procedure. I (H. R.) prefer cefoxitin, 2 g intravenously, every 4 hours from the patient's admission until the patient's discharge from the hospital, usually on postoperative day 2 or 3. Newer cephamycins, cefmetazole, 2 g every 8 hours, or cefotetan, 2 g every 12 hours, can be considered. Oral doxycycline is started on the first postoperative day and continued for 10 days. Although clindamycin and metronidazole demonstrate greater ability to enter abscess cavities and reduce bacterial counts therein, cefoxitin is used to simplify therapy to a single intravenous agent and further assess the efficacy of the laparoscopic surgical procedure; the intravenous antibiotic alone should not be considered the reason for successful therapy. One who pioneered in this area, Henry-Suchet, starts antibiotics during the laparoscopic procedure only after cultures have been taken. The laparoscopic procedure is always performed under general anesthesia. A high-flow CO_2 insufflator is valuable to maintain the pneumoperitoneum and compensate for the rapid loss of CO_2 during suctioning. Hysteroscopy should be performed during the peritoneal insufflation to access and take cultures from the endometrial cavity. A Cohen cannula is then placed in the endocervical canal for uterine manipulation and tubal lavage. A 10-mm laparoscope is inserted through a vertical intraumbilical incision. Lower quadrant puncture sites are made above the pubic hairline and just lateral to the inferior epigastric vessels.

The upper abdomen is examined, and the patient is placed in a 20-degree Trendelenburg position before attention is focused on the pelvis. A Foley catheter is inserted if the bladder is distended. Through the right-sided trocar sleeve, either a blunt probe or a grasping forceps is inserted and used for traction and retraction. Through the left-sided trocar sleeve, a suction-irrigator-dissector (aquadissector) or a suction probe attached to a 50-ml syringe is inserted and used to mobilize omentum, small bowel, rectosigmoid, and tubo-ovarian adhesions until the abscess cavity is entered. Purulent fluid is aspirated while the operating table is being turned to a 10-degree Trendelenburg position. Cultures should be taken from the aspirated fluid; inflammatory exudate should be excised with biopsy forceps; and exudate should be removed near the tubal ostium using a bronchoscope cytology brush.

After the abscess cavity is aspirated, the aquadissector is used to separate the bowel and omentum completely from the reproductive organs and to lyse tubo-ovarian adhesions (aquadissection). Aquadissection is performed by placing the tip of the aquadissector against the adhesive interface between bowel-adnexa, tube-ovary, or adnexa-pelvic sidewall and by using the tip and the pressurized fluid gushing from it to develop a dissection plane that can be extended either bluntly or with more fluid pressure. The 3-mm grasping forceps places the tissue to be dissected on tension so that the surgeon can identify the distorted tissue plane accurately prior to aquadissection. When the dissection is completed, the abscess cavity (necrotic inflammatory exudate) is excised in pieces using a 5-mm biopsy forceps.

It is important to remember that after ovulation, purulent material from acute salpingitis may enter the inner ovary by inoculation of the corpus luteum, which may then become part of the abscess wall. Thus, after draining the abscess cavity and mobilizing the entire ovary, a gaping hole of varying size may be noted in the ovary that heretofore had been intimately involved in the abscess cavity. This area should be well irrigated; it will heal spontaneously, and significant bleeding is rarely encountered.

The next step is to insert grasping forceps into the fimbrial ostia, spreading them to free agglutinating fimbriae. Retrograde irrigation of the tube should be performed with the aquadissector to remove infected debris and diminish chances of recurrence. The fimbrial endosalpinx is visualized at this time, and its quality is assessed for future prognosis.

Tubal lavage with indigo carmine dye through a Cohen-Eder cannula (Eder Instruments Co.) in the uterus should be attempted. With early acute abscesses, the tubes are rarely patent because of interstitial edema. In contrast, when the abscess process has been present for longer than 1 week or the patient was previously treated with an antibiotic, lavage frequently documents tubal patency. Rarely, inspissated necrotic material can be pushed from the tube during the lavage procedure.

The peritoneal cavity is extensively irrigated with lactated Ringer's solution until the effluent is clear. The total volume of irrigant often exceeds 15 liters. ("The solution to pollution is dilution.") As part of this procedure, 2 liters of lactated Ringer's solution is flushed through the aquadissector into the upper abdomen (on each side of the falciform ligament) to dilute any purulent material that may have gained access to these areas during the 20-degree Trendelenburg positioning. The reverse Trendelenburg position is then used for the "underwater" examination. The laparoscope and the aquadissector are manipulated into the deep cul-de-sac beneath floating bowel and omentum, and this area is alternately irrigated and suctioned until the effluent is clear. An underwater examination is then performed to observe the completely separated tubes and ovaries and to document complete hemostasis. At the close of each procedure, at least 2 liters of lactated Ringer's solution is left in the peritoneal cavity to prevent fibrin adherences from forming between operated-upon surfaces during the early healing phase and to dilute the bacteria present.

Without question, the more acute the abscess, the easier will be the dissection. Patient and physician delay often makes the laparoscopic procedure more difficult than it need be. However, even chronic abscesses can be treated successfully by careful blunt aquadissection.

Postoperatively, the patient is usually ambulatory and on a "diet as tolerated" after recovery from anesthesia. Tempera-

ture elevation rarely persists past the first postoperative day. The patient is examined 1 week after discharge, after which all restrictions are removed.

REFERENCES

Ahrenholz DH and Simmons RL: Fibrin in peritonitis. I: Beneficial and adverse effects of fibrin in experimental *E. coli* peritonitis. Surgery 88:41–47, 1980.

Droegemueller WD, Herbst AL, Mishell DR Jr, and Stenchever MA: Comprehensive Gynecology. St Louis, CV Mosby, 1987.

Henry-Suchet J, Soler A, and Loffredo V: Laparoscopic treatment of tuboovarian abscesses. J Reprod Med 29:579–582, 1984.

Hudspeth AS: Radical surgical débridement in the treatment of advanced generalized bacterial peritonitis. Arch Surg 110:1233–1236, 1975.

Jacobson L: Differential diagnosis of acute pelvic inflammatory disease. Am J Obstet Gynecol 138: 1006–1011, 1980.

Jansen RPS: Early laparoscopy after pelvic operations to prevent adhesions: Safety and efficacy. Fertil Steril 49:26–31, 1988.

Landers DV and Sweet RL: Tubo-ovarian abscess: Contemporary approach to management. Rev Infect Dis 5:876–884, 1983.

Reich H and McGlynn F: Laparoscopic treatment of tuboovarian and pelvic abscess. J Reprod Med 32:747–752, 1987.

Rivlin ME and Hunt JA: Surgical management of diffuse peritonitis complicating obstetric/gynecologic infections. Obstet Gynecol 67:652–656, 1986.

Sellors J, Mahony J, Goldsmith C, et al: The accuracy of clinical findings and laparoscopy in pelvic inflammatory disease. Am J Obstet Gynecol 164:113–120, 1991.

Simpson FF: The choice of time for operation for pelvic inflammation of tubal origin. Surg Gynecol Obstet 9:45–62, 1909.

Skau T, Nyström P-O, Öhman L, and Stendahl O: The kinetics of peritoneal clearance of *Escherichia coli* and *Bacteroides fragilis* and participating defense mechanisms. Arch Surg 121:1033–1039, 1986.

Weström L: Incidence, prevalence, and trends of acute pelvic inflammatory disease and its consequences in industrialized countries. Am J Obstet Gynecol 138:880–892, 1980.

FURTHER READINGS

Franklin EW III, Hevron JE Jr, and Thompson JD: Management of pelvic abscess. Clin Obstet Gynecol 16(2):66–79, 1973.

Jansen RPS: Surgery-pregnancy time intervals after salpingolysis, unilateral salpingostomy, and bilateral salpingostomy. Fertil Steril 34:222–225, 1980.

Reich H: Endoscopic management of tuboovarian abscess and pelvic inflammatory disease. *In* Sanfilippo JS and Levine RL (eds): Operative Gynecologic Endoscopy. New York, Springer, 1988, pp 118–132.

Sweet RL and Ledger WJ: Cefoxitin: Single-agent treatment of mixed aerobic-anaerobic pelvic infections. Obstet Gynecol 54:193–198, 1979.

Weström L: Introductory address: Treatment of pelvic inflammatory disease in view of etiology and risk factors. Sex Transm Dis 11:437–440, 1984.

Laparoscopic Myomectomy

REASONS FOR

Indications

Uterine leiomyomas are the most common solid pelvic tumor, occurring in 20% of women older than 35 years of age. Most are asymptomatic. The major indications for myomectomy are:

- Secondary infertility with a past history of second-trimester loss
- Preservation of fertility in women with either hypermenorrhea leading to anemia or a large lower abdominal mass

Except for infertility, the major indications for myomectomy and hysterectomy for fibroids are similar. In many cases, fibroids can be followed with vaginal ultrasound to rule out ovarian neoplasms and rapid increases in fibroid size. Because frank symptoms are unusual, surgery can be avoided. Hysterectomy is the treatment of choice following completion of childbearing when hypermenorrhea leading to anemia or a pelvic mass greater than 12 weeks' gestational size is present.

The most common reason for laparoscopic myomectomy is the patient's decision to forego hysterectomy at all costs, including when it is probably indicated—a strong patient choice for uterine preservation. These women often accept laparoscopic hysterectomy with morcellation and ovarian preservation as an alternative, if counseled properly, because an abdominal incision may be their major concern. In some women, any type of hysterectomy will

not be acceptable, and the surgeon's acceptance of these challenging cases, despite attendant risks, is proportional to his or her developed surgical skills. When these women are older than 40, this "patient choice" surgery should be considered cosmetic, and medical insurance companies should not discriminate against their participating physicians who perform this procedure by forcing them to accept the assignment; rather, a portion of the fee should come from the patient.

It must be emphasized that multiple myomectomy is a more difficult and time-consuming procedure than hysterectomy and is associated with postoperative adhesions and the possibility of a subsequent procedure. Myomectomy by laparoscopy may not be more difficult than an open procedure but is more time-consuming and can be associated with greater blood loss. When laparoscopy is compared with vaginal hysterectomy, laparoscopic advantages of a short hospital stay, rapid recovery, and superior cosmetic result are questionable, especially in relation to cost-effectiveness.

Alternatives

Myomectomy for hypermenorrhea can often be accomplished hysteroscopically using the resectoscope to excise submucous myomas. When two thirds of what looks like a submucous myoma is intramural per ultrasound or clinical assessment, laparoscopic removal should be considered. Laparoscopic excision, even when one half of the myoma is submucous, usually leaves an intact endometrium with little risk of synechia.

Gonadotropin-releasing hormone (GnRH) analogs may reduce the total uterine volume in patients with uterine leiomyomata from 35 to 50%. This reduction in uterine volume is more pronounced in the nonmyoma portion of the uterus (Schlaff et al, 1989). During treatment with depoleuprolide (Depo-Lupron) at a dose of 3.75 mg intramuscularly (IM) once per month, for 3 to 6 months, anemia secondary to hypermenorrhea resolves, and autologous blood donation can be considered prior to a definitive surgical procedure. Packed red blood cells obtained in this manner have a shelf life of 35 days if stored at 1 to 6°C.

Because IM leuprolide, once monthly, reduces uterine volume and the size of the vessels supplying the fibroid and may shrink leiomyomas, women choosing myomectomy should be pretreated for at least 3 months despite the expense. This may be true also for women choosing hysterectomy for the treatment of large myomas, because shrinking the size of the myoma should make vaginal hysterectomy easier. Abdominal hysterectomy, even for large myomas, should be a rare operation in the future.

REASONS AGAINST

Myomectomy Versus Hysterectomy

Myomectomy by any route is a controversial subject. Accepted indications are removal for size or symptoms in women whose fertility is to be preserved. Extensive myomectomies by laparotomy or laparoscopy are not justified in patients who no longer wish to reproduce, since the morbidity and mortality of myomectomy are comparable with those of hysterectomy in these situations. Hysterectomy has additional benefits of eliminating the risk of future regrowth of leiomyomata, removing the cervix and endometrium to eliminate future carcinoma, and leaving the way free for estrogen replacement therapy in the future without need of monitoring the endometrial cavity. For these reasons, hysterectomy is the preferred management for symptomatic leiomyomata when reproduction is not an issue.

Women informed in the lay press of trendy, laser laparoscopic myomectomy to avoid ''unnecessary hysterectomy'' are a fact of life in the current medical marketing era. These requests need to be approached professionally: Risks to the patient of the procedure that they are requesting need to be outlined compared with the benefits that they would receive and the risk-benefit ratios of other procedures (e.g., open laparotomy or hysterectomy).

Myomectomy for Infertility

The performance of myomectomy in a woman undergoing diagnostic laparoscopy for infertility raises the important question of whether or not the fibroids found would in any way interfere with her fertility or capacity to bear a pregnancy to term. Most leiomyomatas do not markedly interfere with fertility or childbearing (Katz et al, 1989). Although more than half of women undergoing myomectomy for infertility conceive (Verkauf, 1992), at least one study concluded that the results of myomectomy to improve fertility are marginal (Berkeley et al, 1983). Thus, benefits of a myomectomy to an asymptomatic infertile woman whose fibroid does not distort the uterine or tubal portion of her reproductive systems cannot be documented by existing literature.

Indeed, risks of laparoscopic myomectomy in infertile women include the creation of uterine adhesions and leaving a weakened uterine wall to rupture during pregnancy. This situation occurs because repair of a uterine defect after myomectomy is much more difficult, even in experienced hands, by laparoscopy compared with the more secure repair through an opened abdominal cavity. A recent American Fertility Society Guideline for Practice concludes that long-term risks and benefits of laparoscopic myomectomy for infertility are not known (American Fertility Society, 1992).

Insistence of Patient

For women who request a myomectomy from their physician, the surgeon is obliged to review all of the aforementioned considerations. If the patient persists in her desire to remove the fibroid, only then is the issue of laparoscopy versus myomectomy by laparotomy appropriate. The issue of insurance coverage is appropriate to review. If an abdominal myomectomy or hysterectomy is indicated and the patient chooses laparoscopy, the insurance company may appropriately consider the surgery "cosmetic" in part (avoiding abdominal scar) and the patient may have to cover a large portion of the cost.

Blood Loss and Postoperative Adhesions

The myomectomies by laparoscopy and laser presented at meetings have all been relatively simple procedures that do not portray problems of blood loss, closure of the myometrium, and removal of the specimen. These myomectomies would take about 20 minutes of open laparotomy time. Closure of the defect, after an intramural myomectomy, is more refined at laparotomy since the uterine peritoneal surface can be brought to close approximation to minimize postoperative adhesion formation. Postoperative adhesions after laparoscopic myomectomy have not been compared with myomectomy by laparotomy, but we suspect that a fundal closure during laparotomy can be accomplished with less ischemic trauma and suture material than by the more clumsy laparoscopy suturing technique.

TECHNIQUE

Enucleation of myomas can be a frustrating, time-consuming experience when attempted laparoscopically. Bleeding problems are common and difficult to resolve. An instrument capable of holding an intramural fibroid on tension during its dissection from surrounding myometrium is essential.

Laparoscopic myomectomy requires a thorough knowledge of electrosurgical and laser techniques for hemostasis, because lower uterine segment tourniquets are not available to reduce intraoperative blood loss. Cutting current through a knife-electrode is used to cut and desiccate (coagulate); coagulation current is used to fulgurate. The knife-electrode tip is used to cut. The flat blade of the electrode is used to tamponade arteriolar bleeding vessels after which cutting current is applied to coagulate them. Diffuse venous bleeding can often be controlled with fulguration, which involves the noncontact application of coagulation current to the tissue through a 1- to 2-mm spark or arc. Cutting with some degree of coagulation is done with cutting or blended current through the broad edge of the knife electrode. Persistent arterial bleeding from small or large vessels requires bipolar desiccation with cutting current. The argon beam coagulator can be used to provide more powerful fulguration; spray coagulation current at 80 W will arc approximately 1 cm through the argon gas with resultant charring and hemostasis. Bipolar electrodes can only desiccate, and a cutting waveform should be selected when using these forceps. An effect similar to blended current is accomplished with the CO_2 laser through the operating channel of an operating laparoscope when used at power settings above 50 W, because a large spot size with diameter from 2 to 4 mm is obtained.

The argon, KTP-532, and Nd:YAG fiber lasers have absolutely no advantage over electrosurgical electrodes for cutting and coagulation and thus do not justify their extreme expense. Fibers cannot be maneuvered into places accessible with the CO_2 laser shot through the operating channel of an operating laparoscope perpendicular to the surgeon's field of vision. Less plume occurs with these lasers because the heat is dispersed into the tissue, causing much greater tissue necrosis.

Vasopressin is not injected myometrially during surgery, because delayed bleeding from the needle puncture sites requires later electrosurgical coagulation. Vasopressin use has been banned in France after fatalities occurred, presumably from cardiac arrhythmias during cervical procedures and myomectomy by *laparotomy*. Electrosurgical hemostasis is often supplemented by the placement of Surgicel inside the defect prior to suture repair. Bulldog clamps inserted through the 10-mm umbilical trocar sleeve can be applied to the infundibulopelvic ligaments for hemostasis in selected cases.

Autologous blood donation for intraoperative transfusion is considered.

Solitary pedunculated myomas can be separated from the uterus after desiccating their pedicle with bipolar forceps and removed from the peritoneal cavity through a culdotomy incision. Adenomyosis may masquerade as an intramural myoma with bulging of the serosa. When encountered, the bulk of the lesion should be removed with an electrosurgical wedge resection; hemostasis should be obtained with fulguration; and the defect should be closed as described later.

Myomectomy, a gross procedure, can be performed entirely with video. Ocular visualization should be considered with finer procedures. The serosa and surrounding myometrial shell are entered with a knife electrode at 25-W cutting current. Arteriolar bleeding is controlled with cutting current desiccation and venous oozing with coagulation current noncontact fulguration at 30 to 40 W. Thereafter, the 5-mm corkscrew (WISAP) is screwed into the myoma, which is pulled outward so that the tip of the aquadissector can be inserted between the fibroid and surrounding myometrial pseudocapsule to aquadissect tissue planes. In some cases, the exposed portion of the fibroid is bivalved at this time using cutting current electrosurgery. Small fibrous adherences between the fibroid and its myometrial shell are divided with electrosurgery or laser and large pedicles, usually at the base, separately desiccated with bipolar forceps. When using CO_2 laser through the operating channel of an operating laparoscope, high-power settings between 50 and 100 W continuous produce large spot sizes that will control most arteriolar and venous bleeding. Throughout the procedure, the aquadissector with single channel and solid distal tip is used to dissect the pseudocapsule cleavage planes, suction-retract myometrium and myoma, and suction smoke.

After removal of the myoma, a myometrial defect of varying size results. Myometrial bleeding is controlled with unipolar fulguration through a knife or hook electrode or argon beamer. Both of these fulguration sources result in shrinkage of the defect. Kleppinger bipolar forceps or microbipolar forceps may also be necessary to obtain complete hemostasis. Thereafter, the defect is repaired with sutures (usually on curved needles) tied outside the peritoneal cavity and slipped down to the defect through a short trapless trocar sleeve with a Clarke knot pusher. Surgicel may be left inside the closed defect. Myometrial dead space in most cases is closed using curved needle suturing techniques to compress the full thickness of exposed myometrium. Although my (H. R.) experience with second laparoscopies after myomectomy is limited, adhesion formation to the operative site has been rare.

The myoma is removed from the peritoneal cavity through a culdotomy incision. Morcellation is too time-consuming with presently available instruments. A wet sponge on ring forceps is inserted behind the cervix to distend the top of the posterior vagina. A probe in the rectum helps to confirm its position and aids in the dissection required if the rectum covers the posterior vagina. The CO_2 laser is used between 60 and 100 W continuous to make a transverse culdotomy incision, without the bleeding that accompanies a vaginal colpotomy incision made with scissors. Often when making the incision laparoscopically, there is a sudden loss of the pneumoperitoneum and field of view. Therefore, there is the potential danger of grasping bowel with a sharp grasper through the vagina after losing sight of where the extracted fibroid is. Following culdotomy, a sponge, pack, or 30-ml Foley balloon should be kept in close contact with the vaginal incision to avoid the loss of pneumoperitoneum and to facilitate the extraction of the large fibroid. The tenaculum or 11-mm corkscrew is inserted through the vagina by maneuvering it around the sponge to minimize loss of pneumoperitoneum. The fibroid is grasped under direct laparoscopic vision. In some cases the fibroid can be pushed into the deep cul-de-sac and held there while a second surgeon identifies it from below and applies the tenaculum. An 11-mm corkscrew device is screwed into the myoma vaginally through the culdotomy incision, and the myoma is put on traction at the incision and further morcellated vaginally with scissors or scalpel if necessary until removal is completed. The incision is closed with interrupted or running 0 Vicryl applied vaginally.

All blood clot is aspirated laparoscopically underwater, usually after displacing the CO_2 pneumoperitoneum with 4 to 5 liters of lactated Ringer's solution. Complete hemostasis is obtained underwater using microbipolar forceps, and copious irrigation/suction is performed until the effluent is clear. At the end of the procedure, 2 to 4 liters of lactated Ringer's solution are left in the peritoneal cavity to separate organs operated on during initial healing. Shoulder pain from CO_2 insufflation is less frequent following displacement of the CO_2 with 2 to 4 liters of Ringer's solution at the close of the procedure. Hyskon is not used because it pulls intravascular fluid into the peritoneal cavity. Normal activity can be resumed within 1 week.

In most cases, a 5-cm intramural fibroid can be removed from the uterus in less than 30 minutes. Another hour may be necessary to obtain complete hemostasis and suture repair the uterus. A 10-cm intramural myomectomy often takes 4 hours to complete. I suspect that a size limit of 15 cm should be considered for myomectomy. I have performed laparoscopic hysterectomy for larger sizes of more than 1000 g.

REFERENCES

American Fertility Society: The American Fertility Society Guideline for Practice: Myomas and reproductive function. Birmingham, AL, American Fertility Society, 1992.
Berkeley AS, DeCherney AH, and Polan ML: Abdominal myomectomy and subsequent fertility. Surg Gynecol Obstet 156:319–322, 1983.
Katz VL, Dotters DJ, and Droegemueller W: Complications of uterine leiomyomas in pregnancy. Obstet Gynecol 73:593–596, 1989.
Schlaff WD, Zerhouni EA, Huth JA, et al: A placebo-controlled trial of a depot gonadotropin-releasing hormone analogue (leuprolide) in the treatment of uterine leiomyomata. Obstet Gynecol 74:856–862, 1989.
Verkauf BS: Myomectomy for fertility enhancement and preservation. Fertil Steril 58:1–15, 1992.

FURTHER READINGS

LEIOMYOMAS AND FERTILITY

Davis JL, Ray-Mazumder S, Hobel CJ, et al: Uterine leiomyomas in pregnancy: A prospective study. Obstet Gynecol 75:41–44, 1990.

UTERINE SIZE REDUCTION

Friedman AJ and Barbieri RL: Leuprolide acetate: Applications in gynecology. Curr Probl Obstet Gynecol Fertil 11:205–236, 1988.
Friedman AJ, Hoffman DI, Comite F, et al: Treatment of leiomyomata uteri with leuprolide acetate depot: A double-blind, placebo-controlled, multicenter study for the Leuprolide Study Group. Obstet Gynecol 77:720–725, 1991.

Laparoscopic Uterosacral Nerve Ablation

Chronic pelvic pain is clinically difficult to eradicate, and often multiple approaches (supportive therapy, surgery) are needed to correct the physical and psychic damage. No operation is always a cure: Even after total hysterectomy there may be some recurrence of pelvic pain, even in patients who had documented uterine pathology (Stovall, 1990). When dysmenorrhea is a component of the pain, anything offering even partial relief will be a step in the right direction for the patient. Interruption of the uterosacral ligament by laser has been described as a simple, conservative, low-risk procedure with good results for half the patients. This concept is presented and examined.

FIGURE 26–1 Uterosacral ligament relationships

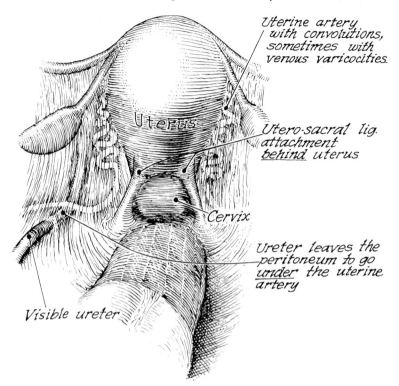

Uterine artery with convolutions, sometimes with venous varicocities.

Utero-sacral lig. attachment behind uterus

Uterus

Cervix

Ureter leaves the peritoneum to go under the uterine artery

Visible ureter

REASONS FOR

Division of nerves to the uterus to relieve dysmenorrhea was described as early as 1899 by Ruggi (Ruggi and Crossen, 1915). Doyle (1955) described a vaginal approach to uterosacral nerve division. In more recent literature, Feste (1985) narrated a laser technique, and Lichten and Bombard (1987) described a laparoscopic uterosacral nerve ablation (LUNA) procedure in which they desiccated the uterosacral ligament with unipolar grasping forceps and divided it with sharp scissors. This procedure can be performed with bipolar coagulation as well.

In patients undergoing laparoscopy with chronic dysmenorrhea as part of their symptoms, division of the uterosacral nerves appears to be of some benefit, which is maintained in approximately 50 to 60% of the patients for at least 12 months (Doyle, 1955; Lichten and Bombard, 1987). The addition of presacral neurectomy to conservative surgery does not appear to result in a greater reduction of pelvic pain than does conservative surgery alone (Candiani et al, 1992).

These benefits need to be considered in terms of the risks of the procedure. Risks can be serious, but they can be avoided with accurate knowledge of the anatomy of the area. If the uterosacral ligament is not properly identified, the ureter, which is lateral to it, can be injured. If the cul-de-sac is not properly identified, or if adherent rectum is misdiagnosed, as it can very easily be, there is real risk of injuring it during transection or desiccation. For these reasons, even though the procedure is technically simple, it is important for the surgeon to identify the uterosacral ligament, distinguish it from the rectum, and positively identify the ureter as being lateral to the ablation site (Fig. 26–1).

Once this is accomplished, uterosacral ablation can be accomplished with relative ease. The uterus is pushed upward and is sharply anteverted with a uterine manipulator to put the uterosacral ligaments on a stretch. A separate grasping forceps can be used to further tent the ligament and draw it away from the underlying ureter and vessels. Bipolar coagulation and sharp division of the desiccated ligament can then be performed. This procedure should be done as close to the uterus as possible (see Atlas, Plate 22) in order to minimize the risk of involvement of the ureter and aberrant uterine vessels. Alternatively, a CO_2 laser can divide the ligament horizontally until there is approximately a 1-cm crater created in the stretched ligament.

REASONS AGAINST

The concept of ablating the uterosacral ligaments when pelvic pathology exists makes no sense. Excision or division of the pathologic problem should reduce or eliminate the pain. Deep fibrotic endometriosis that results from inflammatory fibrosis enveloping reactive endometriosis glands and stroma should be excised as completely as possible from the vesicouterine peritoneal fold, uterosacral ligaments, posterior cervix, posterior vagina, and anterior rectum, because this condition is a major cause of pelvic pain with associated palpable tenderness. If pelvic pain persists for 6 to 12 months thereafter, a second laparoscopic procedure should be considered to excise adjacent lesions that are not visible or palpable during the original procedure. In women with a past history of endometriosis treated surgically but no evidence of recurrent or persistent disease, small uterine "myomas" and uterine dimpled areas should be biopsied. Often what appears to be a myoma will be adenomyosis, differentiated by its friability and yellowish appearance. Myomas maintain their consistency and are much easier to excise completely.

Multiple options are available if no pelvic pathology exists:

- No treatment with patient reassurance during viewing of the procedure on video
- Patient reassurance following a review of surgical procedure during which normal ovarian follicle cysts are drained
- LUNA
- Laparoscopic presacral neurectomy
- Laparoscopic or vaginal hysterectomy

Women who are anxious about cancer, tube blockage due to infection, or endometriosis often respond to a careful review of their normal anatomy documented on video during the laparoscopic procedure. Beard and associates (1977) reported on 18 of 35 women who had no pelvic pathology at laparoscopy. Symptoms disappeared or diminished in five women following an explanation of the findings. Six of nine women with no improvement were symptom free after psychiatric relaxation therapy or sexual counseling for 3 months.

Bleeding during the performance of LUNA has resulted in laparotomy for control in many centers. In one case in my (H. R.) series involving this procedure, the right uterine vein was entered within 2 seconds. This required dissection of the ureter and uterine vessels prior to desiccating the uterine vein. Fortunately, bleeding was controlled by holding the uterus in a sharply antiflex position during the dissection. Although hemostasis was apparent during this dissection, whenever the uterus was relaxed into a neutral position, heavy bleeding would ensue. Thus, I strongly recommend careful examination of the site operated on during the LUNA procedure after removing the intrauterine manipulator and with the patient in a supine position with minimal peritoneal cavity pressure.

Perez reported on laparoscopic presacral neurectomy. Relief pain was achieved in 60 to 70% of 25 patients in Perez's series. This operation on the sympathetic fibers of the inferior hypogastric plexus can be performed with the laparoscope inserted above the pubic symphysis (Perez, 1990) or in the umbilicus (Redwine, 1992). A 1964 review of the world literature on 9937 cases reported 75 to 80% significant relief of dysmenorrhea (Black, 1964). Treatment of secondary dysmenorrhea was successful in 37 to 53% of cases.

To summarize, pelvic pain with laparoscopically discernible pathology should be treated by removal of the offending problem. When normal anatomy is apparent, the five procedures described earlier can be considered. Of the three surgical choices (e.g., LUNA, presacral neurectomy, hysterectomy), only LUNA lacks the necessity for surgical expertise. If it is performed without surgical identification of the ureter and surrounding vessels, there is a risk of injury. This risk should raise great concern regarding the promotion of a procedure with questionable efficacy.

REFERENCES

Beard RW, Belsey EM, Lieberman BA, and Wilkinson JCM: Pelvic pain in women. Am J Obstet Gynecol *128*:566–577, 1977.

Black WT Jr: Use of presacral sympathectomy in the treatment of dysmenorrhea: A second look after twenty-five years. Am J Obstet Gynecol *89*:16–22, 1964.

Candiani GB, Fedele L, Vercellini P, et al: Presacral neurectomy for the treatment of pelvic pain associated with endometriosis: A controlled study. Am J Obstet Gynecol *167*:100–103, 1992.

Doyle JB: Paracervical uterine denervation by transection of the cervical plexus for the relief of dysmenorrhea. Am J Obstet Gynecol *70*:1–16, 1955.

Feste JR: Laser laparoscopy: A new modality. J Reprod Med *30*:413–417, 1985.

Lichten EM and Bombard J: Surgical treatment of primary dysmenorrhea with laparoscopic uterine nerve ablation. J Reprod Med *32*:37–41, 1987.

Perez JJ: Laparoscopic presacral neurectomy: Results of the first 25 cases. J Reprod Med *35*:625–630, 1990.

Redwine DB: Laparoscopic presacral neurectomy. *In* Soderstrom RM (ed): Operative Laparoscopy: The Masters' Techniques. Gaithersburg, MD, Aspen Publishers, 1992, pp 157–160.

Ruggi J and Crossen HS (eds): Gynecology. St Louis, CV Mosby, 1915.

Laparoscopic Pelvic Lymphadenectomy

Harry Reich, M.D.

Nicholas R. Kadar, M.D., Grad IS, MRCOG

REASONS FOR

Laparoscopic lymphadenectomy is proving to be a feasible procedure technically, with benefits of shorter hospital stay and lower morbidity to the patient. Indications for this approach, both male and female, are staging of lesions where a laparotomy may not be necessary for therapy. These lesions include cervical, uterine, ovarian, and prostate cancer.

Querleu and associates (1991) have concluded that it is possible to remove the first-line regional lymph nodes of the cervix for histologic examination. Localized radiotherapy alone, vaginal surgery, or even in some cases cervical cone excision for microinvasive disease can be applied safely without the need for staging laparotomy in cases of negative nodes. Querleu and colleagues believe that laparoscopic lymphadenectomy is a feasible alternative to laparotomy that should be used only by surgeons with considerable expertise in this field.

If CT scanning reveals a node and percutaneous biopsy confirms this finding, a radical procedure may not be indicated in females. However, early stage cervical carcinomas (FIGO stage 1A2) without pelvic metastases can be treated by cervical conization alone. Although laparoscopic node dissection for cervical cancer does not always reach para-aortic or iliac nodes, the risk of "skip metastases," in which these nodes would be positive after skipping the

pelvic nodes, is rare (<2%). Moreover, there is a question whether the poor outcome of patients with para-aortic nodes, regardless of treatment, justifies subjecting all patients to the risks of para-aortic staging by laparotomy.

Presently, in France, Querleu and Dargent (Dargent and Salvat, 1988) start cervical cancer cases laparoscopically with ureteral dissection and lymphadenectomy and marking of the ureters by suture around them. The Schauta radical vaginal hysterectomy is then done. Thus, stage 1B cervical cancer is handled without an abdominal incision.

REASONS AGAINST

There is no doubt that the French (Querleu et al, 1991) and American (Schuessler et al, 1991) experience with pelvic lymphadenectomy in male and female patients has demonstrated that the procedure can be performed by skilled and experienced hands. The arguments in favor of a laparoscopic technique (e.g., shorter hospital stay for these patients to whom life at home is precious, equal efficacy in skilled hands) will be counterbalanced for the foreseeable future by the desire of few oncology surgeons in the United States to develop these laparoscopic skills for the occasional selected patient in (Donato, 1992) whom laparotomy for hysterectomy will not also be indicated. This technique may remain as one documented to be feasible in skilled and experienced hands but not universally applicable for reasons of tradition and training.

HISTORY

Laparoscopic retroperitoneal lymphadenectomy was first introduced in the United States by Salvat from France in August 1988. Dargent and Salvat published their series of more than 100 panoramic retroperitoneal pelviscopic lymphadenectomies for staging of endometrial, cervical, and ovarian cancer in 1988. They performed this procedure by inserting the laparoscope beneath the deep fascia through a midline incision at the pubic hairline. With finger dissection through a midline pubic hairline incision, the deep fascia was located and opened; its underlying areolar tissue was loosened; and a laparoscope with its trocar sleeve was inserted to insufflate the retroperitoneum with CO_2. The bifurcation of the common iliac with external iliac and hypogastric was located on each side; the obturator nerve was identified; and obturator space lymphadenectomy was done.

In November 1988, Reich performed the first transperitoneal laparoscopic pelvic lymphadenectomy to stage ovarian cancer; Querleu in France performed the same procedure 1 week later to stage cervical cancer. In October 1989, Schuessler and Reich did the first male laparoscopic pelvic lymphadenectomy to stage prostate cancer.

Reich's procedure was stimulated by Salvat's August 1988 presentation. A serous cystadenocarcinoma was diagnosed by frozen section in an ovarian mass resembling a benign dermoid cyst, which had just been removed without spillage. An open procedure with hysterectomy, contralateral oophorectomy, lymphadenectomy, and omentectomy was recommended to the patient's husband, the chief of pathology, who suggested a laparoscopic approach because his wife would not accept open incisional surgery or chemotherapy. Laparoscopic hysterectomy, bilateral oophorectomy, omentectomy, and left pelvic lymphadenectomy, up to the aortic bifurcation, were done under laparoscopic guidance for the first time (Reich et al, 1990).

Querleu studied cervical cancer staging by translaparoscopic lymphadenectomy. He reported 39 cervical cancer cases in which he removed between 3 and 22 lymph nodes with no significant morbidity. Laparotomy followed the laparoscopic procedure in 32 of the 39 cases, usually for radical hysterectomy. He found 100% sensitivity and specificity in his series. There were no unexpected metastatic nodes found at laparotomy. He concluded that FIGO stage I, IIA, or proximal IIB cases with negative pathologic staging may be cured by vaginal surgery or by brachytherapy alone without the need for external radiotherapy. On the other hand, radical hysterectomy is avoided when metastatic nodes are present (Potter et al, 1990). The consequent reduction of risks and cost justifies the additional general anesthesia and the short hospital stay of a diagnostic laparoscopy.

Querleu gained access to the retroperitoneal space through an incision in the peritoneum between the round and IP ligaments bilaterally and then did laparoscopic dissection of the external iliac and vessels, umbilical artery, and obturator nerve. The peritoneum was left open for lymph drainage into the peritoneal cavity, and no lymphocysts occurred. His average operating time was 90 minutes.

Reich's initial technique (1989) used three laparoscopic puncture sites including the umbilicus: 10 mm umbilical, 5 mm right, and 5 mm left lower quadrant. The lower quadrant trocar sleeves are placed just above the pubic hairline and lateral to the deep epigastric vessels (and, thus, the rectus abdominis muscle) (Reich, 1989). The rectosigmoid or cecum followed by the ovarian vessel pedicle and its surrounding peritoneum are mobilized upward to gain entrance into the retroperitoneal space at the level of the aortic bifurcation, and nodal tissue is taken. Thereafter, adipose and lymph tissue lateral to the common and external iliac vessels is excised using laser dissection close to the vessels to seal the lymphatic channels. The ureter is retracted medially throughout the dissection. After mobilization of the medial and undersurface of the external iliac vein, the obturator internus fascia of the pelvic sidewall is identified. At the junction of external iliac and hypogastric vein, the obturator nerve, covered with adipose tissue, is identified and exposed. Nodal tissue is then excised, using the external iliac vein as the upper margin of the dissection, the hypogastric vein as a lower margin, and the pubic bone as the inferior margin. Laser is used to divide fibrotic attachments or vaporize arteriolar and venous vessels; when unsuccessful, bipolar forceps are applied. Underwater inspection of the pelvis is performed to detect and control any further bleeding using the Vancaillie microbipolar forceps (Storz) to coagulate through the electrolyte solution, and complete hemostasis is documented.

Obturator lymphadenectomy in men is easier and safer than in women because of a marked reduction in pelvic sidewall vasculature. Schuessler and associates (1991) used this procedure for staging localized prostate cancer in more than 100 men. Their conclusion was that it permits a more accurate staging and therefore counseling of the patient and adds only minimal morbidity to the radiotherapeutic treatment of prostatic cancer. Their technique, which can be applied to women, involves entering the obturator space inferiorly, using the obliterated umbilical fold as a landmark. The obliterated umbilical fold is seen on the anterior abdominal wall, curving into the pelvis where it terminates at the hypogastric artery. The initial incision is made using either laser or scissors just lateral to the obliterated umbilical ligament at the level of the superior pubic ramus. Dissection continues upward to the vas deferens, which is usually desiccated with bipolar forceps and divided to gain better access to the obturator space. The external iliac vein is next identified, and its inferior margin is meticulously dissected. Thereafter, the obturator nerve, which defines the posterior limit of the dissection, is identified. Using biopsy forceps for traction and scissors or laser for division of tissue, the obturator fossa is cleared of nodes and adipose tissue, starting anteriorly just below the pubic ramus and continuing upward to the point where external iliac vein, obturator nerve, and umbilical ligament meet at the commencement of the common iliac vein.

TECHNIQUE FOR GYNECOLOGIC ONCOLOGY

The technique used for pelvic lymphadenectomy is essentially the same regardless of whether the procedure is carried out using a laparotomy incision or laparoscopic visualization. The key ingredients for a successful operation are (1) correct development of the pararectal and paravesical spaces and (2) systematic delineation of the surgical limits of the intended dissection. Although a great deal has been written in the gynecologic literature about the extraperitoneal tissue planes of the pelvis, their anatomic landmarks and a systematic method of developing these spaces are not widely known. To make matters worse, two quite different tissue planes are referred to as the "pararectal space."

Development of the Pararectal and Paravesical Spaces

To gain access to the extraperitoneal tissues for a laparoscopic pelvic lymphadenectomy, the round ligaments are first coagulated and divided close to the internal inguinal rings using the tip of unopened disposable laparoscopic dissecting scissors and a nonmodulated (cutting) monopolar current. The incisions are then continued superficially along the pelvic peritoneum just lateral to the external iliac vessels to the level of the common iliac arteries above the pelvic brim using sharp scissor dissection with the scissors. This point marks the proximal or cephalad limits of the dissection. The left and right peritoneal incisions are then joined by incising the loose peritoneum overlying the front of the cervix above the bladder (the vesicouterine peritoneal fold). The stage is now set to develop the pararectal and paravesical spaces.

If an imaginary line is drawn vertically along the medial leaf of the broad ligament all the way down to the levator floor, the line will first cross the infundibulopelvic ligament, and then, successively, the ureter, the uterosacral ligament, and, finally, the rectal pillars. The pararectal spaces that are used for pelvic surgery are bounded laterally by the internal iliac arteries and medially by the ureters. Prior to the development of these tissue spaces, the ureters lie just above the internal iliac arteries on the pelvic sidewalls; after the pararectal spaces are developed, the ureters mark their medial borders. Therefore, development of the pararectal spaces is an essential step in the identification of the pelvic course of the ureters.

Each pararectal space is developed by first peeling apart the leaves of the broad ligament and separating the loose areolar tissue between them. This is easily done by tenting the medial leaf of the broad ligament with a laparoscopic tissue forceps and then sweeping it medially with the back of the scissors or the suction irrigator (aquadissector). As this maneuver is carried out, an impasse is usually reached at above the level of the ureter and internal iliac artery at which point the areolar tissue is more condensed and will not peel apart any further. This point at the base of the broad ligament marks the roof of the pararectal space. The dense connective tissue forming the roof of the pararectal space cannot be disrupted by simply pulling or pushing on it bluntly, and a separate maneuver is required to open the pararectal space from that used to open the broad ligament. A small opening must first be made in this dense areolar tissue with the point of either the scissors or forceps, following which the instrument can be insinuated into the pararectal space after spreading its tips and used to open the space by pushing on its medial wall in a direction corresponding roughly to the contralateral femoral head. This maneuver develops a bloodless plane that extends from the broad ligament superiorly all the way to the pelvic floor and has the following landmarks: the internal artery laterally, the cardinal ligament anteriorly, and the ureter, uterosacral ligaments, and rectal pillars medially.

It is well to be aware that another avascular tissue plane can be developed medial to each ureter and uterosacral ligament, but lateral to the peritoneum that forms the medial portion of the broad ligament and its inferior extension into the cul-de-sac. The general surgeon calls this plane the pararectal space and uses it for carrying out either anterior or abdominoperineal resection of the rectum for carcinoma. In other words, our colleagues in general surgery never work laterally to the ureter when performing their pelvic operations but leave it attached in its natural position on the lateral pelvic sidewall.

The paravesical space that is to be developed prior to performing a pelvic lymphadenectomy is bordered distally or caudad by the pubic bone, proximally or cephalad by the cardinal ligament, medially by the obliterated umbilical artery (also called the lateral umbilical ligament), laterally by the external iliac vessels, and inferiorly by the obturator fossa. This tissue plane is developed by running the back of the forceps or scissors along the medial border of the external iliac artery down to the pubic bone and then by sweeping it abruptly in a medial direction. When this is done, the dissecting instrument will be applied against the obliterated hypogastric artery, and a bloodless plane will appear between it and the external iliac vessels laterally, all the way down to the obturator fossa. As the obliterated hypogastric artery or lateral umbilical ligament is traced proximally, it becomes the superior vesical artery, which dives deeply down into the pelvis, hugging the lateral aspect of the bladder, and then curves upwards to join the uterine artery and become the internal iliac artery at the pelvic sidewall.

Although it is not an obvious landmark at laparotomy, the obliterated hypogastric artery is easily visible laparoscopically through the peritoneum, where it is crossed by the round ligament, about 1 to 2 cm inferomedial to the internal iliac ring. Therefore, once the round ligaments have been divided lateral to this point, an alternate and perhaps easier way to develop the paravesical space during laparoscopic pelvic lymphadenectomy is simply to grasp the obliterated hypogastric artery with an Endograsp and pull it medially. As the avascular paravesical space begins to open, the dissection is aided by pushing medially on the hypogastric artery at a progressively more proximal point with the convex surface of the forceps.

Surgical Limits of the Dissection

With the pelvic spaces cleanly developed, the next phase of a pelvic lymphadenectomy is the delineation of the limits of the surgical dissection. These are the common iliac artery proximally (cephalad), the psoas muscle laterally, the circumflex iliac vein and pubic bone distally (caudad), the obliterated umbilical artery medially, and the obturator fossa inferiorly (ventrally). In developing the paravesical and pararectal spaces, the proximal, distal, medial, and inferior limits of the dissection have already been delineated. All that remains is to separate the external iliac vessels from the psoas muscle.

Using sharp scissors dissection, the dense areolar tissue attaching the external iliac artery to the psoas muscle is scored very superficially from the proximal to the distal limits of the dissection. This incision must be very superficial to avoid injury to the external iliac vein that lies just below the artery, and a deep incision is in any case not required because the external iliac vessels can be peeled off the psoas muscle easily using blunt dissection with forceps. Very occasionally, some nutrient muscular branches are given off from the lateral aspect of the artery, but this is very much the exception rather than the rule. If present, these vessels must be coagulated or clipped. The visible surface of the artery is first freed all the way down to the circuflex iliac vein, a branch of the external iliac vein that courses outwards and laterally to cross the lower portion of the external iliac artery. Working progressively more deeply (inferiorly), the inferior margin of the artery, and then the external iliac vein are progressively freed from the psoas muscle, and on freeing the vein, the obturator fossa is entered laterally. At this point fatty nodal tissue will come into view, and by continuing the plane of dissection lateral to this tissue, the nodal bundle of the obturator fossa will be mobilized medially. After the external iliac vessels and contents of the obturator fossa are mobilized medially, the lymphadenectomy proper is begun.

Pelvic Lymphadenectomy

The first step is to remove the fatty nodal tissue lying lateral to and in front of the common iliac artery, although sometimes the amount of tissue at this site is very scanty. The nodal tissue is freed by dividing the loose areolar tissue that anchors it to the psoas muscle and common iliac artery, using sharp scissor dissection. The only phase of this dissection requiring special attention is when the uppermost part of the nodal mass is being freed, because an artery is always encountered here on the lateral aspect of the dissection coursing underneath the nodal mass toward the bifurcation

of the aorta, parallel to the superior aspect of the common iliac artery. This vessel has to be either coagulated or clipped.

The external iliac artery and vein are next freed from their areolar investments. Each vessel is completely surrounded by its own distinct areolar sheath, and the two sheaths are fused along the entire course of the vessels. The sheath of the external iliac artery is incised along its dorsal surface from the level of the common iliac artery all the way down to the circumflex iliac vein using scissors. There are never any branches of the external iliac artery in this region, but there is usually a hair-like vessel that crosses the artery obliquely at its midportion superficial to its sheath. This vessel can be coagulated by touching it with the closed point of the scissors using a cutting monopolar current. After opening the artery's sheath, its medial border is grasped with forceps, and the artery is peeled off the inferior surface of its sheath using mostly blunt dissection with the back of the scissors but cutting areolar attachments as needed. The same process repeated on the lateral surface of the artery will free it completely from the underlying vein. At this point, the sheaths of the external iliac artery and vein are still joined along the undersurface of the artery, and the next step is to incise the sheath of the external iliac vein cautiously. *This step requires the greatest care in the entire dissection*, because the edge of the vessel can easily be compressed and merge imperceptibly with the areolar sheath that covers it. However, once a nick has been made in the sheath, the glistening surface of the vein becomes unmistakably clear and distinct from its areolar covering. The same technique of sharp and blunt dissection can then be used to free the vein circumferentially from its sheath as is used to free the artery. The final step in this part of the dissection is to free the inferior border of the vein that is tethered by loose areolar tissue to the pelvic sidewall and obturator fossa. This is done not so much because there are any very noticeable nodes attached to the sheath but rather to gain free access to the obturator fossa.

The external iliac nodes are distributed along the course of the external iliac artery in a cephalic-caudal or "north-south" direction and are attached laterally to the psoas muscle and medially to the sheath of the external iliac artery by loose areolar tissue. Distally, at the level of the circumflex iliac vein, there are quite prominent nodes lying in a lateral-medial or "east-west" direction across the lower part of the external iliac artery. The most lateral part of this nodal bundle is about 2 cm from the artery itself, and there is usually a nutrient branch that has to be coagulated as these nodes are freed from the inferolateral part of the psoas muscle. The medial attachments of these nodes are freed when the external iliac vessels are dissected from their sheaths; all that remains then is to free their lateral attachments to the psoas muscle. As this is done, the iliofemoral and genitofemoral nerves are encountered but can easily be pushed laterally. The nodal tissue and the areolar sheaths of the external iliac vessels to which they are attached can be removed at this point and sent as a separate specimen, or they can be allowed to fall away from the vessels into the obturator fossa and removed later en block with the remainder of the pelvic nodal tissue.

Finally, the obturator fossa and internal iliac vessels are freed. This is best done by retracting the external iliac vessels laterally and teasing out the obturator nerve from the inferiormost part of the obturator nodal bundle using the unopened scissors. Once the nerve is freed, the distal attachment of the nodal bundle can be freed from the pubic bone using scissors, coagulating with a cutting current before dividing the tissues sharply to seal the lymphatics. The nodal bundle is then grasped with forceps, elevated and placed on tension, and then teased off its most ventral attachments below the obturator nerve using a gentle pushing motion with the partly opened scissors. As this nodal tissue is freed in a cephalic direction, residual attachments to the external iliac vein usually need to be freed. Eventually, the internal iliac artery is reached, and the nodal tissue lying anterior, lateral, and medial to it is freed in continuity with the obturator fossa nodal mass. The nodal tissue can be quite adherent in this region because the internal iliac artery does not have an areolar sheath as do the external iliac vessels. With further dissection in a cephalad direction, the crura or bifurcation of the iliac arteries is reached, and this

region must be cleaned with care, ever mindful that the external and internal iliac veins lie just lateral to these structures. Once the attachments of the nodal bundle in this region are divided, the dissection is complete (see Atlas, Plate 31).

Pelvic lymphadenectomy rarely presents any real technical difficulties to the pelvic surgeon who is familiar with the anatomy, is adept at sharp dissection, and takes a systematic approach. As noted, there are two points at which particular care must be taken: on opening the areolar sheath surrounding the external iliac vein, and on cleaning the bifurcation of the iliac arteries. Annoying bleeding can occur at two additional points: the superiolateral aspect of the common iliac nodes and at the inferolateral aspect of the external iliac nodes, where small arteries are constantly present. Finally, an aberrant obturator vein may be present that joins the external iliac vein on its inferior aspect rather than the internal iliac vein, which is usually the case. If present, an aberrant obturator vein has to be clipped and divided to mobilize the external iliac vein completely. If one is mindful of these potential hazards and uses a proper technique of sharp scissor and blunt dissection in a judicious manner, rarely will any significant technical problems be encountered.

REFERENCES

Dargent D and Salvat J: Envahissement Ganglionnaire Pelvien. Paris, Medsi/McGraw Hill, 1988.

Donato DM: Advanced laparoscopic techniques in gynecologic oncology. Contemp Ob/Gyn (Sept.):102–104, 106, 108, 110, 112, 115, 117–118, 1992.

Potter ME, Alvarez RD, Shingleton HM, et al: Early invasive cervical cancer with pelvic lymph node involvement: To complete or not to complete radical hysterectomy? Gynecol Oncol 37:78–81, 1990.

Querleu D, Leblanc E, and Castelain B: Laparoscopic pelvic lymphadenectomy in the staging of early carcinoma of the cervix. Am J Obstet Gynecol 164:579–581, 1991.

Reich H, McGlynn F, and Wilkie W: Laparoscopic management of Stage I ovarian cancer: A case report. J Reprod Med 35:601–604, 1990.

Schuessler WW, Vancaillie TG, Reich H, and Griffith DP: Transperitoneal endosurgical lymphadenectomy in patients with localized prostate cancer. J Urol 145:988–991, 1991.

FURTHER READING

Reich H: New techniques in advanced laparoscopic surgery. Baillieres Clin Obstet Gynecol 3:655–681, 1989.

Laparoscopic Para-Aortic Lymphadenectomy

Joel M. Childers, M.D.

HISTORY

Currently only three reports in the literature describe a series of patients who have undergone laparoscopic pelvic lymphadenectomy. Querleu and associates (1991) described this procedure in staging patients with early carcinoma of the cervix. Schuessler and colleagues (1991) reported their experience with laparoscopic lymphadenectomy in patients with localized prostatic cancer. To date, Childers and associates (1992) are the only ones to report on a series of patients undergoing laparoscopic pelvic and para-aortic lymphadenectomy. This technique was used to stage patients with early and advanced cervical carcinoma. These latter investigators also report two patients with stage I endometrial cancer who were managed by a combined laparoscopic and vaginal approach (Childers and Surwit, 1992). In these patients, a laparoscopic approach was used to inspect the intraperitoneal cavity, obtain pelvic washings, and remove pelvic and para-aortic nodes as well as to assist in the vaginal hysterectomy. A transperitoneal approach to the retroperitoneal space was used in all of these procedures.

In this chapter, I outline the technique of laparoscopic para-aortic lymphadenectomy as it is used in patients with gynecologic malignancies. I have performed more than 100 laparoscopic lymphadenectomies, and in more than half of these patients laparoscopic para-aortic lymphadenectomies were performed. During the last 2 years my technique for this procedure has evolved into the one described here. I currently use this procedure to (1) stage patients with early and advanced cervical carcinoma; (2) stage and convert abdominal procedures to laparoscopically assisted vaginal procedures in patients with endometrial carcinoma; (3) perform restaging procedures on patients with incompletely staged cancers of the cervix, ovary, and uterus; and (4) perform second-look procedures in patients with ovarian carcinoma.

TECHNIQUE

Special instruments such as needle drivers, knot pushers, and stapling devices are not necessary for the lymphadenectomy but are necessary if a laparoscopically assisted vaginal hysterectomy is to be performed (see Indications later). On occasion, the laparoscopic clip applicator may be needed, most commonly for perforating veins on the vena cava.

FIGURE 28–1 Portals for lymphadenectomy

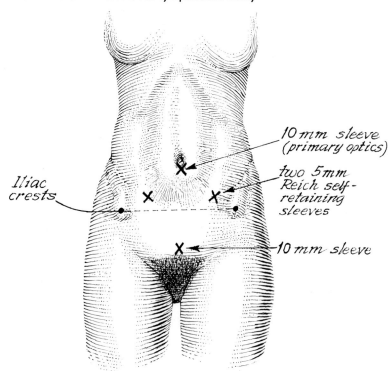

Iliac crests

10 mm sleeve (primary optics)

two 5mm Reich self-retaining sleeves

10 mm sleeve

Instrument Insertions

Gaining access to the intraperitoneal cavity is a procedure well known to most gynecologists. I prefer the technique of direct trocar insertion without the prior establishment of a pneumoperitoneum. This is accomplished by placing a 10- or 11-mm laparoscopic trocar and sleeve through an incision made in the umbilicus. Upward traction on the anterior abdominal wall with the aid of towel clips placed on either side of the umbilicus is important.

If preferred, establishing a pneumoperitoneum can be accomplished first. In this instance, a Veress needle is placed through an incision made in the umbilicus. The pressure should be less than 5 mm Hg in most patients if the Veress needle is properly placed in the intraperitoneal cavity.

In patients with previous abdominal incisions extending through the umbilicus, other sites of insertion for the insufflation needle should be used. I currently favor the left upper quadrant in the midclavicular line a few centimeters below the costal margin for placement of the Veress needle in these patients. Once the pneumoperitoneum is established, the primary trocar may be placed in this site or at McBurney's point on the right or left side. In these cases, it is not advisable initially to place a 10-mm trocar and sleeve. A 5-mm trocar and sleeve should be inserted first with the use of a 5-mm laparoscope for visualization of intraperitoneal adhesions and placement of ancillary trocars. If the surgeon prefers, open laparoscopy can be performed with the use of a Hasson cannula.

Generally, four laparoscopic ports are needed to perform this procedure (Fig. 28–1). The primary port is in the umbilicus and should be 10 mm in size for use of the telescope and camera. The three ancillary ports should be placed under direct laparoscopic visualization. Lysis of adhesions may be required prior to safe placement of these ancillary ports. Two 5-mm trocars and sleeves are placed midway between the umbilicus and the anterior superior iliac crest bilaterally. Care should be taken to avoid the epigastric vessels during placement of these trocars and sleeves. This can be accomplished by either directly visualizing the epigastric vessel through the primary port or by transilluminating the abdominal wall. The third port is placed in the midline above the symphysis and should be 10 mm in size to allow placement of a large spoon forceps for removal of the nodal tissue. Different port sites for para-aortic lymphadenectomy have been suggested based on animal studies. I prefer the location described earlier, because it allows access to the pelvis as well as to the para-aortic area.

Inspection of the Intraperitoneal Cavity

After the laparoscopic ports are in place and before the patient is placed in the Trendelenburg position, it is important to explore the entire intraperitoneal cavity systematically. The cecum and appendix should be visualized as well as the right paracolic gutter. The gallbladder, the surface of the right lobe of the liver, the right hemidiaphragm, the falciform ligament, the greater curvature of the stomach, the anterior wall of the stomach, the left hemidiaphragm with its left ventricular pulsations, the supracolic omentum, the transverse colon, and the infracolic omentum should be carefully inspected. This systematic clockwise inspection continues with evaluation of the descending colon and left paracolic gutter, which leads the surgeon to the pelvis. The pelvis is evaluated after the establishment of the Trendelenburg position. It is helpful, when evaluating the pelvic sidewalls, to grasp the utero-ovarian ligament and to lift the ovary so that the ovarian fossa can be adequately visualized.

Pelvic washings should be taken, and a search for retroperitoneal adenopathy should be performed. Several important landmarks will facilitate this evaluation. The sacral promontory should be identified, and the bowel should be placed in the upper abdomen with the use of graspers inserted through the ancillary ports. The bowel should be placed so that the root of the small bowel can be easily recognized. Pulsation from the aorta should be seen, and the right common iliac artery can be followed in a caudal direction. This aids in identifying the right ureter, the right ovarian vessels, and the bifurcation of the common iliac artery. The round ligaments should be seen traversing from the uterus to the inguinal canal. The epigastric vessels can be seen originating from the external iliac artery in this area as well.

In examining the para-aortic area, the root of the small bowel mesentery can be lifted, and often the second part of the duodenum can be seen. This area from the second part of the duodenum to the inguinal canal should be inspected for obvious adenopathy.

A complete bilateral pelvic and para-aortic lymphadenectomy can be performed through three incisions: one upper incision over the aorta, and lower incisions over the external iliac arteries on either side.

Para-Aortic Lymphadenectomy

When removing the para-aortic nodes, it is important to place the small bowel into the upper abdomen, such that its mesentery can easily be identified and elevated. The Trendelenburg position, a good bowel preparation, and occasionally a lateral tilt of the operating table assist in proper placement of the bowel in the upper abdomen. By mobilizing the mesentery in a caudal and lateral direction, one can often visualize the second part of the duodenum as it crosses the vena cava and aorta. The aorta and right common iliac artery should be identified as well as the ureter on the right side as it crosses the iliac vessels.

The surgeon, on the left side of the patient, performs the procedure with graspers in the lower midline port and scissors in the left lateral port. The assistant holds the camera in the umbilicus and uses graspers in the right lateral port. It is extremely helpful to rotate the camera 90 degrees so that the aorta and vena cava are horizontal on the color monitor.

An incision is made over the aorta above the bifurcation and is extended down the right common iliac to the point where the ureter crosses the iliac vessels. It is also extended up the aorta to the point where the mesentery of the small bowel, or second part of the duodenum, interferes. The peritoneum is lifted with graspers, and dissection is performed laterally toward the psoas muscle. The right ureter is identified and dissected off the underlying areolar tissue.

The grasper in the midline port then lifts the ureter anteriorly, and the dissection is completed laterally until the right psoas and tendon of the psoas are identified completely.

The assistant then places the grasper (in the right lateral port) underneath the ureter and retracts the ureter anteriorly and laterally out of the operative field.

The surgeon then dissects the nodal and fatty tissue off the aorta by creating a plane on the adventitia of the aorta. This is dissected a small distance in a cephalic and caudal direction but is then continued in a lateral direction toward the psoas muscle so that the vena cava is unroofed and the nodal bundle is separated from the aorta and vena cava. Care should be taken to avoid lacerating perforating vessels in this area.

The dissection is then continued cephalad and caudad over the aorta and right common iliac artery by following the plane of the adventitia over these great vessels and using blunt and sharp dissection. Small vessels and lymphatic channels are easily coagulated with the scissors. Large perforating vessels from the vena cava or aorta should be clipped through the 10-mm port in the lower midline.

One end of the nodal bundle should be transected. I have found it easiest to transect the distal end over the right common iliac artery prior to dissecting the more cephalad end. One may clip and cut, but it is easiest to coagulate and cut this nodal and lymphatic tissue laterally. Once the nodal bundle is transected at the caudal end, it is easy to grasp the nodal tissue and dissect it in a cephalic direction, extending the dissection as far as possible and/or necessary. Transection of this cephalic end is again accomplished by clipping and cutting or by coagulating and cutting. The nodal package is then extracted using the spoon forceps through the lower midline port. The operative field is irrigated, and hemostasis is established by using the electrocautery unit when necessary.

The left-sided para-aortic lymphadenectomy is performed by first dissecting in the aortic adventitial plane from the inferior mesenteric artery down to the proximal left common iliac artery. Unlike the right-sided dissection, in which lateral dissection toward the psoas muscle is performed after making the peritoneal incision, lateral dissection on the left side is not performed until after the adventitia of the aorta and common iliac has been cleaned off. This allows the surgeon to dissect laterally in a safe plane below the inferior mesenteric artery and the mesentery of the sigmoid colon. Blunt dissection is continued laterally until the ureter and the ovarian vessels are separated from the psoas muscle. The assistant surgeon places a grasper through the left lateral port into this dissected space. This provides excellent exposure, protecting the ureter and the ovarian vessels from damage during nodal dissection, and creates a "tent" in the peritoneum to prevent small bowel from falling into the operative field. The nodal chain, which is lateral to the arteries on this side, is transected using scissors with electrocautery capability. This is accomplished initially over the proximal common iliac artery by first creating a window beneath the nodal chain. The dissection is continued cephalad until the chain is transected again with electrocautery at the level of the inferior mesenteric artery. After completion of the lymphadenectomy, the site is irrigated and inspected for hemostasis.

The assistant can then use a retractor to retract the ureter caudally to expose the nodal tissue over the right common iliac artery. The nodal tissue can be dissected from this area over the right common iliac artery to include part of the upper external iliac artery and the nodes at the bifurcation of the common iliac artery.

I have found that the easiest access to the nodes at the junction of the hypogastric and external arteries is through the more cephalad Childers peritoneal approach and by retracting the ureter caudally (as described in this section) as opposed to gaining access to this area via the Querleu approach.

INDICATIONS

Cervical Cancer

Patients with cervical cancer who are undergoing this procedure fall into two categories: those who have early cervical cancer and are considered candidates for radical hysterectomy, and those with early or late cervical cancer who are not considered candidates for radical hysterectomy and will receive radiotherapy based on operative findings. The peritoneal incision should be placed appropriately in these two groups of patients.

Patients who are considered possible candidates for radical hysterectomy but who will receive radiotherapy in the presence of extracervical disease should have pelvic lymphadenectomy performed first, with attention drawn to the nodes that are most likely to be positive. These sentinel pelvic nodes should be removed through a Querleu peritoneal incision.

Patients scheduled to have radiotherapy should have nodes sampled high in the radiation field and just outside the field—the high common and low para-aortic nodes. These nodes should be removed through the Childers peritoneal incision.

In addition, many of these patients will require cystoscopy and proctoscopy and examination under anesthesia at the same time. These procedures should be performed prior to the lymphadenectomy, with careful consideration in evacuating as much of the air placed in the rectosigmoid as possible. A dilated rectosigmoid may make the lymphadenectomy difficult.

I currently also take intraperitoneal washings from patients with cervical cancer, knowing that the yield will be low.

Ovarian Cancer

Prior to performing lymphadenectomy on patients with ovarian cancer, careful consideration should be given to the intraperitoneal cavity. First, known sites of prior disease or residual disease after surgical debulking should be thoroughly evaluated; then other areas are sampled. This includes washings from the pelvis, the right and left paracolic gutters, and the right hemidiaphragm, as well as multiple intraperitoneal biopsies. Any remaining omentum is removed if possible. If the results of these specimens prove to be negative, then the lymphadenectomy should be undertaken. In general, the para-aortic lymph nodes in these patients will be sampled through the

Childers peritoneal incision. Lysis of adhesions becomes important in these patients as adhesions may prevent proper placement of the bowel into the upper abdomen, which may not allow access to the nodes. In these patients, the para-aortic lymphadenectomy is taken up to where the ovarian vein enters the vena cava on the right side and to the renal artery and vein on the left side. This currently investigative technique is not described here.

Endometrial Cancer

Patients with stage I endometrial cancer may be managed with hysterectomy as well. We are currently performing laparoscopic staging, intraperitoneal washings, and lymphadenectomy, in addition to laparoscopically assisted vaginal hysterectomy. Preoperatively, these patients receive prophylactic antimicrobial therapy as well as sequential compression devices. They are placed in the dorsal lithotomy position, and a uterine manipulator is placed to aid in the laparoscopically assisted vaginal hysterectomy. Hemoclips are placed across the fallopian tubes to prevent tumor spillage during the procedure. In making the peritoneal incision, the round ligaments are transected, using electrocautery, laterally near the pelvic wall for two reasons. This transection is required for the hysterectomy, and it allows better exposure to the retroperitoneal space. I also ligate and transect the infundibulopelvic ligament for the same reason. This is particularly helpful for gaining access to the common iliac nodes on the left side. The surgeon needs to be familiar with the suturing techniques available.

CONCLUSIONS

The birth of operative laparoscopy in the subspecialty of gynecologic oncology has taken place. This newly developed ability to perform laparoscopic para-aortic lymphadenectomy will undoubtedly entice many gynecologic oncologists to become operative laparoscopists. The role that this technique will play in managing patients with gynecologic malignancies has yet to be determined. Currently the Gynecologic Oncology Group has approved pilot studies using a laparoscopic approach in certain patients with gynecologic malignancies. These studies will be pivotal in determining the place of this technique in our armamentarium. Although currently investigational and still in its infancy, the complication rate appears to be low and the procedure appears to be effective. It is therefore possible that this newly born technique will have a significant impact on the management of some patients with gynecologic malignancies.

REFERENCES

Childers JM, Hatch KD, and Surwit EA: The role of laparoscopic lymphadenectomy in the management of cervical carcinoma. Gynecol Oncol 47:30–43, 1992.

Childers JM and Surwit EA: Combined laparoscopic and vaginal surgery for the management of two cases of Stage I endometrial cancer. Gynecol Oncol 45:46–51, 1992.

Querleu D, Leblanc E, and Castelain B: Laparoscopic pelvic lymphadenectomy in the staging of early carcinoma of the cervix. Am J Obstet Gynecol 164:579–581, 1991.

Schuessler WW, Vancaillie TG, Reich H, and Griffith DP: Transperitoneal endosurgical lymphadenectomy in patients with localized prostate cancer. J Urol 145:988–991, 1991.

GENERAL SURGERY PROCEDURES AND CONTROVERSIES

In the summer of 1987 in Lyons, France, Phillipe Mouret and colleagues successfully performed the first laparoscopic cholecystectomy, an event that revolutionized general surgery (Cuschieri et al, 1991). After 1 year of intense work on animals to refine the technique, François Dubois in Paris performed his first case and was the first person to publish a clinical series (Dubois et al, 1989 and 1990). Similarly, J. Barry McKernan and William B. Saye did the first procedure in the United States in 1988. Eddie Joe Reddick and Douglas Olsen worked with them to develop cholangiography. Working also with James Daniell, a gynecologic laser laparoscopist, this group developed and offered laparoscopic laser cholecystectomy with cholangiography in Nashville, TN, and published the first report in English in 1989 (Reddick et al, 1989). Reddick rapidly developed a training program in laser cholecystectomy for the growing number of interested general surgeons. Laparoscopic cholecystectomy is rapidly replacing open cholecystectomy in the United States. However, reports reveal a bile duct injury incidence of 5 to 10 times that with conventional cholecystectomy (Cameron and Gadacz, 1991; Reddick and Olsen, 1989). As a direct result of increased morbidity, New York State now requires that surgeons do 15 laparoscopic cholecystectomies under supervision before being allowed to do these procedures on their own (Nenner et al, 1992). Nevertheless, most authorities believe that with additional experience and technologic advancement, the injury incidence will be reduced to that with conventional cholecystectomy if not below it.

An attempt to improve the accuracy of the diagnosis of acute appendicitis was also responsible for the introduction of laparoscopy in general surgery (Paterson-Brown et al, 1988). Many general surgeons were first exposed to laparoscopy while assisting gynecologists in the evaluation of young women with atypical right lower quadrant pain. It was soon demonstrated that the appendix could be visualized in as many as 90% of patients.

The field of laparoscopy suddenly exploded, with surgeons and hospitals creating such a demand for laser, video, and laparoscopy equipment that a 6- to 9-month backlog of orders overwhelmed a previously stable industry. This sudden demand also stimulated rapid developments in instrumentation as new manufacturers and surgeons worked together to provide instruments appropriate for surgical procedures. New retractors, clips, staples, suturing devices, trocars, electrosurgical sources, and so forth are pouring out of American ingenuity at the time of this writing.

New procedures are also streaming out as a result of American and European inventiveness in general surgery. Cholecystectomy put the laparoscope into the general surgeon's hands, and as surgeons master this technique, new applications will be devised. Laparoscopic appendectomy and laparoscopic staging procedures for pancreatic and gastric neoplasms are being performed routinely (Chissov et al, 1981; Gotz et al, 1990; Warshaw et al, 1990). Research is under way to develop a mini-access approach for inguinal herniorrhaphy, highly selective vagotomy, colon resection, antireflux procedures, and thoracoscopic lobectomy (Dalmagne, 1991; Salerno et al, 1991). Acknowledging that some elements of this textbook may be obsolete at the time of publication, we have chosen a few of the more developed or obvious surgical uses for laparoscopy. Other uses proposed or under development, such as liver edge tumors and bowel resections, are too early in the development phase for an informed presentation.

We have again asked surgeons more familiar with these operations to present or comment on them. Avram M. Cooperman, M.D., is a professor of surgery at New York Medical College and in private practice in New York City. He presents his elegant technique of cholecystectomy. Charles J. Filipi, M.D., is a clinical professor of surgery at Creighton University, Omaha, with a lifelong scholarly interest in hernia repair. He is a pioneer in laparoscopic applications in general surgery, including cholecystectomy (first animal case in the United States in 1985), hernia, and antireflux procedures. Mark J. Koruda, M.D., and Charles A. Herbst, M.D., are faculty members at the Medical School of the University of North Carolina at Chapel Hill. They pioneered laparoscopy in the Department of Surgery and present thoughtful discussions on the role of laparoscopy for appendectomy in surgery.

The basic principles and surgical techniques for general surgical procedures are no different than for gynecologic ones, and the previous chapters on basic and advanced laparoscopic considerations, hemostasis, lysis of adhesions, resection, and specimen removal apply to general surgeons as well. In this section we present the state-of-the-art of general surgical laparoscopy, with the full and exciting knowledge that if the applications are outdated by the time of publication, the principles and techniques never will be.

REFERENCES

Cameron JL and Gadacz TR: Laparoscopic cholecystectomy (Editorial). Ann Surg *213*:1–2, 1991.

Chissov VI, Maksimov IA, Vinogradov AL, et al: Laparoscopy in the diagnosis of abdominal metastases of stomach cancer. Khirurgiia (Mosk) *11*:13–16, 1981.

Cuschieri A, Dubois F, Mouiel J, et al: The European experience with laparoscopic cholecystectomy. Am J Surg *161*:385–387, 1991.

Dalmagne B: Laparoscopic nissen fundoplication. Conference on Advanced Laparoscopy, St. Vincent's Hospital, Indianapolis, May 21, 1991.

Dubois F, Berthelot G, and Levard H: Cholécystectomy par coelioscopy. Nouv Presse Med *18*:980–982, 1989.

Dubois F, Icard P, Berthelot G, and Levard H: Coelioscopic cholecystectomy: Preliminary report of 36 cases. Ann Surg *211*:60–62, 1990.

Gotz F, Pier A, and Bacher C: Modified laparoscopic appendectomy in surgery: A report on 388 operations. Surg Endosc *4*:6–9, 1990.

Nenner RP, Imperato PJ, and Alcorn CM: Serious complications of laparoscopic cholecystectomy in New York State. NY State J Med *92*:179–181, 1992.

Paterson-Brown S, Thompson JN, Eckersley JRT, et al: Which patients with suspected appendicitis should undergo laparoscopy? BMJ *296*:1363–1364, 1988.

Reddick EJ and Olsen DO: Laparoscopic laser cholecystectomy: A comparison with mini-lap cholecystectomy. Surg Endosc *3*:131–133, 1989.

Reddick EJ, Olsen DO, and Daniell J: Laparoscopic laser cholecystectomy. Laser Med Surg News Adv Feb:38–40, 1989.

Salerno GM, Fitzgibbons RJ, and Filipi CJ: Laparoscopic Inguinal Hernia Repair. St Louis, Quality Medical Publishing, 1991.

Warshaw AL, Gu Z-Y, Wittenberg J, and Waltman AC: Preoperative staging and assessment of resectability of pancreatic cancer. Arch Surg *125*:230–233, 1990.

Cholecystectomy

Avram M. Cooperman, M.D.

Laparoscopic cholecystectomy (LC) has been seized by the public as the least painful way of undergoing cholecystectomy and the quickest way to return to full, unrestricted activity. The criteria for LC include documentation of stones, a nonvisualized gallbladder, and recurrent symptoms compatible with the diagnosis of biliary disease. The operation may be done (acute, chronic) at any time. The indications are identical for open surgery and laparoscopy, and there are few exclusions. A history of abdominal surgery (upper or lower), recent or remote, should not preclude an attempt at LC. The plans and decisions can be altered if the laparoscopic technique proves too difficult. There are no absolute contraindications to LC, but pregnancy and severe bleeding disorders are two relative contraindications. In this chapter, I describe techniques that I have used in more than 900 patients for safe and accurate removal of acute and chronically inflamed gallbladders.

PREPARATION

Preoperative

Most operations are done under general anesthesia, and the patients undergo the requisite preoperative tests that each site or hospital requires. Each patient is kept NPO for 6 to 12 hours prior to surgery and reports to the hospital 2 hours before the scheduled operation.

Operative

A dose of antibiotics effective against biliary organisms is given intravenously, and the patient is positioned with a footboard in place, flat on the table. The patient voids before entering the operating room (ascertained by asking each patient prior to surgery). This strategy avoids the use of a Foley catheter. Nasogastric tubes are not routinely used either. The light source, camera, and insufflator are checked prior to use in each case.

TECHNIQUE

General Comments

Antegrade or retrograde dissection of the gallbladder for acute and chronic cholecystitis may be done safely laparoscopically or by open cholecystectomy. The principles are similar: Accurate identification of the cystic common duct junction and visualization of the common duct above and below the cystic duct are important and independent of the technique. The great advantage of LC is that the surgeon's eye (the laparoscope and camera) is positioned at the liver hilum without traction on any viscus. There is a loss of depth perception, and the distance and relationship of cystic duct and right hepatic duct are not well appreciated from this angle, thus I am not hesitant to reposition the camera to the lateral or fundic port. This location is where the surgeon's eye is accustomed to being and the transfer places it perpendicular, not tangential, to the common duct.

The issue of common duct stones and LC is unresolved. While instrumentation is being developed, some surgeons selectively explore the common duct through the cystic duct or common duct. This method is still cumbersome and can add considerable time to an operation. I prefer endoscopic retrograde cholangiopancreatography (ERCP) prior to surgery if there is any history of pancreatitis, cholangitis, or abnormal liver function tests. The ERCP proves diagnostic and therapeutic if common duct stones are present. I favor intraoperative cholecysto-cholangiograms during surgery. I do this selectively and early in the operation, after ascertaining that the infundibulum is not obstructed by a stone. This procedure defines the anatomy and answers the issue of whether duct stones are present.

The following technique has evolved in more than 900 laparoscopic cholecystectomies. It enables almost all gallbladders to be removed accurately and easily within 10 to 20 minutes. Attention to detail is well rewarded in laparoscopic surgery.

Procedures

The Veress needle is inserted directly through the umbilicus where the skin and fascia are in close proximity after a 1-cm transverse incision is made in the umbilicus and carried to the fascia. The position of the needle in the peritoneal cavity is checked by four tests:

1. Aspirate intraperitoneal air.
2. Inject a few milliliters of saline (it should flow without resistance).
3. Remove the syringe and observe the saline fall into the peritoneum.
4. After starting insufflation, be certain that good flow is established with low pressure.

After abdominal insufflation is achieved, a 10-mm trocar is inserted through the umbilicus. It is directed to the pelvis with little force exerted during its placement. The laparoscope and camera are attached and the abdomen is examined. A thorough exploration is done. The lateral or fundic port (FP) is next placed (Fig. 29–1), usually at the anterior axillary line, 1.5 port lengths below the gallbladder. This procedure allows the instruments to function without repositioning the port. The infundibular port (IP) is placed, medial and superior to the FP. It may be placed close to the FP since there is ample room between ports and gallbladder. This placement allows for unrestricted movements and repositioning of clamps. The operating port (OP) is placed in the upper abdomen near the right xiphoid costal margin. It is helpful if this port is placed at right angles to the laparoscope to enable instrument tips to be visualized without constant camera readjustments (see Atlas, Plate 27). This port *must* be high, near the costal arch. If the falciform ligament is thin, then the port may be placed to the left of it. Keeping out of the falciform ligament is helpful because bleeding from the umbilical vein is avoided and removal of the gallbladder is facilitated.

With upward traction on the fundus through the FP clamp and downward traction on the infundibulum through the IP clamp (ratcheted clamps preferred), the cystic duct is exposed on traction. Repositioning the IP clamp at the gallbladder cystic duct junction will improve cystic duct exposure. Tension on the cystic duct facilitates its dissection.

Few instruments are needed during LC. Downward traction on the infundibulum allows the spatula to dissect and circumscribe the cystic duct (Fig. 29–2). An electrosurgical or laser dissection exposes the adventitia around the duct, particularly at its inferior surface. The spatula then clears the cystic duct on all sides and is passed around the duct. Additionally, the spatula is useful in identifying the cystic duct-common duct junction. The common duct must be visualized above and below the cystic duct entrance. This is the cardinal rule of cholecystectomy (open or closed). If the upper duct is not clearly seen, switching the camera to the FP may expose the duct.

FIGURE 29–1 Trocar placements

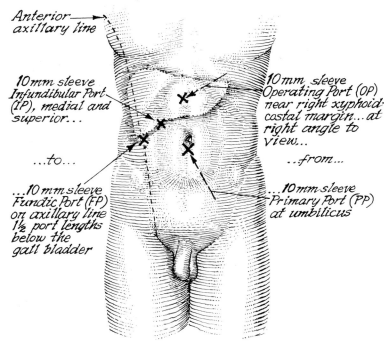

Anterior axillary line

10 mm sleeve Infundibular Port (IP), medial and superior...

10 mm sleeve Operating Port (OP) near right xyphoid-costal margin...at right angle to view...

...to...

...from...

...10 mm sleeve Fundic Port (FP) on axillary line 1½ port lengths below the gall bladder

...10 mm sleeve Primary Port (PP) at umbilicus

FIGURE 29–2 Exposing the cystic duct

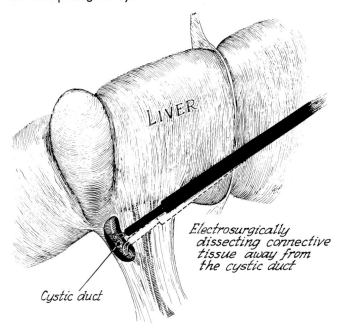

LIVER

Electrosurgically dissecting connective tissue away from the cystic duct

Cystic duct

FIGURE 29–3 Clipping the cystic duct

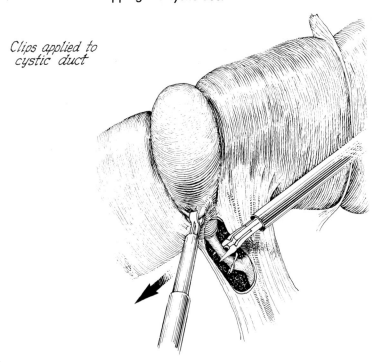

*Clips applied to
cystic duct*

Continued traction on the infundibulum keeps the cystic duct taut and clips are easily applied (Fig. 29–3; see also Atlas, Plate 28). With traction, two to four clips are applied to the cystic duct, which is then transected. The number of clips used depends on the length of cystic duct and on the surgeon's security with the clip placement. A scissors, laser, or electrode divides the cystic duct. Before transecting the duct, the common duct should again be identified above and below the cystic duct.

Upward traction on the infundibulum by pushing with the spatula or scissors will expose the cystic artery (Fig. 29–4). The artery is looped with the spatula at its trunk or its divisional branches. If a small artery is divided, one should look for a posterior divisional artery in the gallbladder fossa. It can be controlled with a cautery or a laser.

FIGURE 29–4 Clipping the cystic artery

*Cystic artery dissected,
and clipped...*

... also...

*...electrosurgically
cut between clips*

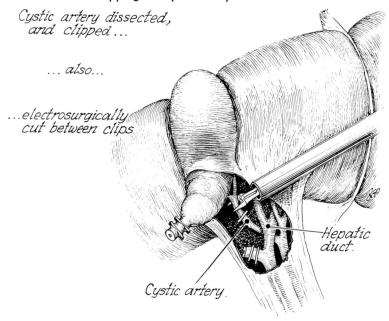

*Hepatic
duct.*

Cystic artery.

Continued repositioning of the IP clamp to keep traction on the gallbladder and its peritoneum is essential (Fig. 29–5). This repositioning allows the cautery or laser to free the gallbladder completely from the liver bed. The surgeon repositions the clamps when needed to maintain traction and exposure. When correct traction is applied, the laser or electricity will "melt" away the peritoneum without causing smoke.

After the gallbladder is freed from the liver bed, I place it between the liver and lateral abdominal wall (Fig. 29–6). The clamps are released from the gallbladder and used to expose the gallbladder fossa. With careful use of the camera, the surgeon can detect bleeding or a bile leak. These are coagulated in the liver bed.

FIGURE 29–5 Gallbladder bed dissection

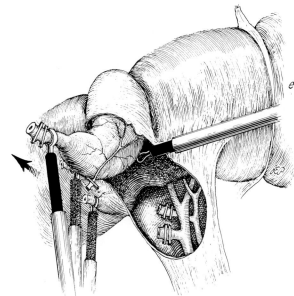
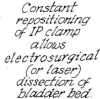

Gallbladder bed dissection:

Constant repositioning of IP clamp allows electrosurgical (or laser) dissection of bladder bed.

FIGURE 29–6 Hemostasis of the gallbladder bed

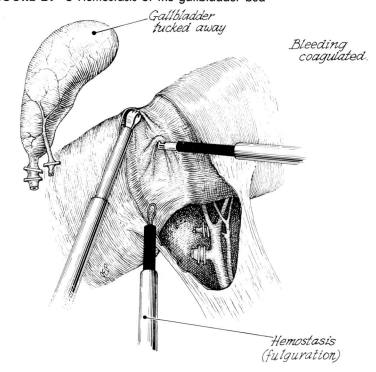

Gallbladder tucked away

Bleeding coagulated.

Hemostasis (fulguration)

FIGURE 29–7 Removal of the gallbladder through a 10-mm port

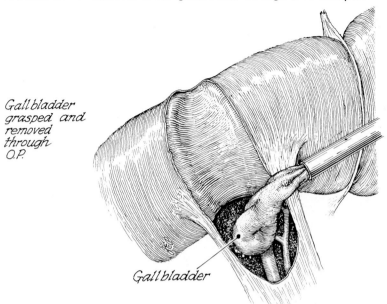

Gallbladder
grasped and
removed
through
O.P.

Gallbladder

FIGURE 29–8 Retrodissection

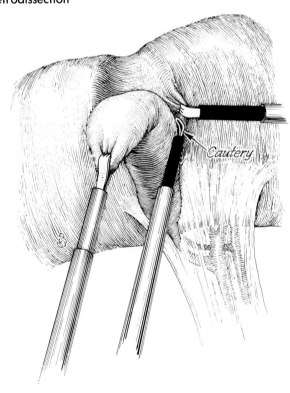

Separation of
Gallbladder
from
liver bed

Cautery

Without repositioning the camera, the gallbladder is grasped at its neck and removed through the OP (Fig. 29–7). A drain may be placed through the FP, if necessary.

If there is severe inflammation in the hilum, exposure and access to the hilar structures may be limited. It may not be possible to dissect the cystic duct and cystic artery antegrade.

In this case, the gallbladder fundus is grasped while the edge of the liver is pushed upward to provide countertraction. The spatula is introduced through the IP and the peritoneum at the top of the gallbladder, and upward pressure on liver edge allows the gallbladder to be teased away from the liver bed (Fig. 29–8).

The fundus of the gallbladder is dissected from the liver bed. The dissection is carried on both sides of the gallbladder to the lower third. Continued traction and countertraction on the gallbladder facilitate its dissection from the liver bed.

When the gallbladder is freed, the cystic duct-common duct junction should be seen clearly and the common duct identified above and below the cystic duct (Fig. 29–9). If this view is not seen, then the camera is shifted to the lateral port by replacing the 5-mm port with a 10-mm port to expose the common duct from this position. The clip applicator is placed around the cystic duct.

Pushing the liver away from the gallbladder and applying downward traction on the gallbladder provides excellent exposure and visualization of the cystic duct. It is then clipped and divided. The cystic artery is isolated, clipped, and divided in a similar manner (Fig. 29–10).

The gallbladder is again removed through the upper midline port. A 10-mm Jackson Pratt drain is usually placed through the tract of the FP to collect any oozing or bile leak.

POSTOPERATIVE MANAGEMENT

The postoperative course for most patients is benign, short, and gratifying. Patients experience modest and varying degrees of pain, both incisional and subdiaphragmatic (referred to the shoulder). Recuperation requires minimal analgesics. A diet is resumed hours after surgery, and patients may be dismissed on the same day or on the next day with return to unrestricted activity within days to 1 or 2 weeks.

FIGURE 29–9 Exposing the cystic duct

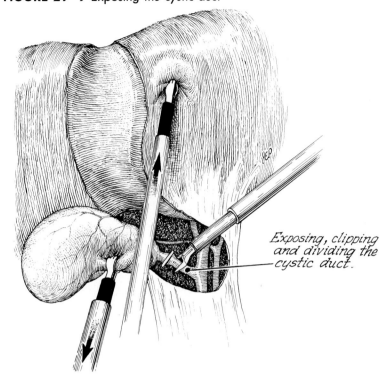

Exposing, clipping and dividing the cystic duct.

FIGURE 29–10 Clipping the cystic artery

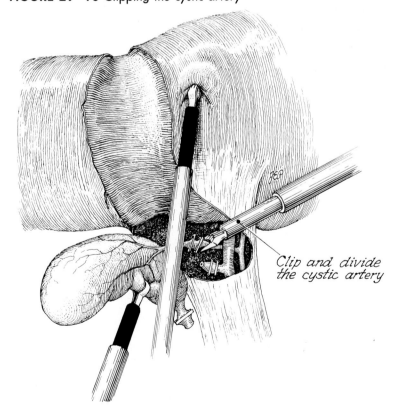

Clip and divide the cystic artery

Laparoscopic Herniorrhaphy

Charles J. Filipi, M.D.

Robert J. Fitzgibbons, Jr., M.D.

Giovanni M. Salerno, M.D.

Each year 500,000 inguinal herniorrhaphies are performed in the United States. An estimated additional 2 million people have unrepaired inguinal hernias. This backlog is attributed to patient reluctance to undergo surgery plus a lack of awareness of potential complications caused by inguinal hernia. The number of work-loss days per year attributable to inguinal hernia is 20 million (Lichtenstein, 1986). The cost in terms of national productivity is high for this disorder. For these reasons, a new and more effective operation with decreased postoperative pain is desirable. In this chapter, we present the history and rationale for laparoscopic herniorrhaphy, technical features of the operation, and early clinical results of the procedure. In addition, we review results of an experimental intraperitoneal prosthetic onlay repair.

HISTORY OF OPEN INGUINAL HERNIORRHAPHY

Surgery for repair of inguinal hernia has been dominated by an extraperitoneal approach. Marcy is credited as being the first person to advocate closure of the internal ring for indirect hernias. Bassini in 1884 popularized a procedure that included apposition of transversalis fascia and the inguinal ligament to close the hernia defect. Halsted, at Johns Hopkins University, independently developed a similar operative approach to inguinal hernia. These procedures were associated with a low operative mortality and a recurrent hernia rate that was one fifth of the rate commonly accepted at the time.

Since the advent of the Bassini repair, numerous variations on the theme of high ligation and inguinal floor reinforcement have been advocated. These variations reflect that the perfect inguinal hernia repair has yet to be discovered.

The recent development of laparoscopic cholecystectomy has introduced general surgeons to the field of therapeutic laparoscopy. Since inguinal hernia is a relatively common condition that general surgeons encounter, it is not surprising that laparoscopic inguinal hernia repair has been considered. There seems to be justification for such an approach because conventional herniorrhaphy is relatively painful and, although excellent results have been reported by highly skilled investigators in single institutions, it is generally accepted that the overall recurrence rate of an inguinal hernia repair is 10% (Rand statistics). In addition, standard herniorrhaphy is associated with a low but nevertheless irreducible rate of testicular complications and damage to cord structures (Condon and Nyhus, 1989).

HISTORY OF LAPAROSCOPIC HERNIA REPAIR

In 1982, Ger described the management of a variety of abdominal wall hernias through a transabdominal approach in patients who underwent laparotomy for other intra-abdominal conditions. Although the Ger procedure for repair of indirect inguinal hernias is similar to the one that Marcy originally described (Fig. 30–1), it differs in two ways. First, the hernia sac is neither dissected, ligated, or reduced. Second, stainless steel Michel staples (3 × 15 mm) are placed with a Kocher clamp across the peritoneal opening of the sac and the underlying tissue to close the sac. Only one recurrence was noted in a series of 13 patients, with the longest follow-up being 44 months. The last patient in Ger's report had the inguinal hernia defect repaired with the staples applied under laparoscopic guidance. The staples were applied with a special stapling device that was inserted through a second laparoscopic cannula. The patient has been followed for 3 years and has shown no evidence of recurrence. Ger, therefore, is credited with performing the first laparoscopic herniorrhaphy in a human.

More recently, Ger published a study on 15 dogs with congenital indirect inguinal hernias (Ger et al, 1990). The purpose of this study was to test his newly conceived laparoscopic approach in the management of inguinal hernias. The first three beagles underwent standard laparotomy and stapling of the peritoneal opening under direct vision; the remaining beagles had closure of the same opening under laparoscopic guidance after creation of a nitrous oxide pneumoperitoneum. Care was taken to leave small gaps between staples to avoid formation of a hydrocele. A prototype stapler (the "herniostat") was developed. Twelve dogs underwent laparoscopic repair of an indirect inguinal hernia, and all were cured. An examination of en bloc inguinal specimens showed that if the staples were properly applied, they "sank" below the peritoneum and disappeared from view. Superficial application of staples resulted in

FIGURE 30–1. Ger hernia repair

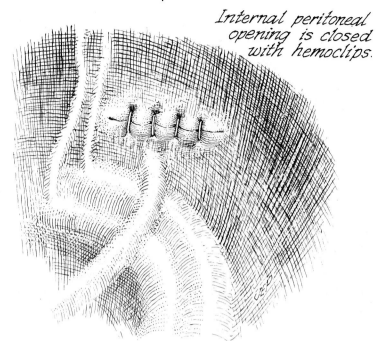

Internal peritoneal opening is closed with hemoclips.

FIGURE 30–2. Male groin anatomy

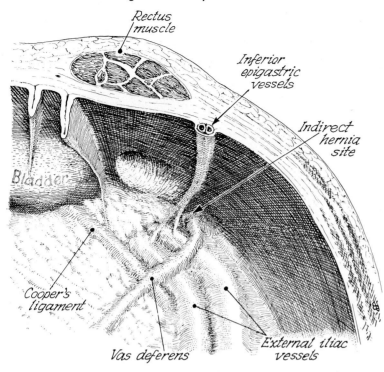

FIGURE 30–3. Male groin anatomy

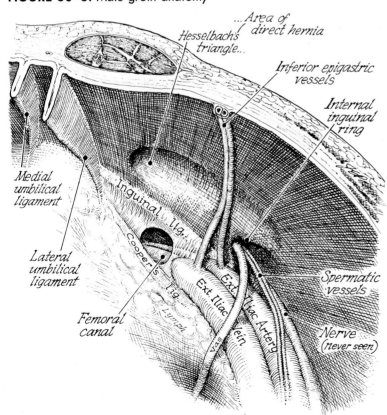

staple migration with loss of effective closure. An examination of the processus vaginalis with probes showed that the sac was obliterated in five cases, and in eight beagles its size was considerably reduced. Ger believed that the following were advantages for laparoscopic repair of a groin hernia:

- Small puncture wounds
- Minimal dissection
- Less chance of injury to the spermatic cord
- Decreased incidence of ischemic orchitis
- Decreased incidence of bladder injury
- Avoidance of ilioinguinal postoperative neuralgia
- Outpatient procedure
- The ability to achieve a very high closure of the peritoneal sac
- Minimal postoperative discomfort
- Faster recovery time
- Simultaneous intra-abdominal diagnostic laparoscopy
- The ability to diagnose and treat bilateral groin hernias without extensive dissection

The anatomy of the inguinal floor as seen laparoscopically is different for general surgeons accustomed to the standard open hernia repair. Bogojavlensky has outlined the laparoscopic landmarks for the right inguinal area (Figs. 30–2 and 30–3). A sagittal section is provided for orientation (Fig. 30–4). Bogojavlensky presented a videotape of laparoscopic herniorrhaphy with mesh at the September 1989 World Congress of Gynecological Endoscopy. Subsequently, he performed 40 herniorrhaphies using laparoscopic techniques and has noted two recurrences. One recurrence was discovered in a patient who had an unrecognized direct and femoral hernia in conjunction with the repaired indirect hernia. A third patient required conversion to standard herniorrhaphy because exposure for a large hernia in an obese patient was inadequate (Personal communication, 1990). Bogojavlensky has used several approaches including an intraperitoneal prosthesis placement, a preperitoneal mesh repair, and mesh plugs for femoral hernias.

The first published report of a laparoscopic hernia repair was in 1990 by the gynecologist Popp (1990). He closed the internal peritoneal opening with extracorporeally tied sutures and covered the area with a dehydrated dura mater patch secured by catgut endosutures. The patient subsequently has done well and has shown no evidence of a recurrence. Popp has also developed a preperitoneal approach for inguinal hernia with the intent of reducing the possibility of postoperative intraperitoneal adhesions.

Corbitt (1991) reported on 20 patients undergoing laparoscopic herniorrhaphy using the ENDO GIA (U.S. Surgical) for amputation of the inverted hernia sac. Prosthetic mesh was placed in the inguinal canal and over the hernia defect prior to closure of the peritoneum. All indirect hernias were repaired successfully, with one exception. Corbitt believed that a concomitant direct inguinal hernia was unrecognized in this case. The length of reported follow-up for these initial patients was 20 months. Careful separation of the cord structures from the sac prior to application of the stapling device is important in this procedure.

FIGURE 30–4. Sagittal section of male pelvis to the right of the midline

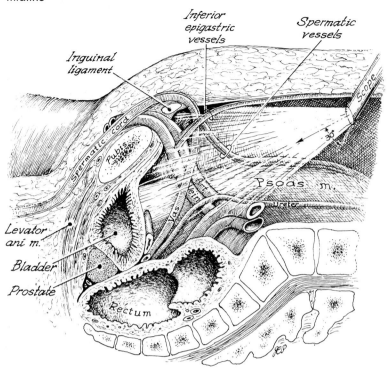

NOTE TO THE READER:

With the 30° laparoscope inserted only a short distance into the abdomen, and its lens very close to the abdominal wall (as shown in the above cut-away diagram), the view is such that the abdominal wall, the epigastric vessels, and the umbilical ligaments appear to be coming up almost directly toward the observer in a greatly foreshortened manner.

In the first issue of the *Journal of Laparoendoscopic Surgery*, Schultz and associates (1990) described preliminary results of laser laparoscopic herniorrhaphy. Their method included laser division of the anterior lateral peritoneal reflection at the indirect sac orifice that provided access to the inguinal canal for placement of polypropylene mesh in the inguinal canal and preperitoneal space. Sheets of mesh were used to reinforce the medial and lateral aspects of the inguinal floor. Indirect sacs were left in situ, and the peritoneum was closed with hemoclips. This repair was applied initially to 20 patients with one recurrence, which was again related to an unrecognized coexisting direct hernia. Subsequent follow-up information revealed that in 67 cases, recurrence had occurred in three additional patients.

Arregui first reported his experience with a laparoscopic preperitoneal mesh hernia repair in 1991 (Arregui and Nagan, 1991) (see Atlas, Plate 30). After having skeletonized the transversalis fascia, femoral and inferior epigastric vessels, spermatic cord, and Cooper's ligament, he covered the inguinal/femoral area with a large nonabsorbable mesh, then he reperitonealized. For indirect hernias, the internal ring is tightened with a suture; and for direct hernias, he loosely approximates transversalis fascia when possible. The mesh was tacked in place with several sutures. The procedure was performed initially in 65 patients without evidence of recurrence after short-term follow-up.

RECURRENT HERNIA

Complications of inguinal herniorrhaphy, such as neuralgia, bleeding, and infection, are well known. The incidence of recurrent hernia has been high (10 to 25%) (Berliner et al, 1978). In the United States, up to 100,000 patients each year develop a recurrent hernia. The recurrence is not only an inconvenience but also the required reoperation is associated with a higher incidence of testicular complications and represents an additional expense for the patient. In addition, the incidence of recurrence increases with each repeat operation.

The proposed causes of recurrent hernias are numerous. Among the most important is excessive tension (usually caused by a lack of understanding of the anatomy and the absence of attention to detail), delay in treatment with a resultant large defect and tissue attenuation, and infection. In some patients collagen synthesis and degradation disorders lead to hernia recurrence (Peacock and Madden, 1974).

The anatomy of the groin is complex, and the subtleties of a good hernia repair are numerous. Clinics specializing in hernia repair report low recurrence rates primarily because of increased experience, intense interest in results, and a familiarity with fine technical points. The operation is a priority, and refinement of technique on the basis of accurate follow-up data has improved results.

NONLAPAROSCOPIC PROSTHETIC MESH REPAIRS

Lichtenstein (1987) has popularized a mesh repair for inguinal hernia with little, if any, tension on the suture line. This repair is accomplished in direct and indirect hernias by introducing polypropylene mesh and suturing its edge to Poupart's ligament and the internal oblique muscle. The absence of tension reduces postoperative discomfort and the incidence of suture pull-out. Patients are allowed to return to work when their discomfort disappears. In Lichtenstein's clinic, this repair has had an associated recurrence rate of 0.25%. This extremely low recurrence rate has not been corroborated by other investigators, although the technique is now widely used.

Several authorities have proposed the preperitoneal approach to inguinal hernia with the use of a prosthesis (Nyhus et al, 1988; Rignault, 1986; Stoppa et al, 1984). For the reported reduction in recurrent hernia incidence with this technique, see Table 30–1.

The techniques vary somewhat. Nyhus and colleagues place a tailored piece of mesh after repairing the direct or recurrent defect (Nyhus et al, 1988). The prosthesis serves as a reinforcement and is sutured securely to Cooper's ligament and transversalis fascia.

Rignault's theory (1986) of repair is different, but the results are also excellent. Instead of repairing the direct or recurrent hernias, a 10 × 12 cm patch of prosthetic material is introduced through a Pfannenstiel incision into the preperitoneal space. The hernia defect is loosely closed, and care is taken to position the prosthesis properly. Mersilene is particularly applicable in this repair because of its flexibility and adhesiveness to surrounding tissue. The spermatic cord is encircled by a keyhole defect in the mesh. Sutures are not necessary to hold the prosthesis. Rignault has written: "By covering the hernia defect and adjacent areas far beyond the limits of the defect with the mesh, the intra-abdominal pressure becomes an efficient means of fixation of the mesh over the site of the hernia rather than a factor in recurrence" (p 468). Indirect hernias can also be treated with this technique. The sac is highly ligated and excised or simply divided at the internal ring.

Stoppa's technique of preperitoneal repair is similar to Rignault's technique, but he makes no attempt to repair direct defects. He introduces a 15 × 15 cm or even larger prosthesis and tacks the mesh in the preperitoneal space. Occasionally, he splits the prosthesis to accommodate the spermatic cord. Because of the successes reported with preperitoneal mesh repairs and the national hernia recurrence rate of 10% (in some series 20% for direct hernias), development of a laparoscopic prosthetic mesh herniorrhaphy seemed warranted.

TABLE 30–1. PREPERITONEAL PROSTHETIC INGUINAL HERNIORRHAPHY

Author	No. of Patients	Recurrence (%)
Nyhus	203	1.7
Rignault	1151*	2.2
Stoppa	572	1.4

*239 were recurrent at a 1.2% rate.

FIGURE 30–5. Laparoscopic hernia repair with staples

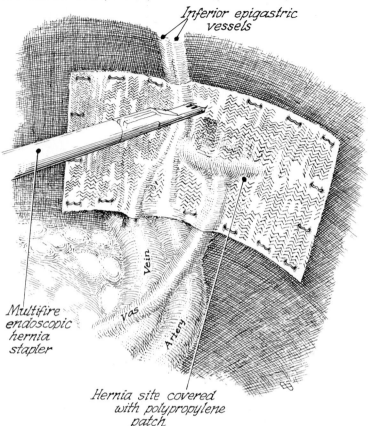

Hernia site covered with polypropylene patch

LAPAROSCOPIC ONLAY MESH REPAIRS

At Creighton University, an investigation has been conducted to study laparoscopic inguinal hernia repair and its effectiveness (Fitzgibbons et al, 1993) using 26 Yorkshire cross-feeder male pigs with indirect inguinal hernias.

Phase I: Inguinal Hernia Repair by Laparotomy

Thirteen pigs underwent abdominal exploration for reduction of the herniated viscus and repair with an onlay of 6 × 5.5 cm polypropylene mesh (Prolene, Ethicon, Inc.). Interrupted sutures fixed the prosthesis to the underlying peritoneum. The inner surface of this patch was modified by suturing a sheet of oxidized regenerated cellulose (Interceed, Johnson and Johnson Products, Inc.) to the mesh with interrupted 5–0 sutures. On the contralateral side or the side with the smaller inguinal hernia defect, if the pig had bilateral hernias, a polypropylene mesh patch without the oxidized regenerated cellulose was placed with a similar technique. Thus, each animal acted as its own control.

Phase II: Inguinal Hernia Repair by Laparoscopy

Eleven herniated male pigs weighing between 25 and 32 kg were used. Under general anesthesia a midline and two additional 10-mm cannulas were introduced into the lower abdomen after a pneumoperitoneum had been established. Prolene mesh with and without Interceed was placed under laparoscopic visualization. Positioning and selection of the prosthesis was similar to that of phase I, but fixation was accomplished using 10-mm stainless steel staples applied by a laparoscopic stapling device (Proximate ES, Ethicon, Inc.) (Fig. 30–5).

All pigs were sacrificed after 6 weeks. At sacrifice, staging of adhesion formation between prosthesis and intraperitoneal organs plus evaluation of the repair was completed. A standard adhesion scale was used (Law and Ellis, 1988), and the percentage of mesh surface area involved with adhesions was recorded.

Results

Data from pigs of the same group were expressed in terms of the mean ± SD. The one-tail Student's t-test was used to compare mean values between the two groups. A difference with a p value of less than .05 was considered statistically significant.

No clinical evidence of hernia recurrence, damage to intra-abdominal organs or cord structures, or signs of infection was noted in any pig. In all pigs, mesh patches were completely covered with granulation tissue and were firmly adherent to the underlying peritoneum. There was no evidence of prosthetic detachment. A histologic examination of the repair revealed peritoneal overgrowth on the abdominal side of the prosthesis.

In the inguinal hernia group (n = 13) repaired by laparotomy with the composite patch (Prolene/Interceed), the average surface area of patch covered by adhesions was significantly less than that of the simple Prolene patches (n = 13) placed on the opposite side. However, at laparotomy, the grade of adhesion associated with Prolene/Interceed patches was not significantly different from that of the Prolene patches.

Inguinal hernias (n = 11) that were laparoscopically repaired with a composite patch presented a lower prosthetic surface area covered by adhesions compared with Prolene prosthetic patches (n = 11). This result was statistically significant. The average grade of adhesion found in the former group was less than that found in the latter group; however, this difference was not statistically significant.

At laparoscopy (n = 11) the average area of the Prolene/Interceed patch or Prolene patch covered by adhesions was lower than that of the 13 pigs that underwent laparotomy placement of a composite patch or Prolene alone. This result was statistically significant.

When grade of adhesions with and without Interceed in the laparoscopic versus laparotomy group was compared, there was improvement with the laparoscopic technique, but the difference noted was not statistically significant.

In all pigs except one, the adhesions observed were between the urinary bladder and the prosthesis. No evidence of intraperitoneal complications was noted in association with applied and lost staples. The average time required to establish pneumoperitoneum, fix the prosthetic patch with staples on both sides, and close the wound was approximately 40 minutes compared with 60 to 90 minutes for the laparotomy group.

FIGURE 30–6. Transabdominal peritoneal laparoscopic hernia repair

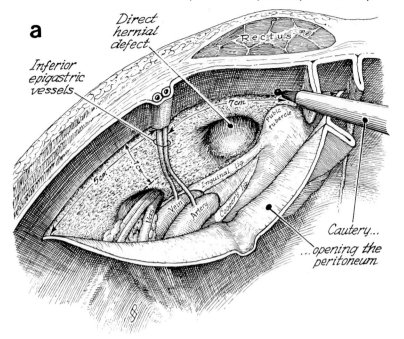

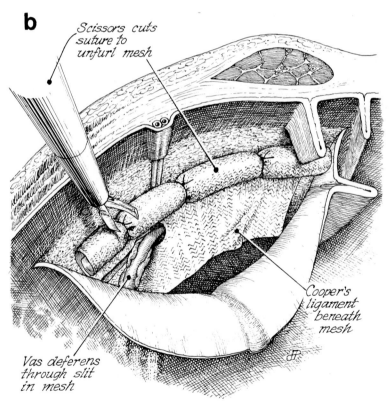

CLINICAL RESULTS

A multicenter clinical trial for laparoscopic herniorrhaphy involving 20 North American and European institutions was initiated in the fall of 1991. Preliminary results in 546 patients have revealed an overall recurrence rate of 1.8% after a mean length of follow-up of 6 months. The learning curve for this procedure is significant, therefore these initial results are considered satisfactory. A postoperative 2.4% incidence of transient thigh pain emphasizes the need to understand the anatomy of the lateral femoral cutaneous nerve. Groin pain was present in 9.3% of patients in the perioperative period. Urinary retention was reported in 3.3% of patients, and cord swelling was reported in 2.7%. There were no complications involving laparoscopy itself, and the mortality rate was 0%.

The most commonly performed procedure in this study was the transabdominal preperitoneal laparoscopic herniorrhaphy (Fig. 30–6; see Atlas, Plates 29 and 30). This procedure is analogous to the Rignault open

FIGURE 30–6 *Continued* Transabdominal peritoneal laparoscopic
hernia repair

c

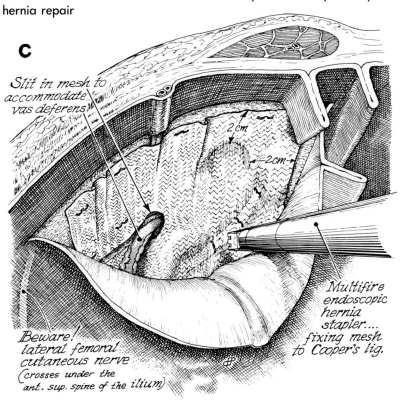

*Slit in mesh to
accommodate
vas deferens*

2cm

2cm

*Beware!
lateral femoral
cutaneous nerve
(crosses under the
ant. sup. spine of the ilium)*

*Multifire
endoscopic
hernia
stapler....
fixing mesh
to Cooper's lig.*

d

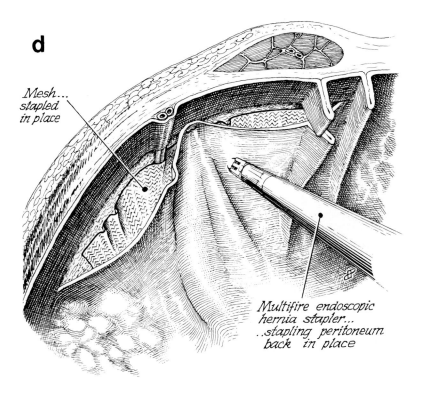

*Mesh...
stapled
in place*

*Multifire endoscopic
hernia stapler...
..stapling peritoneum
back in place*

FIGURE 30–7. McKernan extraperitoneal hernia repair

preperitoneal repair. McKernan, who is one of the multicenter investigators, performed 76 extraperitoneal mini access herniorrhaphies without evidence of recurrence at 6-month follow-up (Fig. 30–7).

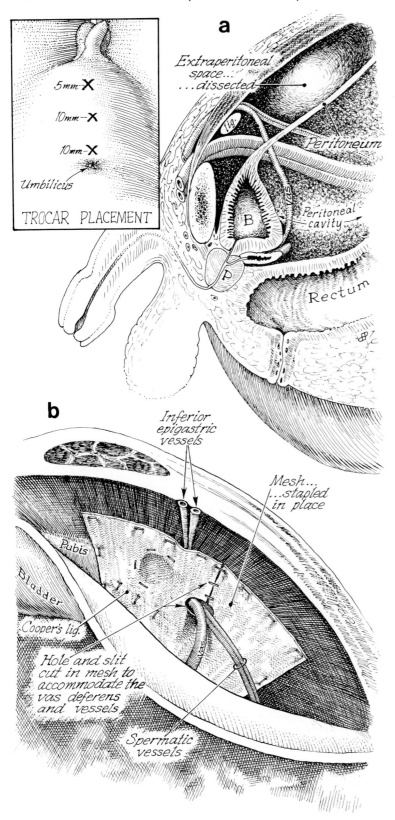

The intraperitoneal onlay mesh repair was performed in 157 patients with a 1.3% recurrence rate at 6 months (Fig. 30–8). With large direct hernias the onlay technique results in early recurrence and we consider the method to be contraindicated for this condition. With an improved adhesion barrier on the inner surface of the polypropylene patch and use of local anesthesia with sedation rather than general anesthesia, this procedure may become the operation of choice for indirect hernia. It is easy to perform; there is no tension on the repair; and no tissue dissection is required.

FIGURE 30–8. Intraperitoneal onlay mesh hernia repair

a

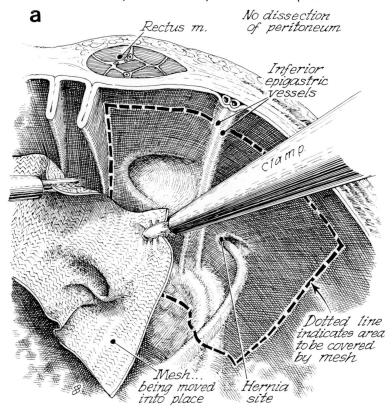

b

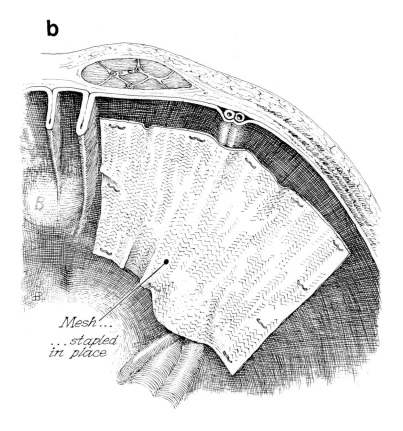

SUMMARY

Inguinal hernia repair has evolved from a crude procedure associated with a high recurrence rate to a variety of complex repairs associated with an improved, but nonetheless significant, recurrence rate. Various laparoscopic herniorrhaphy techniques are now being investigated with the hope that they will be technically easy and associated with less pain, minimal disability, and an early return to work. If this repair is proved safe and is widely used, it is our belief that the national hernia recurrence rate will improve.

REFERENCES

Arregui ME and Nagan RF: Laparoscopic repair of inguinal hernias with mesh using a preperitoneal approach. Presented at Conference on Advanced Laparoscopy, St. Vincent's Hospital, IA, May 20, 1991.

Berliner S, Burson L, Katz P, and Wise L: An anterior transversalis fascia repair for adult inguinal hernias. Am J Surg 135:633–636, 1978.

Condon RE and Nyhus LM: Complications of groin hernias. *In* Nyhus LM and Condon RE (eds): Hernia. Philadelphia, JB Lippincott, 1989, pp 253–269.

Corbitt JD: Laparoscopic herniorrhaphy. Surg Laparosc Endosc 1:23, 1991.

Fitzgibbons RJ Jr and Filipi CJ: Laparoscopic hernia repair: Onlay mesh techniques. Surg Clin North Am, Vol 73, 1993.

Ger R, Monroe K, Duvivier R, and Mishrick A: Management of indirect inguinal hernias by laparoscopic closure of the neck of the sac. Am J Surg 159:370–373, 1990.

Law NW and Ellis H: Adhesions formation and peritoneal healing on prosthetic materials. Clin Mat 3:95–101, 1988.

Lichtenstein IL: Hernia Repair Without Disability: A Surgical Atlas Illustrating the Anatomy, Technique, and Physiologic Rationale of the "One-Day" Hernia and Introducing New Concepts, Tension-Free Herniorrhaphies. St. Louis, Ishiyaku Euroamerica, 1986.

Lichtenstein IL: Herniorrhaphy. A personal experience with 6,321 cases. Am J Surg 153:553–559, 1987.

Nyhus LM, Pollak R, Bombeck CT, and Donahue PE: The preperitoneal approach and prosthetic buttress repair for recurrent hernia: The evolution of a technique. Ann Surg 208:733–737, 1988.

Peacock EE and Madden JW: Studies on the biology and treatment of recurrent inguinal hernia. II: Morphological changes. Ann Surg 179:567–571, 1974.

Popp LW: Endoscopic patch repair of inguinal hernia in a female patient. Surg Endosc 4:10–12, 1990.

Rignault DP: Preperitoneal prosthetic inguinal hernioplasty through a Pfannenstiel approach. Surg Gynecol Obstet 163:465–468, 1986.

Schultz L, Graber J, Pietrafitta J, and Hickok D: Laser laparoscopic herniorrhaphy: A clinical trial with preliminary results. J Laparoendosc Surg 1:41–45, 1990.

Stoppa RE, Rives JL, Warlaumont CR, et al: The use of Dacron in the repair of hernias of the groin. Surg Clin North Am 64:269–285, 1984.

Laparoscopic Appendectomy

Mark J. Koruda, M.D.

Charles A. Herbst, Jr., M.D.

Acute appendicitis is the most common emergency surgical disease of the abdomen in the United States (Storer, 1984). The annual incidence of this disease is between 1.5 and 2 per 1000 between the ages of 17 and 64 (Sleisenger, 1979), and countless prophylactic appendectomies are performed concurrently with elective abdominal operations (Eiseman et al, 1983).

If not diagnosed at an early stage, appendicitis can progress to perforation, which may lead to wound infection; pelvic, subphrenic, and intra-abdominal abscesses; and diffuse peritonitis, fecal fistula, pylephlebitis, and intestinal obstruction (Condon, 1981). The development of gangrenous or perforated appendicitis increases morbidity fivefold and mortality sixfold (Blind and Dahlgren, 1986; Condon, 1981). To avoid these potentially lethal complications in patients with appendicitis who are not operated on expeditiously, most surgeons accept, albeit begrudgingly, diagnostic error rates in the range of 15 to 30% (Berry and Malt, 1984; Buchman and Zuidema, 1984; Hobson and Roseman, 1964; Lewis et al, 1975; Pass and Hardy, 1983; Scher and Coil, 1980). A 15 to 20% incidence of normal appendices following open appendectomy is acceptable to minimize missing a perforated appendix. But this figure is approximately 40% in select groups of patients and is associated with a 5 to 10% incidence of morbidity—and even rarely mortality

(Chang et al, 1973; Lewis et al, 1975; Pieper et al, 1982). A correlation exists between the rate of perforation and diagnostic accuracy, with the best accuracy associated with the highest perforation rate (Berry and Malt, 1984).

Surgeons with preoperative diagnostic accuracies in excess of 85% are criticized because they are thought to risk increased morbidity and mortality in patients with appendicitis in whom the operation is delayed (Pass and Hardy, 1983). This "accepted" 15% rate of diagnostic inaccuracy is increased in specific groups such as children in whom history and physical examinations are difficult to interpret or sexually active women of childbearing age in whom gynecologic pathology may cause the symptoms (Cunningham and McCubbin, 1975; Gomez and Wood, 1979). The incidence of misdiagnosis in children is from 20 to 40%; and for women in the fertile age group, the rate is as high as 46% (Chang et al, 1973).

In addition to the risk of subjecting individuals to unnecessary surgery, other consequences of "negative" appendectomies include an average hospital stay of 5.9 ± 5.6 days, a loss of time from work or school of 19.1 ± 8.8 days, and an average complication rate of 15% (Blind and Dahlgren, 1986; Chang et al, 1973; Jerman, 1969; Lau et al, 1984). Mortality following a negative result on appendectomy has been reported to range from 0.65 to 2 per 1000 operations (Barnes et al, 1962; Howie, 1966).

A "negative" appendectomy is not a benign procedure.

Many nonsurgical diseases such as acute mesenteric adenitis, urinary tract infection, yersiniosis, regional enteritis, *Campylobacter* enteritis, salpingitis, and acute gastroenteritis have signs and symptoms that may mimic appendicitis (Gilmore et al, 1975; Moore and Davidson, 1984; Olinde et al, 1984). This extensive differential diagnosis increases the difficulty of making an accurate preoperative diagnosis of appendicitis. Despite advances in other areas of surgical diagnosis, there is still no laboratory test (or combination of tests), radiologic examination, or physical finding with sufficient specificity and sensitivity to diagnose appendicitis preoperatively. The diagnostic accuracy is not significantly improved by hematologic tests such as white blood cell counts and differentials, erythrocyte sedimentation rates (Bolton et al, 1975; Raftery, 1976; Sasso et al, 1970), or abdominal roentgenograms (Jenkins and Lee, 1970; Soter, 1973). Similarly, the presence or absence of fever, and pain and tenderness in the right lower quadrant, will not necessarily distinguish patients with appendicitis from those with benign self-limiting diseases (Pass and Hardy, 1983).

White and associates (1975) reported a reduction in unnecessary appendectomies in infants and children by using an approach of intensive in-hospital observation with frequent physical examinations. Despite these findings, this approach may be associated with inordinate delay, allowing the appendicitis to progress to perforation (Berry and Malt, 1984; Buchman and Zuidema, 1984; Puylaert et al, 1987).

High-resolution ultrasonography with graded compression has shown some potential in assisting in the diagnosis of acute appendicitis but still has shortcomings. Most American and European studies give high sensitivity (80 to 89%) and specificity (94 to 100%) for high-resolution ultrasonography in diagnosing acute appendicitis (Abu-Yousef et al, 1987; Jeffrey et al, 1987; Kang et al, 1989; Karstrup et al, 1986; Puylaert, 1986). However, other studies have not been as impressive, with sensitivities as low as 58% and specificities as low as 86% (Puylaert et al, 1987; Takada et al, 1986). False-negative results range from 3 to 24%, and false-positive results range from 0 to 3% (Abu-Yousef et al, 1987; Jeffrey et al, 1987; Kang et al, 1989; Puylaert, 1986; Takada et al, 1986).

REASONS FOR

Diagnostic laparoscopy is perhaps the most useful modality in the management of patients with questionable appendicitis. In an early study, laparoscopy was performed on 32 pediatric patients in whom appendicitis was suspected, but clinical findings were insufficient to establish the diagnosis (Leape and Ramenofsky, 1980). Twelve patients were spared operation by laparoscopy, thus decreasing the negative appendectomy rate to 1%. However, two patients in whom the diagnosis of appendicitis was missed at laparoscopy underwent subsequent appendectomy because of persistent symptoms.

Deutsch and associates (1982) performed diagnostic laparoscopy in 36 women aged 15 to 44 with the diagnosis of appendicitis prior to surgery. As a result of the laparoscopy, surgery was cancelled in one third of the cases. More recently, Paterson-Brown and colleagues (1988) reduced the negative appendectomy rate to 7.5% with preoperative laparoscopy compared with 22% without it.

Diagnostic laparoscopy facilitates prompt and appropriate care for patients with the suspected diagnosis of appendicitis. Even when patients present with classic history and physical findings, laparoscopy can reduce the unnecessary appendectomy rate by up to 50%. Failure to visualize the appendix at laparoscopy occurs approximately 20% of the time (Anteby et al, 1975; Leape and Ramenofsky, 1980), and false-positive results also occur. Therefore, caution is advisable when diagnostic laparoscopy is available since application in patients who would not have otherwise been explored may negate the improved diagnostic accuracy of laparoscopy (Whitworth et al, 1988).

With diagnostic laparoscopy, a "negative" appendectomy can be very useful to the female patient, since the thorough abdominal and pelvic exploration possible at laparoscopy can positively establish the reason for her symptoms, such as unsuspected endometriosis or tubal infection.

Since the overall complication rate associated with a *negative* appendectomy (15%) is not significantly different from appendectomies performed for *nonperforated* appendicitis, morbidity from this procedure appears to be related more to the laparotomy itself and not to appendiceal pathology; thus the *laparotomy*, not the *appendectomy*, is the source of postappendectomy complications. Laparoscopy has a complication rate of less than 3% and a mortality rate of 0.1 per 1000 laparoscopies (Chamberlain, 1980). If appendectomies can be performed safely using laparoscopic techniques, the high complication rate associated with negative appendectomies may be obviated.

The laparoscopic appendectomy was first described by the German pelviscopist Semm in 1982 (Semm, 1982, 1983). Schreiber (1987) reported his early experience with laparoscopic appendectomy in 70 women aged 15 to 65. Acute appendicitis was present in only 24% of his cases, and 10% were described as "suppurative." He reported only one complication (1.4%) in which cecal perforation occurred secondary to heat damage.

Gotz and associates (1990) reported the greatest experience with laparoscopic appendectomy to date. In 30 months, the clinical indication for appendectomy was given in 431 consecutive patients. Conventional appendectomy was performed because of the surgeon's preference in 38 patients. Laparoscopic appendectomy was attempted in 388 patients and was successful in 97%. In their first 50 cases, 12 patients (3%) were converted to conventional appendectomy because of adhesions, adiposity, bleeding, perforation, and abscess. Operative time was 15 to 20 minutes. Histopathology revealed that 74% were acute appendicitis (8 gangrenous, 43 phlegmatous, 5 perforated), and 12% were "negative." There were only two complications—abscesses following perforated and phlegmatous appendicitis. No wound infections occurred. The authors updated their report to include 625 cases (Pier et al, 1991). These reports demonstrate a significant improvement in the morbidity associated with conventional appendectomy.

These early experiences with laparoscopy illustrate its potential in improving the diagnosis and treatment of acute appendicitis. Technical expertise in operative laparoscopy is essential. All the authors describe a higher incidence of failures and complications early in their series (Phillips, 1977). However, in *experienced* hands, laparoscopy clearly can assist in the early diagnosis of appendicitis and can also improve the morbidity associated with appendectomy for the perforated, nonperforated, and the "negative" appendix.

REASONS AGAINST

U.S. surgeons' embracement of laparoscopic cholecystectomy since its introduction at the American College of Surgeons in October 1989 has quickly led to a search for other applications of this tool in general surgery. One of the most obvious areas is laparoscopic appendectomy for acute appendicitis. Semm (1982) and Gotz and associates (1990) described the techniques. Laparoscopy is a unique approach, but in the case of appendectomy, is it a technique in search of an operation? Should laparoscopic appendectomy be performed *routinely*, even when signs and symptoms point clearly to appendicitis; or should laparoscopic appendectomy be performed at all or only in *selected* cases, in which laparoscopy is used as a diagnostic tool as well as a therapeutic approach indicated by findings? Only carefully conducted clinical trials will answer these questions, but in the meantime what arguments should guide our use of laparoscopic appendectomy now?

There is no evidence to suggest that acute appendicitis is better managed by laparoscopic appendectomy compared with an open appendectomy through a right lower quadrant abdominal incision. A gridiron incision is strong and is not much longer than the combined scars required by three trocar sites. A laparoscopic approach may allow better visualization, especially of the pelvis, and a smaller scar in the obese patient in which exposure is a problem. The need for general anesthesia, operating time, and the risk of infection of the surgical site appears about equal. Ability to irrigate and completely evacuate exudate in suppurative or early perforated appendicitis may be better with laparoscopy because of better exposure of the pelvis. However, retrocecal or a walled-off perforated appendix is better approached as an open case because of exposure limitations with laparoscopy. The advantage of laparoscopy, therefore, lies not so much in performing appendectomy as much as in its potential diagnostic benefit by possibly eliminating an unnecessary appendectomy.

Laparoscopic examination as a diagnostic tool in these select groups of patients, followed by laparoscopic appendectomy when indicated, has been reported to reduce the incidence of normal appendixes (Leape and Ramenofsky, 1980; Paterson-Brown et al, 1988; Reiertsen et al, 1985; Whitworth et al, 1988). These reports, however, must be interpreted carefully because laparoscopy results are sometimes combined with the entire experience, and these reports usually assume that all equivocal cases would have had open appendectomy rather than a period of observation and reevaluation, which is usually the case. For example, Leape and Ramenofsky (1980) performed laparoscopy in 32 patients with equivocal clinical and laboratory findings out of a total of 119. They reported a 1% negative appendectomy rate, with one false-positive result and two false-negative results—a 9% error rate for laparoscopy. Jersky and associates (1980) performed diagnostic laparoscopy followed by appendectomy in 27 patients, with one false-positive result and two false-negative results—an 11% error rate. Incomplete visualization of the appendix in 15 to 29% of patients adds further uncertainty to the reliability of the procedure (Leape and Ramenofsky, 1980; Whitworth et al, 1988). Nevertheless, patients who might benefit most from diagnostic laparoscopy include children and sexually active women.

Therefore, the emphasis of laparoscopic appendectomy should be on the potential diagnostic capabilities of the technique rather than its therapeutic uses until controlled trials prove otherwise. Any patient who presents with periumbilical pain that settles in the right lower quadrant (RLQ), nausea, anorexia, slight fever, slight leucocytosis, and RLQ tenderness—clear signs and symptoms of appendicitis—should have open appendectomy through an RLQ gridiron incision. Also included should be the patient in whom perforation or abscess is strongly suspected. Any patient who has equivocal findings, especially women in the second to fourth decades, could first undergo diagnostic laparoscopy to determine the cause of the abdominal symptoms. If appendicitis is present, laparoscopic appendectomy should be performed. If another surgical process is identified, appropriate laparoscopic or open surgery should be employed as warranted. If the appendix cannot be visualized because of omental adhesions, or retrocecal location, and symptoms persist, open appendectomy should be performed. If the appendix appears normal and there is no other explanation for the symptoms, further observation is indicated. Most will not require surgery.

TECHNIQUE

Semm (1982) has described laparoscopic appendectomy for postoperative appendiceal adhesions in infertile patients, elongated appendixes extending into the small pelvis, endometriosis, and subacute-chronic appendicitis. His technique follows the classic operative steps that McBurney describes (Fig. 31–1), including separate ligation of the appendiceal stump and appendiceal artery followed by a pursestring suture to invert the appendiceal stump into the cecum.

De Kok (1977) and Fleming (1985) reported a laparoscopic technique during which the appendix is visualized, then delivered through a small stab wound near McBurney's point. Thereafter, routine appendectomy is performed at skin level, outside the peritoneal cavity. Acute appendicitis was present in four of Fleming's cases.

Gangal and Gangal (1987) described a novel approach to laparoscopic appendectomy using a band applicator that is usually reserved for female sterilization (Falope's ring). Prior to developing their appendiceal procedure, they had experience using banding to treat trocar perforation of the colon successfully. For appendectomy, the appendix is divided 1 cm from the cecum, and this stump is immediately banded. Thereafter, a second band is placed on the mesoappendix and the free appendix is removed from the peritoneal cavity through one of the trocar sheaths. In 73 cases, this banding procedure worked well, without need to invert or bury the appendiceal stump.

Appendectomy is most frequently performed in our gynecologic practice for endometriosis or extensive adhesions involving pelvic organs.

FIGURE 31–1 Appendectomy: McBurney-Semm method

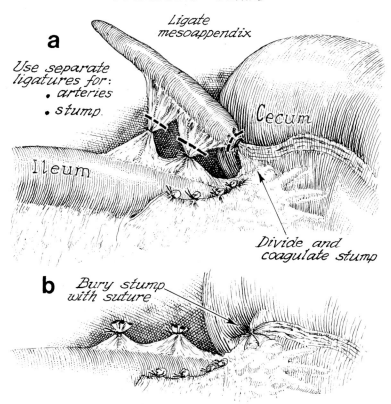

FIGURE 31–2 Appendectomy: Reich method

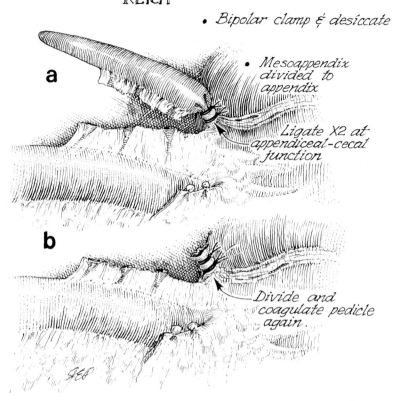

REICH

- *Bipolar clamp & desiccate*

- *Mesoappendix divided to appendix*

Ligate X2 at appendiceal-cecal junction

a

b

Divide and coagulate pedicle again.

The Reich technique is to divide all adhesions surrounding the appendix, mesoappendix, cecum, and terminal ileum. The mesoappendix is then desiccated with bipolar forceps (cutting current) (Fig. 31–2). The mesoappendix is then divided using scissors or a CO_2 laser. Following isolation of the appendiceal-cecal junction, bipolar desiccation is used 1 cm from this junction to sterilize and fuse the tissue in this area. Thereafter, two or three Endoloops (Ethicon) are placed at the appendiceal-cecal junction. The appendix is then divided in the desiccated area with the CO_2 laser. Next an operating laparoscope is used with a biopsy forceps in the operating channel to remove the appendix from the peritoneal cavity. Copious irrigation in the area of the appendix is then performed to ensure complete hemostasis, and at least 2000 ml of lactated Ringer's solution is left in the peritoneal cavity at the close of the procedure.

Treatment of appendiceal abscess or ruptured appendix is very similar to that described in the section on laparoscopic treatment of tubo-ovarian and pelvic abscess. Acute adhesions are very easy to lyse, using mainly aquadissection and traction with a grasping forceps. At the close of the procedure, the peritoneal cavity is alternately irrigated and suctioned until the effluent is clear throughout the peritoneal cavity as determined by an underwater examination.

REFERENCES

Abu-Yousef MM, Bleicher JJ, Maher JW, et al: High-resolution sonography of acute appendicitis. AJR Am J Roentgenol *149*:53–58, 1987.

Anteby SO, Schenker JG, and Polishuk WZ: The value of laparoscopy in acute pelvic pain. Ann Surg *181*:484–486, 1975.

Barnes BA, Behringer GE, Wheelock RC, and Wilkins EW: Treatment of appendicitis at the Massachusetts General Hospital (1937–1959). JAMA *180*:122–126, 1962.

Berry J and Malt RA: Appendicitis near its centenary. Ann Surg *200*:567–575, 1984.

Blind PJ and Dahlgren ST: The continuing challenge of the negative appendix. Acta Chir Scand *152*: 623–627, 1986.

Bolton JP, Craven ER, Croft RJ, and Menzies-Gow N: An assessment of the value of the white cell count in the management of suspected acute appendicitis. Br J Surg *62*:906–908, 1975.

Buchman TG and Zuidema GD: Reasons for delay of the diagnosis of acute appendicitis. Surg Gynecol Obstet *158*:260–266, 1984.

Chamberlain G: Gynaecological laparoscopy. Ann R Coll Surg Engl *62*:113–115, 1980.

Chang FC, Hogle HH, and Welling DR: The fate of the negative appendix. Am J Surg *126*:752–754, 1973.

Condon RE: Appendicitis. *In* Sabiston DC (ed): Textbook of Surgery: The Biological Basis of Modern Surgical Procedure, 12th ed. Philadelphia, WB Saunders, 1981, pp 1048–1064.

Cunningham FG and McCubbin HJ: Appendicitis complicating pregnancy. Obstet Gynecol *45*:415–420, 1975.

de Kok HJ: A new technique for resecting the non-inflamed not-adhesive appendix through a mini-laparotomy with the aid of the laparoscope. Arch Chir Neerlandicum *29*:195–198, 1977.

Deutsch AA, Zelikovsky A, and Reiss R: Laparoscopy in the prevention of unnecessary appendicectomies: A prospective study. Br J Surg *69*:336–337, 1982.

Dunn EL, Moore EE, Elerding SC, and Murphy JR: The unnecessary laparotomy for appendicitis—can it be decreased? Am Surg *48*:320–323, 1982.

Eiseman B, Moore EE, and Dunn EL: Incidental operative procedures. *In* Delaney JB and Varco RL (eds): Controversies in Surgery II. Philadephia, WB Saunders, 1983, pp 293–303.

Fleming JS: Laparoscopically directed appendicectomy. Aust N Z J Obstet Gynaecol *25*:238–240, 1985.

Gangal HT and Gangal MH: Laparoscopic appendicectomy. Endoscopy *19*:127–129, 1987.

Gilmore OJ, Browett JP, Griffin PH, et al: Appendicitis and mimicking conditions: A prospective study. Lancet *2*(7932):421–424, 1975.

Gomez A and Wood M: Acute appendicitis during pregnancy. Am J Surg *137*:180–183, 1979.

Gotz F, Pier A, and Bacher C: Modified laparoscopic appendectomy in surgery: A report on 388 operations. Surg Endosc *4*:6–9, 1990.

Hobson T and Roseman LD: Acute appendicitis—when is it right to be wrong? Am J Surg *108*:306–312, 1964.

Howie JGR: Death from appendicitis and appendectomy—an epidemiological survey. Lancet *2* (7477):1334–1337, 1966.

Jeffrey RB Jr, Laing FC, and Lewis FR: Acute appendicitis: High-resolution real-time US findings. Radiology *163*:11–14, 1987.

Jenkins D and Lee P: Radiology in acute appendicitis. J R Coll Surg Edinb *15*:34–37, 1970.

Jerman RP: Removal of the normal appendix: The cause of serious complications. Br J Clin Pract *23*:466–467, 1969.

Jersky J, Hoffman J, Shapiro J, and Kurgan A: Laparoscopy in patients with suspected acute appendicitis. S Afr J Surg *18*:147–150, 1980.

Kang W-M, Lee C-H, Chou Y-H, et al: A clinical evaluation of ultrasonography in the diagnosis of acute appendicitis. Surgery *105*:154–159, 1989.

Karstrup S, Torp-Pederson S, and Roikjaer O: Ultrasonic visualisation of the inflamed appendix. Br J Radiol *59*:985–986, 1986.

Lau W-Y, Fan S-T, Yiu T-F, et al: Negative findings at appendectomy. Am J Surg *148*:375–378, 1984.

Leape LL and Ramenofsky ML: Laparoscopy for questionable appendicitis. Can it reduce the negative appendectomy rate? Ann Surg *191*:410–413, 1980.

Lewis FR, Holcraft JW, Boey J, and Dunphy JE: Appendicitis: A critical review of diagnosis and treatment in 1,000 cases. Arch Surg *110*:677–684, 1975.

Moore MH and Davidson JRM: *Campylobacter* enteritis in the acute surgical ward. N Z Med J *97*:219–220, 1984.

Olinde AJ, Lucas JF Jr, and Miller RC: Acute yersiniosis and its surgical significance. South Med J *77*:1539–1540, 1984.

Pass HI and Hardy JD: The appendix. *In* Hardy JD (ed): Hardy's Textbook of Surgery. Philadelphia, JB Lippincott, 1983, pp 558–564.

Paterson-Brown S, Thompson JN, Eckersley JRT, et al: Which patients with suspected appendicitis should undergo laparoscopy? BMJ *296*:1363–1364, 1988.

Phillips JM: Complications in laparoscopy. Int J Gynaecol Obstet *15*:157–162, 1977.

Pieper R, Kager L, and Nasman P: Acute appendicitis: A clinical study of 1018 cases of emergency appendectomy. Acta Chir Scand *148*:51–62, 1982.

Pier A, Gotz F, Bacher C, and Thevissen P: Laparoscopic appendectomy in 625 cases: From innovation to routine. Surg Laparosc Endosc *1* (1):8–13, 1991.

Puylaert JBCM: Acute appendicitis: US evaluation using graded compression. Radiology *158*:355–360, 1986.

Puylaert JBCM, Rutgers PH, and Lalisang RI: A prospective study of ultrasonography in the diagnosis of appendicitis. N Engl J Med *317*:666–669, 1987.

Raftery AT: The value of the leucocyte count in the diagnosis of acute appendicitis. Br J Surg *63*:143–144, 1976.

Reiertsen O, Rosseland AR, Hoivik B, and Solheim K: Laparoscopy in patients admitted for acute abdominal pain. Acta Chir Scand *151*:521–524, 1985.

Sasso RD, Hamma EA, and Moore DL: Leukocytic and neutrophilic counts in acute appendicitis. Am J Surg *120*:563–566, 1970.

Scher KS and Coil JA: The continuing challenge of perforating appendicitis. Surg Gynecol Obstet *150*:535–538, 1980.

Schreiber JH: Early experience with laparoscopic appendectomy in women. Surg Endosc *1*:211–216, 1987.

Semm K: Advances in pelviscopy surgery. Curr Probl Obstet Gynecol *5*(10):1–42, 1982.

Semm K: Endoscopic appendectomy. Endoscopy *15*:59–64, 1983.

Sleisenger M: Acute appendicitis. *In* Beeson B, McDermott W, and Wyngaardent JB (eds): Cecil's Textbook of Medicine. Philadelphia, WB Saunders, 1979, pp 1579–1583.

Soter CS: The contribution of the radiologist to the diagnosis of acute appendicitis. Semin Roentgenol *8*:375–388, 1973.

Storer EH: Appendix. *In* Schwartz SI (ed): Principles of Surgery. New York, McGraw-Hill, 1984, pp 1245–1250.

Takada T, Yasuda H, Uchiyama K, et al: Ultrasonographic diagnosis of acute appendicitis in surgical indication. Int Surg *71*:9–13, 1986.

White JJ, Santillana M, and Haller JA Jr: Intensive in-hospital observation: A safe way to decrease unnecessary appendectomy. Am Surg *41*:793–798, 1975.

Whitworth CM, Whitworth PW, Sanfillipo J, and Polk HC Jr: Value of diagnostic laparoscopy in young women with possible appendicitis. Surg Gynecol Obstet *167*:187–190, 1988.

Emergency Room Laparoscopy

REASONS FOR

Peritoneal lavage was introduced in 1965 by Root (Root et al, 1965) and is now indicated for blunt or sharp injury to the abdomen and for some cases of undiagnosed hypotension to rule out intra-abdominal hemorrhage. A 2- to 3-mm cannula is inserted through an incision into the abdominal wall. This incision is similar to Hasson's "open laparoscopy" technique (Hasson, 1974). The lavage needle then allows a catheter to instill some saline, which is aspirated and studied for the presence of blood, bowel content, or exudate. If the peritoneal lavage is negative, the assumption is made that intra-abdominal injury has not occurred, and exploration is not performed.

The use of laparoscopy for these emergency situations was suggested in the 1970s (Carrnevale et al, 1977; Gazzaniga et al, 1976), but these surgeons used the standard 10-mm laparoscopes in these emergency room procedures. Laparoscopic instruments are also available in 4- to 5-mm diameters. Making a slightly larger incision than for the cutdown for peritoneal lavage, but using the identical instruments, a 5-mm laparoscopic trocar and sleeve can be introduced into the abdomen under the same conditions as peritoneal lavage. The advantage of laparoscopy is the rapidity with which the abdominal contents can be visualized. Blood can quickly be identified or ruled out.

Using such small equipment and modified technique, Berci and associates (1983) and Sherwood and colleagues (1980) studied 129 such procedures and found that 72 cases (56%) were negative, 33 cases (25%) had moderate hemoperitoneum (clots only, no active bleeding seen) requiring observation only with no surgery, and 24 patients (19%) had massive hemoperitoneum requiring exploratory laparotomy. Thus, surgery was averted in the 25% of patients who had moderate hemoperitoneum but who would have been considered positive by lavage. Only one of these patients required subsequent laparotomy 8 days later for a sealed perforation of the sigmoid colon. These physicians considered that the findings were more rapid and less equivocal than would have occurred with peritoneal lavage.

As general surgeons become more comfortable with using laparoscopy for cholecystectomy, it may become an obvious and logical step to bring smaller optics to the emergency room where they can be used for rapid evaluation of patients in whom peritoneal lavage would be indicated:

- History of blunt abdominal trauma or stab wound
- Unexplained hypotension
- Equivocal signs of an acute abdomen
- Mental obtundation

The indications could extend to patients with undiagnosed peritonitis, in which again the presence of a ruptured viscus or blood could rapidly be ruled in or out for exploratory surgery. It is unlikely that more refined diagnoses, such as the differentiation between appendicitis and pelvic inflammatory disease, could be made under emergency room conditions without general anesthesia, since these painful conditions require more thorough exploration of the relaxed abdomen than emergency room conditions would allow.

It can be anticipated that in the next decade surgeons currently in training will explore the potential benefits of emergency room laparoscopy to aid in their more rapid diagnosis of the acute abdomen in the emergency room.

REASONS AGAINST

Emergency room laparoscopy implies a diagnostic procedure under local anesthesia to look for peritoneal cavity pathology. If a treatable condition is present, the patient would then be admitted to the hospital and transferred to the operating room for definitive surgery.

Emergency room diagnostic laparoscopy relegates the laparoscope to diagnostic purposes only. It does not take into consideration the enormous possibilities for laparoscopic treatment following diagnosis. A thorough visualization is not presently possible under local anesthesia. Thus, not only is diagnosis compromised but also treatment following diagnosis requires that the patient be transferred to another part of the hospital, induction of general anesthesia, and a probable laparotomy.

Today, most of the causes of an acute abdomen can be treated laparoscopically. For general surgeons, acute appendicitis, acute cholecystitis, perforated viscus, bowel obstruction secondary to adhesive bands, and trauma can all be treated laparoscopically. Pier and colleagues (1991) reported 625 cases of laparoscopic appendectomy, 70% of which were acute, with 10 gangrenous and 9 perforated. Mouiel and Katkhouda (1991) have suture-repaired eight perforated duodenal ulcers, popularizing the techniques of total truncal vagotomy and Taylor's truncal posterior vagotomy and anterior seromyotomy. Mouret and Marsaud (in press) have treated ruptured

appendicitis and bowel obstruction. I (H. R.) have repaired ruptured unprepared rectosigmoid after evacuating a large pelvic abscess, and I have treated three cases of diverticular abscess by extensive laparoscopic débridement. Gynecologic emergency room visits most frequently result from acute pelvic inflammatory disease, ectopic pregnancy, and ruptured physiologic ovarian cysts, which are all manageable by operative laparoscopy. Torsion and rupture of endometriomas or dermoids are rare but also treatable causes.

In summary, the emergency room is not the place to install a laparoscope. Accurate diagnosis demands a thorough exploration, and this can be performed only under general anesthesia, to be followed by laparoscopic treatment in many centers. Most present-day emergency room physicians do not have the training to assess peritoneal cavity pathology adequately. I fear that emergency room laparoscopy could soon be followed by office laparoscopy at increased cost to our health care system with little associated benefit.

REFERENCES

Berci G, Dunkelman D, Michel SL, et al: Emergency minilaparoscopy in abdominal trauma: An update. Am J Surg 146:261–265, 1983.

Carrnevale N, Baron N, and Delany HM: Peritoneoscopy as an aid in the diagnosis of abdominal trauma: A preliminary report. J Trauma 17:634–641, 1977.

Gazzaniga AB, Stanton WW, and Bartlett RH: Laparoscopy in the diagnosis of blunt and penetrating injuries to the abdomen. Am J Surg 131:315–318, 1976.

Hasson HM: Open laparoscopy: A report of 150 cases. J Reprod Med 12:234–238, 1974.

Mouiel J and Katkhouda N: Laparoscopic truncal and selective vagotomy. In Zucker KA (ed): Surgical Laparoscopy, Vol 13. St. Louis, Quality Medical Publishing, 1991, p 263.

Mouret P and Marsaud H: Appendectomies per laparoscopic technique and evaluation. Surg Endosc (in press).

Pier A, Gotz F, Bacher C, and Thevissen P: Laparoscopic appendectomy in 625 cases: From innovation to routine. Surg Laparosc Endosc 1:8–13, 1991.

Root HD, Hausner CW, McKinley CR, et al: Diagnostic peritoneal lavage. Surgery 57:633–637, 1965.

Sherwood R, Berci G, Austin E, and Morgenstern L: Minilaparoscopy for blunt abdominal trauma. Arch Surg 115:672–673, 1980.

COMPLICATIONS

It has been said that there is no field of medicine as intensely self-analytical as obstetrics. A compulsion for compiling and reviewing statistics has dramatically altered maternal and infant mortality and is now concerned with morbidity of the newborn. Laparoscopy was born into this tradition, with detailed analysis by individuals, universities, hospitals, and national organizations of their experiences richly abundant in the past 2 decades of literature. This section includes the results of this self-study, with the incidence and management of major complications as they have been experienced.

Survey Data: Mortality and Morbidity

In the United States, nearly half a million women undergo sterilization annually and have done so for 20 years. With such a large experience, major sequelae of the procedure should have been detected and reported. It is reassuring that this has not often occurred. Rather, interested scientific groups such as National Institutes of Health, Centers for Disease Control, and American Association of Gynecological Laparoscopists have conducted prospective and retrospective surveys to detect and evaluate possible subtle changes in the woman's immediate complications to determine their low incidence. In this chapter we review the results of these studies.

TABLE 33-1.	LAPAROSCOPIC COMPLICATIONS: AMERICAN ASSOCIATION OF GYNECOLOGICAL LAPAROSCOPISTS SURVEY—1973*

	No.	Rate per 1000 Laparoscopies
Diagnostic	9988	
Operative	21,173	
Total	31,161	
Laparotomies required for (total)	147	5.0
Mesosalpingeal tears	55	3.0†
Known bowel coagulation	30	1.4†
Other vascular accidents	15	0.5
Other bowel injuries	9	0.3†
Miscellaneous reasons	38	1.0
Pregnancies		
At time of surgery	6	0.3
Established after surgery	18	1.0
Deaths (total)	8	0.3; 0.13‡
Survey data	2	0.1
Data from word-of-mouth reports	6	—
Other complications requiring hospitalization	59	
Cardiac arrests	10	0.3
Failed laparoscopies	201	6.0

*Adapted from Hulka JF, Soderstrom RM, Brooks PE, and Carson SL: Complications Committee of the American Association of Gynecological Laparoscopists Second annual report, 1973. In Phillips JM and Keith L (eds): Gynecological Laparoscopy: Principles and Techniques: Selected Papers and Discussion from the First International Congress of the American Association of Gynecological Laparoscopists in New Orleans, Louisiana. New York, Stratton International, 1974, pp 427–432.

†Based on operative laparoscopies only, excluding diagnostic ones.

‡Based on an estimate of 60,000 laparoscopies performed in 1973.

As laparoscopy became widespread in the United States in the 1970s, Phillips organized the American Association of Gynecological Laparoscopists (AAGL) to disseminate information regarding this new technique to practitioners (Phillips et al, 1981). As chairman of the Complications Committee, I (J. F. H.) participated in annual surveys of the membership to determine the cause and possible prevention of complications. Results of the 1973 complications survey gave physicians the first approximation of the nature and incidence of laparoscopic complications (Table 33–1).

In 1976 the Royal College of Obstetricians and Gynaecologists began a national survey in the United Kingdom prospectively collecting data concerning all laparoscopies performed and by August 1977 had collected information on 50,247 cases. The British physicians summarized these findings about complications in their 1978 report *Gynaecological Laparoscopy* (Chamberlain and Brown, 1978) (Table 33–2).

TABLE 33–2. **NATURE AND RATE OF LAPAROSCOPIC COMPLICATIONS: UNITED KINGDOM SURVEY***

Complications	No.	Rate per 1000 Laparoscopies
Anesthetic Complications		
Anesthetic	38	0.8
Cardiac arrhythmias	20	0.4
Cardiac arrest	9	0.2
Failed Procedures		
Failed laparoscopy	376	7.5
Failed abdominal insufflation	178	3.5
Failed vaginal insufflation	2	0.0
Burns		
Bowel burn	27	0.5
Skin burn	13	0.3
Other burns	10	0.2
Direct Trauma		
Damage to pelvic organs	172	3.4
Bowel	90	1.8
Urinary tract	11	0.2
Hemorrhage		
Pelvic blood vessels and tubal mesentery	134	2.7
Abdominal wall	125	2.5
Mesentery of bowel	54	1.1
Pelvic sidewall and ovarian vessels	43	0.9
Infection		
Abdominal wound	26	0.5
Pelvic infection	25	0.5
Urinary tract	24	0.5
Chest infection	11	0.2
Other Complications		
Other	156	3.1
Damage to pelvic organs not due to laparoscopy procedures	132	2.6
Late complications	41	0.8
Lost foreign body	29	0.6
Chest pain	13	0.3
Deep vein thrombosis	10	0.2
Pulmonary embolism	8	0.2
Deaths	4	0.1

*Adapted from Chamberlain G and Brown JC (eds): Gynecological Laparoscopy: Report on the Confidential Enquiry into Gynaecological Laparoscopy. London, Royal College of Obstetricians and Gynecologists, 1978.

TABLE 33–3. COMPARISON OF AMERICAN ASSOCIATION OF GYNECOLOGICAL LAPAROSCOPISTS (AAGL) AND UNITED KINGDOM (UK) SURVEY DATA*

Procedure	Rates	
	AAGL Data	UK Data
Sterilization		
Complications requiring laparotomy per 1000 cases	3.7	12.1
Bowel burn per 1000 cases	0.5	0.6
Deaths per 100,000 cases	2.5	10.4
Diagnostic Procedures		
Complications requiring laparotomy per 1000 cases	4.6	6.6
Bowel burn per 1000 cases	NA†	0.4
Deaths per 100,000 cases	5.2	4.9

*Adapted from Chamberlain G and Brown JC (eds): Gynaecological Laparoscopy: Report on the Confidential Enquiry into Gynecological Laparoscopy. London, Royal College of Obstetricians and Gynecologists, 1978.
†NA = not available.

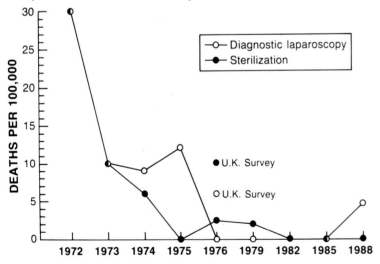

FIGURE 33–1 Mortality from 1972 to 1988 taken from AAGL survey data (with 1976 U.K. data added)

For comparisons of the retrospectively gathered AAGL data with the prospectively collected United Kingdom data see Table 33–3.

In the late 1970s, the Centers for Disease Control (CDC) assumed the task of surveillance of sterilization procedures within their charge of scrutinizing the reproductive health of the United States and has worked closely with the AAGL and the American College of Obstetricians and Gynecologists. A prospective collection of surgical and follow-up data concerning all forms of sterilization, including laparoscopy, was begun in 1978 as the Collaborative Review of Sterilization (CREST) study; data comparing different sterilization techniques are not available yet but should provide important information concerning the comparative efficacy and safety of all sterilization methods.

MORTALITY

Since 1973 the AAGL has sent survey forms to its membership with strictly anonymous return cards. The high degree of trust in the confidentiality of sensitive information such as deaths has led to impressively honest reporting by the membership (Fig. 33–1). The relative accuracy of these data is illustrated by the similarity with the British mortality rates from their prospective study in 1976, added to Figure 33–1.

The most recent mortality surveillance data emerging from the CDC indicate that anesthetic complications account for almost one third of the recent deaths associated with laparoscopy in the United States. Of these, general anesthesia without intubation is prominently associated with deaths. Three deaths from bowel burns after unipolar coagulation were also reported as probably preventable, since equally efficacious alternative laparoscopic sterilization methods are now available. Three deaths from large vessel laceration included one injury each inflicted by a trocar, a Veress needle, and a scalpel at the time of skin incision. Their estimate of the annual death rate from all causes for laparoscopic sterilization in the United States is 4 to 6 per 100,000, which is a figure in close agreement with estimates of the previous surveys. This continuing documentation of low mortality rates from laparoscopic sterilization justifies quoting the last paragraph of the United Kingdom survey report:

> Both the British and the American Surveys make one important observation: The documented death rate from elective laparoscopy sterilization is much less tha(n) the documented recurrent annual risk of death associated with oral contraception. Further, sterilization is a single incident in a woman's life and usually never repeated but taking oral contraception is a recurrent event going on for perhaps 20 years. Elective laparoscopic sterilization thus emerges as a safe alternative for a permanent method of sterilization.
>
> (Chamberlain and Brown, 1978, p 153.)

MAJOR COMPLICATIONS

Major complications are defined as those requiring laparotomy for management. The annual incidence of major complications, as compiled by the annual AAGL surveys, appears in Figure 33–2. Again, the 1976 United Kingdom survey rates are added to the figure. As the nature of major complications was identified, techniques were modified to minimize hazards. For example, bleeding from mesosalpingeal vessels during sterilization emerged as a major complication preventable by not dividing the tube, but coagulating only or by using an occlusive device. Bowel injuries continue to be prominent complications and are discussed further.

COMPLICATIONS OF OPERATIVE LAPAROSCOPY

The AAGL has surveyed its membership to assess the incidence of complications during operative laparoscopy. The membership reported 36,928 procedures in 1988 (Peterson et al, 1990b). The most frequent indication was endometriosis (13,336 procedures), and pelvic pain (41%) was as frequent a complaint as infertility (40%). Two deaths were reported from complications of bowel injury. A serious complication rate of 15.4 per 1000 was reported from persistent β-hCG after ectopic pregnancy, prolonged hospitalization for hemorrhage or bowel injury,

FIGURE 33–2 Major complications from 1972 to 1988 taken from AAGL survey data (with 1976 U.K. data added)

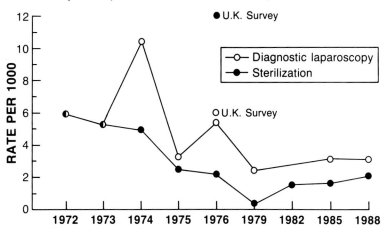

| TABLE 33–4. | COMPLICATIONS ASSOCIATED WITH OPERATIVE LAPAROSCOPY* |

Complication	No.	Rate per 1000 Procedures
Hospitalization >72 hr	154	4.2
Persistent human chorionic gonadotropin titer elevation after ectopic pregnancy (1914 ectopic cases reported)	121	63.2
Hospital readmission	115	3.1
Unintended laparotomy to manage		
Hemorrhage	96	2.6
Bowel or urinary tract injury	59	1.6
Nerve injury†	18	0.5
Spill of unsuspected ovarian cancer cysts (5075 adnexal mass cases reported)	3	0.6
Death (rate per 100,000 procedures)	2	5.4

*From Peterson HB, Hulka JF, and Phillips JM: American Association of Gynecologic Laparoscopists, 1988 membership survey on operative laparoscopy. J Reprod Med 35:587–589, 1990.

†Brachial plexus injury or foot-drop.

and so forth. This compares with the complication rate of 3.1 per 1000 diagnostic procedures and illustrates the continued need to monitor and analyze laparoscopic complications. For complications of operative laparoscopy from the 1988 survey, see Table 33–4.

A repeat AAGL survey of operative laparoscopy in 1991 revealed a 1.5-fold increase in procedures performed (56,536 cases) compared with 1988. There was a twofold increase in managing ectopic pregnancies and myomectomies by laparoscopy, but the complication rates did not rise notably.

MANAGEMENT OF MAJOR COMPLICATIONS

Bowel Injury

Bowel injury occurs in approximately three cases per 1000 laparoscopies. Although these injuries were just thought to be unipolar burns, recent evaluations of this problem have led to the current impression that most bowel injuries are trocar or Veress needle injuries, with bowel burns accounting for about 0.5 per 1000 laparoscopies.

In a definitive review of the management of unipolar bowel burns, Wheeless (1978) reported on 38 patients, of whom 33 were known to have injury occurring at surgery. With conservative management by observation alone, 27 of these patients did not require surgery. Of the six who did undergo laparotomy, only two were found to have leaking perforation in the ilium; in the remaining four no bowel lesions were found. Thus, of 33 bowel burns, only two (under 10%) resulted in leakage. The implications of this finding are that with bowel injuries, particularly of the large intestine, conservative observation may be elected. If any sign of peritonitis occurs, immediate laparotomy will be necessary.

Thermal injury with a bipolar technique is quite different from the unipolar, being sharply limited to the area of current flow and heat generated between the forceps. In contrast to the unipolar, in the bipolar lesion the burn seen is the extent of the burn. If the burn is relatively small, observation can again be successfully elected. If the burn is severe, excising it and suturing the defect (if small) or simple end-to-end anastomosis (if the lesion involves more than half of the bowel lumen) will suffice. These procedures can be safely performed within 12 hours of the injury if a general surgeon is not available, although surgery under the same anesthesia as for the laparoscopy is, of course, preferred. If perforation and peritonitis have occurred after use of the bipolar technique, the precautions that Wheeless outlines are pertinent, except for the wide margin of excision.

Large Vessel Injuries

Injury to a large vessel is an acute emergency requiring an immediate laparotomy to save the patient's life. The hazard of major blood vessel injury is the principal reason for recommending that laparoscopists be trained in an operating room with full laparotomy potential, should this unfortunate accident occur. Penfield (1978) has collected anecdotes involving more than 100 injuries of the large vessels during 10 years in the United States. Assuming that approximately 2 million women have undergone laparoscopy within this time period, this would suggest one such injury for every 20,000 laparoscopies performed. One of the deaths detected by the CDC in 1980 was because of an unrecognized vascular injury; the 5 to 6 liters of blood were all retroperitoneal, unseen by the laparoscopist.

The first step in management of this problem is to put out an emergency call for a vascular surgeon. The next step is to consider leaving the trocar or needle in place to make identification in a retroperitoneal hematoma more feasible. If it is a major aortic tear, an immediate laparotomy (without preparation) and pinching off the aorta above the tear with fingers are extreme but lifesaving measures to prevent excessive blood loss and maintain cerebral and renal perfusion. The spinal canal can sustain this anoxia for 30 to 40 minutes, after which lower limb paralysis will result if the vascular surgeon has not placed an appropriate clamp around the vessel.

REFERENCES

Chamberlain G and Brown JC (eds): Gynaecological Laparoscopy: Report on the Confidential Enquiry into Gynaecological Laparoscopy. London, Royal College of Obstetricians and Gynaecologists, 1978.

Hulka JF, Peterson HB, Phillips JM, and Surrey M: Operative laparoscopy: AAGL 1991 Membership Survey. J Reprod Med *38*, 1993 (in press).

Penfield AJ: Vascular injuries and their management. *In* Phillips JM (ed): Endoscopy in Gynecology. Downey, CA, American Association of Gynecologic Laparoscopists, 1978, pp 299–302.

Peterson HB, Hulka JF, and Phillips JM: American Association of Gynecologic Laparoscopists' 1988 membership survey on operative laparoscopy. J Reprod Med *35*:587–589, 1990b.

Phillips JM, Hulka JF, Hulka B, and Corson SL: 1979 AAGL membership survey. J Reprod Med *26*:529–533, 1981.

Wheeless CR Jr: Gastrointestinal injuries associated with laparoscopy. *In* Phillips JM (ed): Endoscopy in Gynecology. Downey, CA, American Association of Gynecologic Laparoscopists, 1978, pp 317–324.

FURTHER READINGS

ACOG Committee on Gynecologic Practice: Tubal sterilizations. ACOG Newslett *26*:8, 1982.

Hulka JF: Complications of laparoscopy. Curr Probl Obstet Gynecol *4*:1–63, 1980.

Hulka JF, Soderstrom RM, Brooks PG, and Corson SL: Complications Committee of the American Association of Gynecological Laparoscopists second annual report, 1973. *In* Phillips JM and Keith L (eds): Gynecological Laparoscopy: Principles and Techniques: Selected Papers and Discussion from the First International Congress of the American Association of Gynecological Laparoscopists in New Orleans, Louisiana. New York, Stratton Intercontinental, 1974, pp 427–432.

Peterson HB, DeStefano F, Rubin GL, et al: Deaths attributable to tubal sterilization in the United States, 1977 to 1981. Am J Obstet Gynecol *146*:131–136, 1983.

Peterson HB, Hulka JF, and Phillips JM: American Association of Gynecologic Laparoscopists' 1988 membership survey of laparoscopic sterilization. J Reprod Med *35*:584–586, 1990a.

Late Complications of Sterilization

An unexpected complication of sterilization is pregnancy. In this chapter, we review method failure and subsequent pregnancies as they have been investigated in two major prospective studies in the United States. Some of these poststerilization pregnancies are ectopic, a quite serious complication; we illustrate one method of preventing it. A number of women experience various symptoms following sterilization. We examine several studies of the "post-tubal syndrome" in England and the United States, as well as the changes in the woman's health status, including possible endocrine changes following sterilization.

TABLE 34–1.	METHOD FAILURES AT 12 MONTHS BY LIFE TABLE ANALYSIS*	
Method	**Rate per 100 Women-Years**	
Electrocoagulation	0.26	
Silastic band	0.47	
Spring clip	0.18	

*From Bhiwandiwala PP, Mumford SD, and Feldblum PJ: A comparison of different laparoscopic sterilization occlusion techniques in 24,439 procedures. Am J Obstet Gynecol 144:319–331, 1982.

TABLE 34–2.	RISK OF ECTOPIC PREGNANCY FOLLOWING STERILIZATION METHODS*		
Method	**Intrauterine No.**	**Ectopic No.**	**Rate of Ectopics to Total Pregnancies (%)**
Pomeroy	657	145	18
Unipolar, coagulation, division	107	76	41
Unipolar, coagulation only	61	57	48
Bipolar, coagulation, division	46	37	44
Bipolar, coagulation only	151	61	29
Silastic ring	180	33	15
Spring clip	24	1	4
Total	1226	410	33

*From Phillips JM, Hulka JF, Hulka B, and Corson SL: 1979 AAGL membership survey. J Reprod Med 26:529–533, 1981.

SUBSEQUENT PREGNANCIES

The efficacy of sterilization techniques was not and could not be addressed in the American and British surveys. The correct approach is to follow prospectively a large number of women undergoing sterilization to detect the true incidence of pregnancy subsequent to this event. This was done extremely well in Baltimore by Johns Hopkins University in the early years of electrocoagulation and once again by the University of North Carolina at Chapel Hill in the evolution of the spring clip and subsequent pregnancies. Both studies had more than 90% follow-up on more than 1000 patients each. Since then, data concerning subsequent pregnancies have been difficult to evaluate because of lower levels of follow-up, even with correction using life table analyses. The most recent comparative efficacy report available, based on 24,439 sterilizations performed and analyzed by Family Health International (formerly the International Fertility Research Program), reveals varying pregnancy rates for three types of sterilization procedures (Table 34–1).

The Centers for Disease Control's prospective Collaborative Review of Sterilization (CREST) study has suggested a much higher pregnancy rate for all methods, approaching 8 per 100 pregnancies within 3 years of sterilization. (The clip pregnancies in the CREST study and those reviewed histologically by the author (J. F. H.) have been mostly applications on the ampulla or incompletely across the isthmus.) For these reasons, the latest Patient Evaluation Pamphlet on Sterilization (ACOG Committee on Patient Education, 1991) of the American College of Obstetricians and Gynecologists states:

> More than 99 of every 100 women who have this procedure will not become pregnant, but you should be aware that the procedure does not guarantee sterility. Although the risk of failure is low, sometimes the procedure does not work.

ECTOPIC PREGNANCIES

Ectopic pregnancy is a rare but very serious late complication of sterilizations and their failures. The 1979 AAGL survey, for the first time, presented data in which sufficient numbers of pregnancies were reported to justify analysis (Table 34–2). As discussed in Chapter 11, bipolar coagulation is associated with a high proportion of subsequent pregnancies being ectopic.

Women with less tissue damage (from Pomeroy, band, and spring clip sterilizations) had a decreased relative risk of ectopic pregnancy. As described in Chapter 6, these ectopic pregnancies may be attributable to fistulas connecting the uterine cavity to the peritoneal cavity following extensively destructive techniques, permitting sperm to fertilize an ovum and lodge in the distal segment of the tube (Fig. 34–1). This reasoning suggests leaving a longer segment of isthmus with all forms of sterilization to minimize the possibility of uteroperitoneal fistula (Fig. 34–2).

FIGURE 34–1 Uteroperitoneal fistula

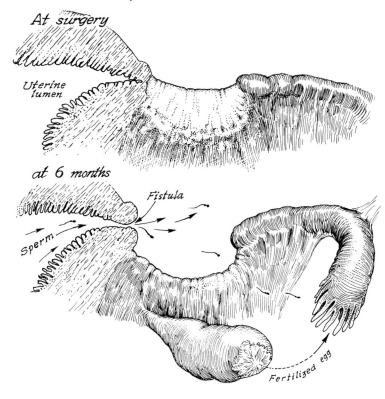

FIGURE 34–2 Preventing a fistula

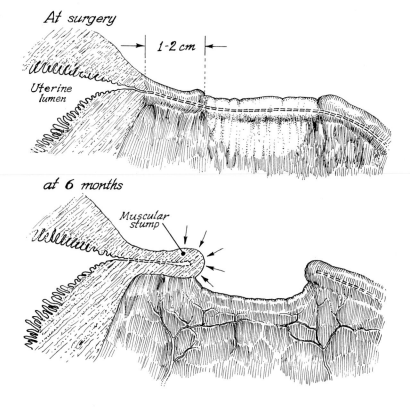

POST-TUBAL SYNDROME

An estimated 6 million women in the United States have undergone tubal sterilization as an elective procedure. Hundreds if not thousands of these women are presenting themselves to their gynecologists with symptoms of menometrorrhagia and pain and are being labeled "post-tubal syndrome" as a justification to perform hysterectomy. Pathologic examination of the specimen usually reveals no findings.

The possibility of a cause-and-effect relationship between extensive laparoscopic coagulation and uterine bleeding was first raised in England by Neil and associates (1975), who found markedly increased complaints of irregular bleeding and pain among laparoscopically coagulated women compared with wives of men who had had vasectomies. Rioux (1977) thoroughly reviewed the entire field and correctly pointed out that all of the reports to date had serious epidemiologic methodology errors in selection of control groups for comparison. He urged that this defect be answered by a long-term prospective study of women undergoing tubal sterilization, comparing them with another identical group of women who did not undergo sterilization. The possibility of conducting such a prospective study is currently receiving close attention by the National Institutes of Health and the Centers for Disease Control. An important contribution in this area of concern was made by Family Health International (Bhiwandiwala et al, 1982) in a report of menstrual disturbances following different methods of sterilization (Fig. 34–3). The study found no association between subsequent menstrual changes and any particular method of sterilization.

Another report from England analyzed sequelae to sterilization among 17,032 women who were prospectively followed for contraception (Vessey et al, 1983). In this ongoing study, 2243 women had undergone sterilization, and 3551 had husbands who had undergone vasectomy. There was no difference between wives of vasectomized husbands and women undergoing sterilization with respect to hospital referral leading to hysterectomy, dilatation and curettage, or admission for psychiatric disorder. There was a slight excess of hospital referrals for menstrual disorders in sterilized women, especially among those who had coagulation, but these differences were not significant.

In 1989, two prospective studies of menstrual sequelae to sterilization were reported by Shain and colleagues and by Rulin and associates (Rulin et al, 1989; Shain et al, 1991). Among 227 sterilized women, Shain and colleagues reported more initial menorrhagia, menstrual irregularity, and dysmenorrhea among women undergoing bipolar coagulation or Pomeroy ligation compared with women who had undergone mechanical tubo-occlusion, 132 wives of vasectomized husbands, and 87 nonsterilized women. A larger collaborative study of 1213 sterilized versus 601 comparison groups reported by Rulin and others reveals only an increase in dysmenorrhea among sterilized women. Changes in sexuality among sterilized women were reported by Shain and colleagues in 1991. During a 5-year follow-up period, all groups showed a gradual decline of satisfaction and interest, although the sterilized women had a significant rise in coital frequency in the first year.

ENDOCRINE CHANGES

In a related issue, the possibility of sterilization's altering ovarian function has been observed by Radwanska and associates (1979); Radwanska and colleagues (1982); and Donnez and associates (1981) (Fig. 34–4). In these studies, women who had undergone Pomeroy, electrocoagulation, or spring clip sterilization were compared with normal controls with respect to midluteal progesterone levels. These patients were all asymptomatic and did not represent a post-tubal syndrome. The normal level of plasma progesterone (among women who became pregnant in the cycle studied) was 17 to 18 ng/ml, whereas those who had undergone coagulation or Pomeroy sterilizations had an average of 9 to 10 ng/ml. Clip patients had normal average levels of 15 to 17 ng/ml. The authors postulated that extensive destruction of the vasculature with Pomeroy or coagulation caused a subtle interference in adequate luteal function, which did not occur with less extensive vascular damage such as with the clip. However, other studies of human endocrine function failed to show significant changes in luteal function after sterilization or even hysterectomy. A carefully designed study of endocrine function after bilateral salpingectomy and hysterectomy in monkeys also failed to reveal significant alterations in endocrine function (Castracane et al, 1979).

Rock and colleagues (1981) reported the presence of endometrial implants in the proximal stump of the tube as an asymptomatic incidental finding (see Atlas, Plate 27). Such an implant might occasionally cause menstrual pain, although this has yet to be documented or reported. Findings of endometriosis in women undergoing anastomosis after sterilization have similarly not been reported as either significant or symptomatic.

The conclusion to be drawn at the moment is that neither endocrine nor symptomatic changes after sterilization have been consistently reported and that the post-tubal syndrome remains to be documented.

FIGURE 34–3 Menstrual flow following sterilization by different methods

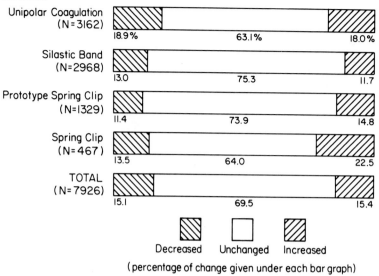

(percentage of change given under each bar graph)

FIGURE 34–4 Progesterone levels following sterilization by different methods

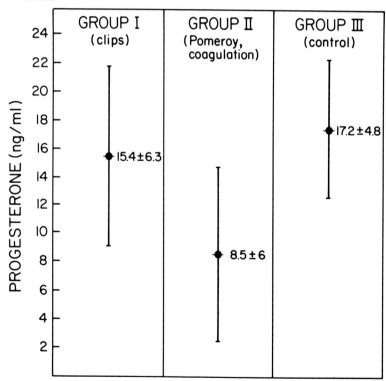

REFERENCES

ACOG Committee on Patient Education: Sterilization for women and men. APO11, April 1991. Washington, DC.

Bhiwandiwala PP, Mumford SD, and Feldblum PJ: A comparison of different laparoscopic sterilization occlusion techniques in 24,439 procedures. Am J Obstet Gynecol 144:319–331, 1982.

Castracane VD, Moore GT, and Shaikh AA: Ovarian function in hysterectomized Macaca fascicularis. Biol Reprod 20:462–472, 1979.

Donnez J, Wauters M, and Thomas K: Luteal function after tubal sterilization. Obstet Gynecol 57:65–68, 1981.

Neil JR, Noble AD, Hammond GT, et al: Late complications of sterilisation by laparoscopy and tubal ligation: A controlled study. Lancet 2:699–700, 1975.

Radwanska E, Berger GS, and Hammond J: Luteal deficiency among women with normal menstrual cycles, requesting reversal of tubal sterilization. Obstet Gynecol 54:189–192, 1979.

Radwanska E, Headley SK, and Dmowski P: Evaluation of ovarian function after tubal sterilization. J Reprod Med 27:376–384, 1982.

Rioux J-E: Late complications of female sterilization: A review of the literature and a proposal for further research. J Reprod Med 19:329–340, 1977.

Rock JA, Parmley TH, King TM, et al: Endometriosis and the development of tuboperitoneal fistulas after tubal ligation. Fertil Steril 35:16–20, 1981.

Rulin MC, Davidson AR, Philliber SG, et al: Changes in menstrual symptoms among sterilized and comparison women: A prospective study. Obstet Gynecol 74:149–154, 1989.

Shain RN, Miller WB, Holden AEC, and Rosenthal M: Impact of tubal sterilization and vasectomy on female marital sexuality: Results of a controlled longitudinal study. Am J Obstet Gynecol 164:763–771, 1991.

Vessey M, Huggins G, Lawless M, and Yeates D: Tubal sterilization: Findings in a large prospective study. Br J Obstet Gynecol 90:203–209, 1983.

FURTHER READINGS

Alvarez-Sanchez F, Segal SJ, Brache V, et al: Pituitary-ovarian function after tubal ligation. Fertil Steril 36:606–609, 1981.

Corson SL, Levinson CJ, Batzer FR, and Otis C: Hormonal levels following sterilization and hysterectomy. J Reprod Med 26:363–370, 1981.

Hargrove JT and Abraham GE: Endocrine profile of patients with patients with post-tubal-ligation syndrome. J Reprod Med 26:359–362, 1981.

Richards IS: Menstrual function following tubal sterilization. AVS Biomed Bull 2:1–6, 1981.

Shain RN, Miller WB, Mitchell GW, et al: Menstrual pattern change 1 year after sterilization: Results of a controlled, prospective study. Fertil Steril 52:192–203, 1989.

Templeton AA and Cole S: Hysterectomy following sterilization. Br J Obstet Gynecol 89:845–848, 1982.

Laparoscopic Management of Complications

Veress needle and trocar-induced vascular and viscus injury can be life-threatening complications of laparoscopic surgical procedures. Perforation of the bowel or large vessels during initial trocar placement is a known rare risk of laparoscopy beyond the control of the surgeon. These injuries cannot be completely eliminated since trocar insertion is a blind procedure involving forceful thrust of a sharp instrument into the abdomen. An open laparoscopy approach will not reduce the risk of bowel trauma when bowel is fused to the anterior abdominal wall beneath the entry site. One quarter of the respondents to a survey of certified Canadian gynecologists had experienced at least one case of sharp trocar or needle injury, with half the cases requiring laparotomy for correction (Yuzpe, 1990). Advanced laparoscopic surgery such as lysis of adhesions involving bowel will result in bowel injury just like lysis at laparotomy. In this chapter we present the management of these complications, with emphasis on what can be managed laparoscopically.

VESSEL INJURY

Injury to a large vessel (aorta or iliac vessels) usually signifies the need for immediate laparotomy (Bergqvist and Bergqvist, 1987). However, fatal cases have been reported in which the bleeding progressed slowly into the retroperitoneal space and was not diagnosed by the surgeon at the time of laparoscopy. The increased intra-abdominal pressure (10 to 15 mm Hg) caused by insufflation of CO_2, the decreased venous pressure from the Trendelenburg position, and retroperitoneal hematoma formation may tamponade a large vessel injury. As soon as the pressure gradients return to normal, bleeding may start and can lead eventually to hypovolemic shock.

To avoid this deadly complication, it is essential to examine the course of the large vessels at the start and finish of the endoscopic procedure. When an injury has occurred, it is usually possible to detect a defect in the peritoneum overlying the site of retroperitoneal entry. This allows the operator to differentiate between a Veress needle (small round) or a trocar injury (triangular). If one is absolutely certain that the Veress needle is the causative agent, consideration may be given to not intervening immediately and observing the patient in an intensive care unit instead.

If a hematoma is present, its overlying peritoneum is opened using laparoscopic scissors or a CO_2 laser. The hematoma is evacuated by alternating suctioning with irrigation (aquadissection) in the retroperitoneal space. Bleeding vessels in areolar and adipose tissue are desiccated. Laparotomy should be performed if there is any evidence of hematoma expansion or persistent bleeding. At laparotomy, exploration is done by a vascular surgeon. The aorta and common iliac vessels should be isolated with vascular tourniquets (Dacron tape) prior to exploring the area of the suspected laceration.

Epigastric Vessels

Injury to the deep epigastric vessels can be avoided by observing them directly with the laparoscope, because one can usually see its venae comitantes adjacent to the obliterated umbilical ligaments of the anterior abdominal wall (see Figs. 30–2 and 30–3). The deep epigastric artery with its two veins comes off the external iliac artery near its transition into the femoral artery and lies in the medial peritoneal fold of the internal inguinal ring; the round ligament curls around these vessels on entrance into the inguinal canal. Superficial epigastric vessels are noted by transillumination. Direct observation and transillumination should be performed in every case. As the deep epigastric vessels lie beneath the lateral margin of the rectus muscle, lateral insertion also avoids muscle bleeding.

If bleeding ensues from a second puncture site, rotating the second puncture sleeve through 360 degrees often results in vessel tamponade. Thereafter, pressure on this spot for 5 to 10 minutes may control the bleeding. During this time, intraperitoneal manipulation can be performed through another second puncture site. If this procedure does not control the bleeding, long Kleppinger bipolar forceps through the operating channel of an operating laparoscope are used to desiccate the vessels above the parietal peritoneum cephalad and caudad to the trocar. If a subfascial hematoma is present at the end of the procedure, the peritoneum at one side of the hematoma, usually in the flank, is opened and the hematoma is evacuated by alternating irrigation with suction until clear effluent is obtained.

Although bipolar desiccation has never failed in our experience, other methods are available. Tamponade of the vessel at the site of injury can be obtained by inserting a Foley catheter through the second puncture cannula, removing the cannula after inflating the Foley, and bringing the distended Foley balloon into pressurized contact with the laceration. The balloon is held in this position by a hemostat clamped to the Foley catheter on the skin.

Suture occlusion of the vessels can be considered. A Keith straight needle can be inserted into the peritoneal cavity on one side of the vessel and out on the other to perform ligation. Large curved needles can be used at full thickness through the abdominal wall under laparoscopic observation.

Ovarian or Uterine Vessels

Bipolar desiccation is capable of controlling any bleeding from ovarian or uterine vessels. Collateral circulation to the pelvic organs ensures that ischemic changes will not occur.

VISCUS INJURY

Gastrointestinal injuries may occur during laparoscopic surgery, and the surgeon should be familiar with their management, in many cases without laparotomy, regardless of specialty training. Treatment of gynecologic conditions such as rectal endometriosis and ovarian remnants requires special understanding.

Stomach

The routine use of an orogastric tube is recommended to eliminate the possibility of a trocar injury to the stomach. However, if such an injury occurs, as diagnosed by a laparoscopic view of the inside of the stomach, treatment should consist of extending the trocar incision into a minilaparotomy (leaving the trocar in the stomach as a marker) for a two-layer closure. A laparoscopic approach would be a pursestring suture or a figure-of-eight suture in the seromuscular layer surrounding the defect and nasogastric tube drainage for 2 days.

Bowel

TROCAR INSERTION INJURY. Perforation of the intestine occurs either at Veress needle or umbilical trocar insertion or during surgery. Injury by Veress needle probably occurs more often than is diagnosed and goes unnoticed. This Veress needle injury is not usually serious because it occurs most often where intestinal loops are adherent to the anterior abdominal wall and the perforation seals off promptly. Expectant management is recommended for this type of mishap, and exploratory laparotomy is not recommended. Air insufflation of an intestinal loop occurred eight times in 500 procedures from one series (Ruddock, 1957; Vilardell et al, 1968). The emanation of foul-smelling gas through the pneumoperitoneum needle is a helpful diagnostic sign.

Injury during insertion of the first-puncture trocar (usually umbilical) may represent a diagnostic challenge, and recognition of this complication at the time of laparoscopy is crucial. A segment of bowel (usually transverse colon) can adhere to the abdominal wall and result in trocar injury in about one case in 4000. The trocar can pierce through the entire lumen of the bowel. The bowel remains fixed around the sleeve of the trocar during the entire procedure; thus the accident may not be noticed unless the operator carefully examines the entire abdominal cavity. Again, recognition of the complication at the time of laparoscopy is most important. If perforation of the transverse colon is suspected, the trocar sleeve and the laparoscope inside it are retracted slowly. If pierced, the bowel lumen will come into view during this maneuver. The recommended treatment is minilaparotomy for suture repair of the perforation or resection of the bowel segment. In some cases if an experienced laparoscopic surgeon is available, a laparoscopic suture or a laparoscopic stapler (ENDO GIA 30) can be used to close the defect. If the perforation has occurred in a bowel segment other than the transverse colon, it may be beneficial to leave the trocar in situ until the affected segment is identified and clamped. Colostomy is rarely indicated.

Small bowel perforation occurs most often at laparoscopic surgery while inserting umbilical or lower quadrant trocars in cases involving extensive small bowel adhesions. The perforation is not usually recognized until later in the procedure, after omental and small bowel adhesions are freed from the anterior abdominal wall. If the omentum and small bowel adhesions are not freed from the anterior abdominal wall, these perforations may not be recognized at all. Thus, the surgeon who encounters extensive adhesions surrounding the umbilical puncture should consider a higher primary puncture site. The left costal margin in the midclavicular line is usually satisfactory, giving a panoramic view of the entire peritoneal cavity. Thereafter, the adhesions can be freed down to and just beneath the umbilicus, at which time it becomes possible to reestablish the umbilical portal for further work. If CO_2 insufflation is not obtainable through the umbilicus, a Veress needle puncture in the left ninth intercostal space, anterior axillary line, can be done.

After a small bowel perforation has been recognized, it can be repaired transversely with interrupted 3–0 Vicryl, silk, or polydioxanone (PDS) on a tapered SH needle tied either externally or with intracorporeal instruments. Sterile milk is instilled into the bowel lumen prior to the closing of the last suture to detect leakage from the laceration and occult perforations near the small bowel mesentery.

INJURY DURING ENDOSCOPIC SURGERY. Injury during surgery occurs most often at the level of the rectosigmoid. Detection and careful inspection of the lesion are again the most important factors. Superficial lesions can be managed by careful postoperative observation. Defects involving the full thickness of the wall require surgical repair by an experienced surgeon, either laparoscopically or by laparotomy. Resection with or without colostomy is rarely indicated.

Superficial thermal injuries to bowel noted during surgery can be treated prophylactically with a laparoscopically placed pursestring suture. The suture should be placed beyond the thermally affected tissue.

FIGURE 35–1 Bowel repair

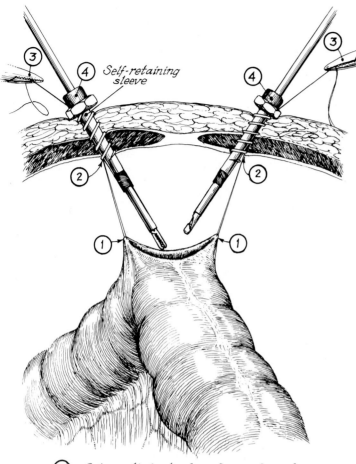

Self-retaining
sleeve

(1) Sutures tied at edge of wound and
brought out through sleeve

(2) Sleeve removed, suture remains in track,
sleeve re-inserted next to suture

(3) Elevate sutures to see wound.
Hold under tension outside abdomen
with hemostats as "stay-sutures."

(4) Two sleeves allow two instruments
to suture wound.

LARGE BOWEL INJURY. In the bowel-prepared patient, injury to the anterior rectum can usually be repaired laparoscopically. Full-thickness penetration of the rectum may occur during the excision of rectal endometriosis nodules. After excision of the nodule and identification of the rent in the rectum, a single or double-layered repair is done using 3–0 silk, Vicryl, PDS, or the ENDO GIA 30. Stay sutures are placed at the transverse angles of the defect and brought out through the lower quadrant trocar sleeves, which are then replaced in the peritoneal cavity over the stay suture (Fig. 35–1). After closure, povidone-iodine (Betadine) solution is injected into the rectum through a Foley catheter with a 30-ml balloon, and an underwater examination is done to check for any leaks, which, if seen, are then reinforced. I have had no late sequelae following five such procedures (Reich et al, 1991).

Concerning the unprepared bowel, the decision whether to repair laparoscopically depends on the amount of fecal spillage present. If a large amount of fecal contamination occurs, laparotomy followed by repair should be considered. Otherwise, laparoscopic suture closure, followed by copious irrigation until the effluent clears, should be satisfactory. There is little indication for colostomy during the repair of bowel injuries noted during the course of a laparoscopic procedure.

The practice of performing a colostomy during treatment of bowel injury began following the 1944 report of Ogilvie, who reported significant reductions in mortality following treatment of colon injuries during World War II. In fact, in 1943, the Surgeon General of the United States issued an order that all colon injuries sustained in battle should be treated by performing a colostomy (Office of the Surgeon General, 1943). In 1951, Woodhall and Ochsner reported their experience with primary repair without colostomy: their mortality rate fell from 23% to 9% with primary repair. In 1979, Stone and Fabian reported the first well-controlled prospective randomized study on primary closure of traumatic colon perforations. Morbidity for the randomized colostomy group was 10-fold higher, and the average hospital stay was 6 days longer. Similar results were obtained by George and colleagues (1989) and by Burch and associates (1986). Thus, we find little indication for colostomy during the repair of bowel injuries noted during the course of a laparoscopic procedure.

SMALL BOWEL LACERATION. Small bowel perforation during small bowel adhesiolysis surgery for pain is common, occurring in more than 25% of these procedures. These adhesions are the result of multiple previous surgeries in most cases. Despite the application of traction and countertraction to each adhesion, bowel punctures are inevitable as these adhesions are carefully cut.

Following recognition of a small bowel perforation, it can be repaired as described earlier (see Fig. 35–1).

PERITONITIS AFTER UNRECOGNIZED OR DELAYED PERFORATION. Delayed bowel injury can result from traumatic perforation that is not recognized during the procedure (Veress needle or trocar puncture or laceration during adhesiolysis or excision) or from thermal damage from any source. Rarely, delayed injuries can occur from perforation of mechanically devascularized bowel or from hemorrhagic ischemic necrosis after mesenteric venous thrombosis. Bowel perforation after thermal injury usually presents 4 to 10 days following the procedure. With traumatic perforation, symptoms usually occur within 24 to 48 hours, although their occurrence up to 11 days later has been reported (Penfield, 1985). At surgery for delayed bowel perforation, gross appearance of traumatic and electrical injuries is the same; the perforation is usually surrounded by a white area of necrosis (Levy, 1985). Microscopic examination of the lesions reveals the persistence of dead amorphous tissue without polymorphonuclear infiltrate following electrical burns. With puncture injuries, there is rapid and abundant capillary ingrowth, white cell infiltration, and fibrin deposition at the injury site (Levy et al, 1985). Wheeless (1978) has outlined well the management of delayed bowel perforation with peritonitis. Treatment consists of a bowel resection of all necrotic tissue with end-to-end anastomosis, copious lavage, antibiotics, and minidose heparin therapy (preferably supervised by a general surgeon).

OTHER COMPLICATIONS

Bladder

The second-puncture trocar can perforate the bladder, especially in a patient who has had previous pelvic surgery. A reliable diagnostic sign is the sudden appearance of gas in the Foley catheter drainage bag. Thus, when bladder identification cannot be made, because no bladder distention occurs during the surgery, consideration should be given to inserting a Foley catheter to observe for gas.

The most important factor in treatment is early detection. Treatment consists of placing an indwelling catheter for 7 to 10 days and prophylactic antibiotics. If the defect is large from manipulation through the trocar sleeve during laparoscopic surgery, it should be closed with a figure-of-eight suture through the surrounding bladder muscularis and a second suture to close the overlying peritoneum. A watertight seal should be documented by filling the bladder with blue dye solution (Reich and McGlynn, 1990).

Postoperative urinary retention can occur, especially with the use of large amounts of fluid for irrigation and hydroflotation. Urine can accumulate rapidly in the bladder in the drowsy patient who is recovering from anesthesia. The Foley catheter should not be removed at the end of operative procedures lasting for longer than 2 hours. Foley catheter removal should be delayed until the patient is awake in the short-stay unit and is aware that the catheter is in place, usually 1 hour postoperatively. At this time, a useful protocol is to administer 25 mg of bethanechol chloride (Urecholine). If spontaneous voiding does not occur within 3 hours after the catheter is removed, straight catheterization is performed and the patient is administered another 25 mg of bethanechol chloride. This regimen has successfully avoided urinary retention during the past 2 years on our service.

Ureter

An intravenous pyelogram (IVP) should be obtained if postoperative flank or pelvic pain presents after adnexal surgery. Thermal injury to a ureter will result in ureteral narrowing and hydroureter. Treatment during the early phase is often possible by the placement of a ureteral stent for 3 to 6 weeks. Intraoperatively, ureteral integrity can be checked by injecting 5 ml of indigo carmine solution intravenously. Elimination of the dye begins soon after the injection, usually appearing in the urine within 5 to 10 minutes in average cases.

Incisional Hernia

Failure to close fascial defects from incisions greater than 7 mm can lead to incisional hernia of the anterior abdominal wall requiring future surgery. If possible, incised fascia should be located, with the help of skin hooks, and repaired.

Infection

Infection is exceedingly rare following laparoscopic surgery, especially when 2 liters of Ringer's lactate solution are left in the peritoneal cavity at the close of the procedure and underwater examination is used to evacuate all blood clots. There is a theoretical risk that bacterial infection can be disseminated throughout the peritoneal cavity during extensive use of aquadissection and underwater surgery. However, bacteria grow poorly in Ringer's lactate solution.

Umbilical incision infections are usually prevented by burying the knot below the deep fascia. Incision infection is detected by pain, swelling, and erythema of the overlying skin. Treatment should consist of warm compresses, drainage, and appropriate antibiotic therapy. Lower quadrant incision infection rarely occurs, especially following closure without suture. We have experienced only one rectus muscle infection requiring drainage in more than 2000 procedures.

Dissemination of Cancer

A similar theoretical risk exists for dissemination of cancer cells in cases of cyst aspiration. In our experience, no recurrence has occurred with two early ovarian serous cystadenocarcinomas or four endometrial adenocarcinomas treated laparoscopically. Hysterectomy performed 1 month after laparoscopic myomectomy diagnosed as sarcoma was negative for residual disease. When a suspicious lesion is excised, consideration should be given to leaving 1 liter of sterile water in the peritoneal cavity at the close of the procedure to lyse free cells. However, this usually results in a marked increase in urinary output, and the patient should be observed carefully for any sign of urinary retention postoperatively.

Cutaneous seeding of gallbladder cancer has been reported after laparoscopic cholecystectomy (Drouard et al, 1991). Thus, cysts or organs with possible malignant excrescences should not be pulled through tight incisions. The LapSac is ideal for these cases, and cysts should be placed in it prior to their aspiration and later removal.

Fluid Overload

Fluid overload is possible when one is using large amounts of fluid during a lengthy procedure. Fortunately, most long laparoscopic surgery procedures are performed on relatively healthy patients. Also, the fluid used is in physiologic balance with body fluids. Absorption from the peritoneal surfaces during and after the laparoscopic procedure is mainly excreted through the kidneys. Loosely approximately umbilical and lower quadrant incisions provide an easy exit for excess fluids. When the patient's intra-abdominal pressure rises, leakage from umbilical and lower quadrant incisions is common and usually ceases within 12 hours. No wound infections have been encountered despite this seepage.

Pulmonary edema is a possibility and has occurred in four of our last 1000 cases. Treatment is with furosemide (Lasix), 40 mg IV, and supplemental oxygen. Sufficient oxygen saturation is monitored with a pulse oximeter (SaO_2). Through most long laparoscopic procedures, lactated Ringer's solution should be infused at 4 to 5 ml/kg/hr, which in a 70-kg woman results in 280 to 350 ml of fluid per hour.

Subcutaneous and Subfascial Emphysema and Edema

Other complications relate to distribution of fluid in tissue and potential spaces outside the peritoneal cavity. (Accumulation of fluid in tissue is edema; accumulation of gas in tissue is emphysema.) Areas commonly affected usually follow the path of subcutaneous emphysema: the subcutaneous and subfascial spaces. Often both subcutaneous emphysema and edema exist concurrently, with edema more prominent in the dependent areas.

Manipulation of instruments often loosens the parietal peritoneum surrounding their portal of exit into the peritoneal cavity. CO_2 then infiltrates the loose areolar tissue of the body, and crepitant areas can sometimes be palpated in the shoulder and facial regions. This swelling subsides within a few hours following the end of the procedure. Subfascial edema of the labia can often be expressed through the lower-quadrant incisions by pressure on the labia. Similar pressure on the anterior abdominal wall will push CO_2 from the umbilical incision during or following the procedure.

When this fluid-gas mixture affects the vulva, marked vulvar swelling can occur, and an indwelling Foley catheter may be necessary overnight. Facial edema, including periorbital and scleral edema, is proportional to the length of the procedure and the degree of Trendelenburg position. It rapidly resolves within 2 to 4 hours postoperatively, usually by the time of discharge from the outpatient department. In rare cases, pleural effusion may be present and should be ruled out with an upright abdominal x-ray when persistent upper abdominal "gas pain" is present.

REFERENCES

Bergqvist D and Bergqvist A: Vascular injuries during gynecologic surgery. Acta Obstet Gynecol Scand 66:19–23, 1987.

Burch JM, Brock JC, Gevirtzman L, et al: The injured colon. Ann Surg 203:701–711, 1986.

Drouard F, Delamarre J, and Capron JP: Cutaneous seeding of gallbladder cancer after laparoscopic cholecystectomy (Letter). N Engl J Med 325:1316, 1991.

George SM Jr, Fabian TC, Voeller GR, et al: Primary repair of colon wounds. A prospective trial in nonselected patients. Ann Surg 209:728–734, 1989.

Levy BS, Soderstrom RM, and Dail DH: Bowel injuries during laparoscopy: Gross anatomy and histology. J Reprod Med 30:168–172, 1985.

Office of the Surgeon General: Circulation Letter, no. 178. October 23, 1943. Washington, DC.

Ogilvie WH: Abdominal wounds in the Western Desert. Surg Gynecol Obstet 78:225–238, 1944.

Penfield AJ: How to prevent complications of open laparoscopy. J Reprod Med 30:660–663, 1985.

Reich H and McGlynn F: Laparoscopic repair of bladder injury. Obstet Gynecol 76:909–910, 1990.

Reich H, McGlynn F, and Budin R: Laparoscopic repair of full-thickness bowel injury. J Laparoendosc Surg 1:119–122, 1991.

Ruddock JC: Peritoneoscopy: A critical clinical review. Surg Clin North Am 37:1249–1260, 1957.

Stone HH and Fabian TC: Management of perforating colon trauma: Randomization between primary closure and exteriorization. Ann Surg 190:430–436, 1979.

Vilardell F, Seres I, and Marti-Vicente A: Complications of peritoneoscopy: A survey of 1455 examinations. Gastrointest Endosc 14:178–180, 1968.

Wheeless CR Jr: Gastrointestinal injuries associated wih laparoscopy. In Phillips JM (ed): Endoscopy in Gynecology. Downey, CA, American Association of Gynecologic Laparoscopists, 1978, pp 317–324.

Woodhall JP and Ochsner A: The management of perforating injuries of the colon and rectum in civilian practice. Surgery 29:305–320, 1951.

Yuzpe AA: Pneumoperitoneum needle and trocar injuries in laparoscopy: A survey on possible contributing factors and prevention. J Reprod Med 35:485–490, 1990.

APPENDIX A INSTRUMENTS AND EQUIPMENT FOR LAPAROSCOPY

Harry Reich, M.D.

Instrument/Equipment	Manufacturer/Order Number*
Scopes (R. Wolf)	
10-mm 0-degree Panoview	8934.401
10-mm 0-degree Panoview laserscope	8912.401
Adapter to convert laserscope to operative laparoscope	8911.315
Light cord	8064.558
5-mm 0-degree Panoview telescope	8935.401
5-mm 25-degree hysteroscope Panoview	8989.401
Outer sheath	8989.151
5-mm Laparoscopy Set (Short Set) (R. Wolf)	
5-mm Blunt sawtooth scissors	8383.46
5-mm Hooked scissors (to cut suture)	8383.02
5-mm Metzenbaum scissors	Jarit 600-202
5-mm Pointed Metzenbaum scissors	ENDOlap F260.43
5-mm Blunt Metzenbaum scissors	ENDOlap F260.43B
5-mm Biopsy forceps (single tooth)	8383.10
5-mm Atraumatic grasping forceps (ureter)	8383.03
5-mm Atraumatic ovarian grasper	8383.322
5-mm Cyst grasper	8383.324
5-mm Atraumatic grasper (fallopian tube)	8383.142
5-mm Microscissor	Storz 26169-S
5-mm Microscissor	8382.02
5-mm Fimbria holder	8383.41
5-mm Single-tooth grasping forceps	8383.033
5-mm Multi-tooth grasping forceps	8383.032
5-mm Babcock clamp	Stryker 250-10-207
5-mm Allis forceps	Stryker 250-10-206
5-mm Atraumatic Allis forceps	Jarit 600-113
Manhes instruments	Storz
Single-puncture blunt sawtooth scissors	8384.021
Atraumatic grasper for bowel	WISAP 7651-D
Dorsey bowel clamp	American Surgical 1001A
Left-angle dissector	Stryker

Order numbers listed without a manufacturer pertain to the R. Wolf Co.

Appendix continued on following page

Harry Reich, M.D. *Continued*

Instrument/Equipment	Manufacturer/Order Number*
Entry and Closure	
No. 3 knife handle	
No. 11 and No. 15 blades	Bard Parker
Disposable pneumoperitoneum needle/SURGINEEDLE 120 mm	U.S. Surgical 172015
Extra-long Veress needle	8302.15
10-mm Olympus trocar	Olympus A5228
Reich 5.5-mm self-retaining trocar sleeve	8351.02
Reich trocar	8351.122
5-mm Blunt probe (to expel CO_2)	8383.76
Silastic tubing with Luer-Lok connector	2043.51
Hunt/Reich disposable secondary trocar	Apple 900-800
10-mm Hunt/Reich disposable trocar	Apple 900-860
12-mm Hunt/Reich disposable trocar	Apple 900-850
Javid clamps (second-puncture site approximator) with collodion	Baxter V. Mueller CH7950
Toothed Adson forceps	
Suture scissors	
Uterine and Vaginal Manipulators	
Cohen cannula	8378.00
Valtchev uterine mobilizer	Conkin Surgical VUM-4
Humi	Unimar Inc. 6001
Hulka controlling tenaculum	8371.00
Blunt curettes	Sims 3 or 4
Vaginal access sheath	Cook OB/GYN
Trans Anal Endoscopic Micro Surgery System	R. Wolf
Basic element	8840.20
200-mm length rectoscopy tube with obturator	8840.04
Adapter with viewing window and illumination insert	8840.25
Rectal probe (No. 81 French)	Reznik CM24-517
Lateral vaginal retractor	Euro/Med or Simpson/ Basye
Sponge forceps	
Greenberg self-retaining retractor	Codman
Laparoscopic Suturing Set (R. Wolf)	
5-mm Needle holder	8383.53 or 8383.533
3-mm Needle holder	8383.52
Curved needle driver	Cook OB/GYN
Standard (3-mm or 5-mm)	
Oblique (right or left)	
Curved needle holder	WISAP
Clarke Suture Passer (knot pusher)	Marlow Surgical
Micro	MP781
Macro	MP782
Endoloop (chromic gut ligature)	Ethicon EL10G
Semm Adapter (Endo Loop)	8383.78
Ethicon Suture	Ethicon
4–0 PDS	Z-420
5–0 Vicryl	D7676
2–0 Vicryl (tapered SH needle)	J-317
3–0 Vicryl (tapered SH needle)	J-316
0 Vicryl (CT-2)	J-333
10 Vicryl (CT-1)	J-339

*Order numbers listed without a manufacturer pertain to the R. Wolf Co.

Appendix continued on opposite page

Harry Reich, M.D. *Continued*

Instrument/Equipment	Manufacturer/Order Number*
Laparoscopic Minimally Invasive Retractors	
Portsaver Endoscopic Retraction System	Laparomed
ERS Clip percutaneous cannula needle assembly	
Standard tooth	ERS1000S
Fine tooth	ERS100F
Portsaver Endoscopic Retraction System Snare	ERS1200B
Aquadissection Set-up	
Aqua-Purator (pump)	WISAP
Suction irrigator handpiece	WISAP 1614
Bottle puncturer	WISAP 1634
1000-ml lactated Ringer's solution bottles	Baxter Healthcare
Niagara High-Flow Irrigator System	Cabot Med 005652-901
IrrigaTORR High Pressure Irrigation System	O.R. Concepts Inc.
Medi-Vac CRD Suction System	Baxter Healthcare
Electrodes and Irrigators	
5-mm Vancaillie microbipolar forceps	Storz 26177
5-mm Microbipolar irrigator	8383.091
Suction coagulator	8383.73
Kleppinger syringe-style forceps	8383.24
Kleppinger insert (broad paddle)	8383.11
Bipolar cord	8108.01
Unipolar cord	8106.00
5-mm Needle electrode	Storz 26177C
Knife/hook electrodes (adaptable to hand controls)	Kirwan Surgical
EPM-1 Endpoint Monitor (for Bipolar)	Electroscope
Irrivac-Irrigator/Evacuator (for microbipolar)	Dexide 200-01
Pump Vac Plus	Marlow 88-2050
Myomectomy	
5-mm Corkscrew	WISAP 7655MB
11-mm Corkscrew	WISAP 7672MB
Surgicel	Johnson & Johnson
Laparoscopic Stapling Equipment for Hysterectomy Procedure (U.S. Surgical)	
ENDO GIA 30 (size 3.5)	Reorder 030813
ENDO GIA 30 (size 30 vascular)	Reorder 030811
Multifire ENDO GIA	
Disposable loading units (size 3.5)	Reorder 030807
Disposal loading units (size 30 vascular)	Reorder 030805
ENDO CLIP ML applier	Reorder 176615
12-mm Trocar	Reorder 171036
Other Useful Stapling Instruments	
AcuClip	Origin OMS-A8
Operating Room Table Equipment	
Allen stirrups	Allen Medical Systems
Bilateral ulnar pads (Zimfoam laminectomy arm cradle set)	Zimmer
Stierlen-Maquet shoulder braces	Siemens Med. Systems E.N.R. 1002.09C

*Order numbers listed without a manufacturer pertain to the R. Wolf Co.

Appendix continued on following page

Harry Reich, M.D. *Continued*

Instrument/Equipment	Manufacturer/Order Number*
Video Equipment (R. Wolf)	
Dual auto/iris light projector	5150.00
Camera system	5377.10
Beam splitter 50/50	5257.523
C mount direct coupler	5261.27
Sony TV monitor	5366.36
Video cassette recorder	Panasonic 7300
Digital Photographer Unit	Stryker 240-50-210
High-Flow Insufflators	
Electronic Laparoflator (9.9 l/min flow rate)	Storz 26012C
Wolf Insufflator (6-1 flow rate)	2054.60
Electric Insufflator-Clearview (20 1/min)	I.C. Medical ICM200
Electrosurgical Generators	
Wolf Bipolar generator	2351.001
Generator	Aspen Lab
Force 2	Valley Lab
Force 4	Valley Lab
Argon beam coagulator (Beamer Two: 2 l/min flow)	Beacon Lab
Disposable hand-control pencil	Beacon Lab 4020
Laparoscopic electrodes, 28 or 36 cm	
CO_2 Laser	
LaserSonics Alumina 780 Laser	Haraeus LaserSonics
Sure Shot Laparoscope Coupler	I.C. Medical 00131
Clear View EBS (smoke evacuator)	I.C. Medical ICM 350
Intra-Abdominal Plume Eliminator Tubing Set	I.C. Medical ICMT005
Disposable filter and water trap	I.C. Medical ICM006-000
Coherent 6000L	Coherent Laser
Coherent coupler	Coherent Laser
Miscellaneous	
LapSac (5 × 8 or 2 × 5 cm)	Cook OB/GYN
EndoBag	Dexide 250-20
Instrument pouch	3M/Medical-Surgical 1018
PAM no-stick cooking spray (instrument lubricant)	Boyle-Midway
Dust Away Plus (pressurized burst cleaning system)	Photoco

*Order numbers listed without a manufacturer pertain to the R. Wolf Co.

Manufacturers, Addresses, and Phone Numbers

Allen Medical Systems, 5198 Richmond Rd., Bedford Heights, OH 44146-1331; 800-433-5774 or 216-765-0990
American Surgical Instruments, P.O. Box 157, Butler, MD 21023; 301-374-9596
Apple Medical, 93 Nashaway Rd., Bolton, MA 01740; 508-779-2926
Aspen Lab, 7211 S. Eagle St., Englewood, CO 80112; 800-552-0138
Bard Parker. *See Becton Dickinson.*
Baxter Healthcare, 1435 Lake Cook Rd., Deerfield, IL 60015; 708-940-5000
Baxter V. Mueller, 1425 Lake Cook Rd., Deerfield, IL 60015; 800-323-9088
Beacon Lab, Unit D, 2150 W. 6th Ave., Broomfield, CO 80020; 800-955-2150
Becton Dickinson, Acute Care Division, 1 Becton Dr., Franklin Lakes, NJ 07417-1880; 800-333-4813
Boyle-Midway Household Products, 220 7th St. SE, Canton, OH; 216-456-8257
Cabot Medical, 2021 Cabot Blvd. W., Langhorne, PA 19047; 215-752-8300
Codman & Shurtless, Inc., Park Drive, Randolph, MA 02368; 617-961-2300
Coherent Laser, 3270 W. Bayshore Rd., Palo Alto, CA 94303; 800-635-1313

Conkin Surgical Instruments, P.O. Box 6707, Station A, Toronto, Ontario, Canada M5W 1X5; 416-922-9496

Cook OB/GYN, P.O. Box 271, Spencer, IN 47460; 800-541-5591 or 812-829-6500

Davol, Inc., P.O. Box 8500, Cranston, RI 02920; 401-463-7000

Dexide, 7509 Flagstone Dr., Fort Worth, TX 76118; 800-645-3378

Electroscope, 4880 Riverbend Rd., Boulder, CO 80301; 303-444-2600

Ethicon, P.O. Box 151, Somerville, NJ 08876-5106; 800-888-9234

Euro/Med, 8561 154th Ave. NE, Redmond, WA 98052-3557; 800-848-0033

Heraeus LaserSonics, 475 Cottonwood Dr., Milpitas, CA 95035-7434; 408-954-4000

I.C. Medical, Inc., 2340 W. Shangri La, Suite 3, Phoenix, AZ 85029; 602-943-6162

Jarit, 9 Skyline Dr., Hawthorne, NY 10532; 914-592-9050

Johnson & Johnson, Patient Care Division, 501 George, New Brunswick, NJ 08903; 800-526-2459 or 201-524-0400

Kirwan Surgical, P.O. Box 35, Rockland, MA 02370

Laparomed Corp., 9272 Jeronimo Rd., Unit 109, Irvine, CA 92718; 714-768-1155

Marlow Surgical, 1810 Joseph Lloyd Pkwy., Willoughby, OH 44094; 800-992-5581

Olympus, 4 Nevada Dr., New Hyde Park, NY 11042; 800-548-5515

O.R. Concepts, Inc., 200 N. Oak St., Roanoke, TX 76262; 800-826-3723

Origin Medsystems, Inc., 1021 Howard Ave., San Carlos, CA 94070; 415-508-9900

Panasonic, 1 Panasonic Way, Secaucus, NJ 07094; 201-348-7000

Photoco Inc., 4347 Cranwood Pkwy., Cleveland, OH 44128; 216-581-0880

Reznik, 7337 N. Lawndale Ave., Skokie, IL 60076; 708-673-3444

Siemens Medical Systems, 84 Inverness Circle E., Englewood, CO 80112; 800-333-8646

Simpson/Basye, 430 Ayre St., Wilmington, DE 19804; 302-995-7191

Karl Storz Endoscopy-America, 10111 W. Jefferson Blvd., Culver City, CA; 800-421-0837 or 910-232-3578 or 910-340-6372

Stryker Endoscopy, 210 Baypointe Pkwy., San Jose, CA 95134; 800-624-4422 or 408-435-0220

3M Medical/Surgical Division, St. Paul, MN 55144-1080; 800-752-8086

Unimar Inc., 475 Danbury Rd., Wilton, CT 06897-2126; 800-243-6608

U.S. Surgical, 150 Glover Ave., Norwalk, CT 06856; 800-321-0263

Valley Lab, 520 Longbow Dr., Boulder, CO 80301; 800-255-8522

WISAP, 14227 Sand Lane, Tomball, TX 77375; 800-233-8448

Richard Wolf Medical Instruments Corporation, 353 Corporate Woods Parkway, Vernon Hills, IL 60061; 708-913-1113

Zimmer, P.O. Box 708, Warsaw, IN 46581-0708; 800-382-1212

Index

Note: Page numbers in *italics* refer to illustrations; page numbers followed by (t) refer to tables.